Maternal and Infant Drugs and Nursing Intervention

Maternal and Infant Drugs and Nursing Intervention

Editors

Elizabeth J. Dickason, R.N., M.A.
Associate Professor
Queensborough Community College

Martha Olsen Schult, R.N., M.A.
Associate Professor
Queensborough Community College

Elaine Muller Morris, R.N., M.A.
Assistant Professor
Queensborough Community College

Contributors/Consultants

Paul A. Michelson, M.S.
Assistant Clinical Professor of Pharmacy
Northeastern University, Boston

Stephen R. Kandall, M.D.
Chief, Department of Neonatology
Beth Israel Medical Center, New York

McGraw-Hill Book Company
New York   St. Louis   San Francisco   Auckland   Bogotá   Düsseldorf
Johannesburg   London   Madrid   Mexico   Montreal   New Delhi
Panama   Paris   São Paulo   Singapore   Sydney   Tokyo   Toronto

MATERNAL AND INFANT DRUGS AND
NURSING INTERVENTION

Copyright © 1978 by McGraw-Hill, Inc. All rights reserved. Printed in the United States of America. No part of this publication may be reproduced, stored in a retrieval system, or transmitted, in any form or by any means, electronic, mechanical, photocopying, recording, or otherwise, without the prior written permission of the publisher.

3 4 5 6 7 8 9 0 MUMU 7 8 3 2 1 0

This book was set in Caledonia by Creative Book Services, subsidiary of McGregor & Werner, Inc. The editors were Sally J. Barhydt and Timothy Armstrong; the designer was Elliot Epstein; the production supervisor was Robert C. Pedersen. The drawings were done by George Ramponeau and J & R Services, Inc.
The Murray Printing Company was printer and binder.

Library of Congress Cataloging in Publication Data

Main entry under title:

Maternal and infant drugs and nursing intervention.

Includes index.
1. Obstetrical pharmacology. 2. Obstetrical nursing.
I. Dickason, Elizabeth J. II. Schult, Martha Olsen. III. Morris, Elaine Muller. DNLM: 1. Obstetric nursing. 2. Pediatric nursing. 3. Drug—Administration and dosage—Nursing texts. 4. Drug therapy—In infancy and nursing texts. 5. Drug therapy—In pregnancy—Nursing texts. WY157 M4235
RG528.M37 615'.7 77-19105
ISBN 0-07-016788-5

Contents

Preface

Some of the drugs which have been taken by women of childbearing age have adversely affected their infants. As a result, there is an awakened concern about the effect of every drug given to women during pregnancy and lactation as well as those given to newborn infants. Initial studies of drug effects on laboratory animals have often proved to be inapplicable to the human mother and fetus. In addition, there is a time lag between identification of problems and general application of information, e.g., the discovery of adverse effects of heavy maternal sedation on newborn recovery.

Nurses who wish to remain up-to-date find a variety of conflicting views on drug utilization during pregnancy. Physiologic variables affecting drug use are rarely applied, and custom often rules. For this reason Chapters 1 and 7 review drug impact on the developing human infant first during fetal development and then during the perinatal period and into early infancy.

Dysmorphogenesis is discussed by phases of pregnancy, since drug effects differ as the fetus matures. New discoveries of certain long-term carcinogenic effects and altered hormonal states have focused attention on drugs long thought to be safe because no observable anomaly appeared at birth. Tables on drug effects on the fetus and infant during pregnancy and lactation are included, as is an extensive bibliography.

One of the major problems of pharmacologic effects during pregnancy and the perinatal period is that the drug dosage and action cannot be accurately adjusted to compensate for the changing maternal metabolism and, at the same time, adjusted for the rapidly growing fetus. In addition, the placental role in screening, metabolizing, or transferring drugs is just beginning to be understood.

The period of postnatal development includes such rapid changes that drug dosage cannot be calculated as if the child were a miniature adult. Incomplete development of body enzymes, organs, and metabolic pathways alter in unexpected ways the metabolism and excretion of drugs in small children. For example, certain drugs speed up maturation processes, while others interfere with excretion of waste products. In addition, metabolites of several drugs have been shown to be harmful even when the parent drugs are considered "safe." The transitional period is of such importance to the newborn that a chapter on resuscitation, transitional effects of maternal drugs, and therapy of drug withdrawal is included.

Because drug utilization during normal pregnancy should be minimal, a number of nonpharmacologic methods of alleviating minor discomforts are included. Nurses would do well to encourage the reduction of drug utilization whenever possible. Pregnant women should receive only prescribed drugs and then only when benefit outweighs the risk. However, a number of complications during pregnancy do require pharmacologic therapy. In these cases, the nurse must be alert to drug precautions for each problem. Therefore, a section introducing each major complication in relation to drug requirements precedes tables of selected, most commonly used drugs.

Because the field is changing so rapidly, we have indicated trends in the use of drugs and have had repeatedly to acknowledge the tentative nature of many conclusions. In compiling drug descriptions, we found that the reasons for precautions during pregnancy were not always given, although manufacturers placed a disclaimer about use in pregnancy in their literature. Therefore, we have had to rely on reports of current research, and our conclusions often had to remain tentative. Drug descriptions and dosages have been checked with standard pharmacologic references, such as *AMA Drug Evaluation*, Goodman and Gilman's *The Pharmacological Basis of Therapeutics*, Martin's *Hazards of Medication*, American Hospital Formulary Service, and *Physicians Desk Reference*, and extensive references are used. Nurses are encouraged to check current research into drug effects on the fetus and the newborn, and particularly pertinent references are starred with an asterisk.

The nurse who takes this problem affecting fetal and infant well-being seriously should seek current information as it is made available in order to provide better care for mothers and infants. The purpose of this handbook is to alert the nurse to drug problems while focusing attention on assessment and observation of drug effects. Nursing interventions are provided for situations in which drugs are necessary for mother or infant.

Acknowledgments

We gratefully acknowledge the assistance and generous support of our consultants, Stephen R. Kandall, M.D., and Paul A. Michelson, M.S. A special note of recognition and thanks for excellent secretarial assistance must be given to Deena M. Ryan, Catherine Musgrave, and Sylvia Rockness.

Elizabeth J. Dickason
Martha Olsen Schult
Elaine Muller Morris

Maternal and Infant Drugs and Nursing Intervention

1

The Problem of Drug Use During Pregnancy

Elizabeth J. Dickason

Nurses who are aware of possible adverse drug effects on the growing fetus and newborn must be concerned about their role in administering drugs to pregnant women, lactating women, and newborns. The need for a handbook has arisen out of this concern to provide safe care for maternity patients and newborns.

Since the 1960s, when the teratogenic effects of thalidomide and rubella were first noted, contradictory statements have appeared in the literature concerning the adverse effects of certain commonly used drugs. The result has been confusion, disbelief about new claims, or fear of all pharmacologic therapy.

As the authors prepared this handbook, they noted the problems that nurses face in administering drugs in maternity and infant care. These problems are compounded by various interpretations of drug studies, inadequate sources of information about drugs, uneven dissemination of such information, and difficulty in understanding the meaning of the benefit-to-risk ratio.

The Collaborative Study of the National Institute for Neurologic Diseases and Stroke found that among 50,000 women studied, 900 different drugs were prescribed or taken without prescription during pregnancy. The average number of drugs taken per patient in other recent studies (Fofar and Nelson, 1973) varied from four to nine. Thus, if a malformation should occur, determining the causative agent or agents would be difficult. However, in an attempt to isolate causative agents, birth-defect registries have recently been established in several countries, and drug-related defects are being recorded through careful monitoring. The refinement of statistical methods has enabled the cause of many defects to be assigned at the present time to (1) the individual drug alone, (2) a combination of maternal illness plus drug, (3) environmental pollutants, (4) multifactorial genetic inheritance, (5) multifactorial inheritance plus drug, or (6) still unknown factors.

Currently, as a result of research, many drugs have been approved for use in therapeutic doses for treating the pregnant woman. Unfortunately, a larger number of other drugs have not been studied adequately and remain on "effect unknown" or "suspect" lists. In addition, even drugs cleared for use may turn out to produce long-term adverse effects.

INTERPRETATION OF DRUG STUDIES

Most studies of drug effects on the fetus must be done on laboratory animals and the results extrapolated to human beings. Doses given to lab animals are often nearly lethal, being proportionately much higher than doses that would be given to humans. When malformations result, the offending drug is labeled *teratogenic*, and publicity in the media usually follows.

To balance these findings (which often eliminated useful drugs), prospective and retrospective studies of large numbers of women throughout pregnancy have been undertaken in the last 5 years. Based on these studies, it has been found that, at present, there are few clearly teratogenic agents (see Table 1-1). The problem lies in the fact that most adverse effects result unpredictably under the influence of multiple factors. When an individual case or series is reported, all influential factors should be considered. All conflicting reports need to be closely analyzed and methods of statistical reporting examined before final conclusions are drawn (Heinonen et al., 1977).

Table 1-1   Agents Which Are Confirmed Teratogens

PHYSICAL	BIOLOGICAL
Ionizing radiation, high doses	Viruses
	Rubella
	Cytomegalovirus
DRUGS	Herpesvirus hominis
Thalidomide	Toxoplasma
Antineoplastic drugs	Syphilis
Tetracyclines	
Steroid hormones	CHEMICAL
Androgens	Mercury
Diethylstilbestrol	Lead
Oral progestogens	

INADEQUATE INFORMATION

Nurses who seek information from their usual sources, nursing texts, and the *Physician's Desk Reference (PDR)* will find few specific references to pregnancy and the newborn period. Recently children have been called "therapeutic orphans" by Shirkey because of the lack of attention to their unique differences in handling drugs. In the existing therapeutic situation, pregnant women, their fetuses, and newborn infants are also "orphans," for many drugs listed in the *PDR* have disclaimer notices such as "not yet proven to be safe during pregnancy," "safety and efficacy in the pediatric age group has not been established," or "the physician should weigh risks against benefits before prescribing." These notices are inserted to protect the manufacturer when data are not sufficient to conclude that there is no risk. When no disclaimer is given, clues that indicate a lack of data are the absence of dosage information for infants or for children under 12 years of age or the absence of statements about precautions during pregnancy.

Wilson surveyed the *PDR* and found that for 22 percent of the medications listed, some reference to children was given, i.e., the dose for children was given, the dose was given only for older children (over 12 years of age), or there was a disclaimer about any use for children at all. Pregnant women fared only slightly better: 39 percent of the medications had a disclaimer noted for pregnancy, and in 13 percent, a caution about use during breast-feeding was given (J. T. Wilson, 1975). This lack of information in one of the most commonly used drug references available to nurses emphasizes the problem of obtaining the data needed to make informed judgments for drug administration to mothers and their children.

UNEVEN DISSEMINATION OF INFORMATION

It is not unusual for a drug to be prescribed by a physician in spite of fairly widely accepted precautions. In some cases, circumstances may have been considered and the choice made as being the best one available. In other situations, however, the physician may not be familiar with current research on a particular drug. An example is the continued use of diuretics during pregnancy for edema of the lower extremities. Diuretics can mask symptoms of preeclampsia and are thought not to be therapeutic at the present time, unless given only in short test doses. Many nurses do not feel secure enough in their knowledge of drug use to challenge an order. In some situations, they may challenge an order on the basis of inadequate information without understanding the benefit-to-risk ratio which has been considered by the physician. In these situations, when asked to administer a questionable drug, the nurse can consult the hospital pharmacist as an objective resource person.

BENEFIT-TO-RISK RATIO

The benefit-to-risk ratio is important to consider because nurses necessarily are involved in a teaching role with patients. This term implies that an *informed* choice has been made that, even though there is some possibility of harm, the value of the drug to the mother outweighs the risk to the fetus. This choice is made by the physician, who must take responsibility for it.

At the same time, because of the growing fears of the public, this benefit-to-risk ratio should be discussed with the patient, who has a right to understand the problems in therapy before being given the drug. A corollary to this statement is made by McCrory: "Whenever a pregnant woman takes a drug she should do it with educated awareness of the choice she is making between a therapeutic benefit to her and a toxicity risk to her unborn baby." McCrory defines risk of toxicity as follows: "Undesirable risk can be defined, for our purposes, as existing whenever drug ingestion by the pregnant mother can lessen the infant's health potential by fetal exposure without clear evidence that the drug contributes to maternal protection from a known health hazard" (McCrory, 1973).

An example of weighing benefit against risk is the use of phenytoin for the epileptic woman. When taken together, phenytoin and barbiturates have apparently resulted in a higher incidence of anomalies, mainly cleft lip and palate and congenital heart defects (Waziri et al., 1976). The Collaborative Study found that the incidence of these anomalies was about two and one-half times greater for women taking phenytoin during early pregnancy than for nonexposed women. However, no one knows the risk of spontaneous abortion or the anomalies that might occur with omission of the drug and the resultant increase in convulsions. The dilemma is a real one, and the choice is usually made to administer phenytoin.

TERATOGENS

An agent toxic to cell differentiation or growth is called a *teratogen*. In 1969, the World Health Organization expanded the definition to include not only agents causing structural defects but also those causing growth retardation and biochemical and behavioral effects lasting into the newborn period and perhaps longer. This group includes agents which have been shown to be carcinogenic in later childhood. The expanded definition has supported reexamination of routinely used obstetric drugs as well as more rigorous testing for newly developed drugs. Wilson identifies environmental effects on fetal development as an action-reaction sequence, dependent on a wide range of factors. Genetic susceptibility, dosage level and duration, day of development, maternal health and nutrition, placental functioning, and numerous other factors are influential in determining whether or not a specific teratogenic agent does, in fact, have an injurious effect on the developing human fetus. He defines teratogenic action as "one or more mechanisms that cause cells to die, change their rates of proliferation or biosynthesis or otherwise fail to follow their prescribed course in development" (J. G. Wilson, 1977, p. 358).

Structural Damage

It is known that some bacteria, viruses, heavy metals, radiation, and other pollutants have caused fetal organ deformity. Until thalidomide so clearly demonstrated its specific time-

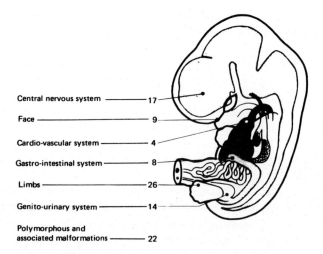

Central nervous system — 17
Face — 9
Cardio-vascular system — 4
Gastro-intestinal system — 8
Limbs — 26
Genito-urinary system — 14
Polymorphous and associated malformations — 22

Figure 1-1   Distribution of congenital defects (%) in humans. (*After Tuchman-Duplessis, Drug Effects on The Fetus: ADIS Press, Sydney, 1976; by permission of author and publisher.*)

related effects on the embryo, very little thought or lab testing for effect on pregnancy was given to seemingly safe prescription drugs. In fact, it took 5 years of thalidomide effects to focus public attention on the damage caused by this ordinarily innocuous drug. Fortunately, enough became known to remove the drug from the world market. [The effects lingered for several years, as some women took the leftover pills in home medicine cabinets, unaware of the research or forgetful of the drug name (Smithells, 1973).]

Severe structural damage is usually incompatible with life, and the small embryo is aborted. But teratogenic drugs have target organs, it seems, and timing can be all-important. When the cell differentiation is taking place, usually during just a few crucial days, insult may delay, distort, or divert development of one group of cells (Fig. 1-1). Before 8 weeks of development, major anomalies can occur with only one or two doses of a teratogen.

Behavioral and Biochemical Defects

Changes in the fetus or newborn resulting from biochemical distortion are harder to identify. Such distortion may inhibit growth and change future behavior. An example is the effect of supplemental female hormones on male children of a group of diabetic mothers who, during their entire pregnancies, received estrogen and progesterone. No anatomic changes were noted, but behavioral development at 6 years and at 16 years showed measureable differences in athletic coordination and lower interest in usual male child activities (Yalom, 1973). The influence of extra female hormones on the male fetus did not appear to change gonads or genitalia structurally but perhaps influenced future production of testosterone. Currently, additional research is in progress, since the initial sample was small.

Biochemical function is altered by maternal ingestion of drugs which affect the fetus as they do the mother. Fetal thyroid growth will be inhibited if the mother ingests iodides (found in some cough syrups) or takes antithyroid medication, for iodides inhibit uptake of iodine in the thyroid. The result is a temporary neonatal goiter, a condition which can be treated in the newborn.

The fetus is known to experience withdrawal symptoms in utero as well as after birth. Thus, maternal narcotic ingestion influences fetal activity and recovery after birth but long-term effects have not yet been fully determined.

Long-Range Carcinogenic Effects

Estrogen, particularly diethylstilbestrol (DES), has been implicated in causing vaginal adenocarcinoma in a small number of female children whose mothers were treated during the first 18 weeks of pregnancy (Herbst, 1975). At birth, no observable defects, growth retardation, or behavioral effects were noted. Adenocarcinoma is a very rare condition, especially in early puberty. When cases began to occur and histories were taken, the common element was found to be the DES treatment 10 to 15 years before. Obstetricians then made a search through their records to locate women who had received such treatment before giving birth to female children. Each was asked to bring in her child for examination. Some girls demonstrated advanced cases and some exhibited only early changes, but fortunately, the incidence was less than had been feared. Currently, each surviving girl is being followed for any untoward developments in the future, and male children of these mothers are being extensively studied. This DES effect emphasizes the problem of therapeutically prescribed drugs during pregnancy that is, the impossibility of predicting long-range adverse effects on the infant.

Assignment of Causation

Wilson has identified four categories into which all adverse environmental influences on fetal health can be placed (J. G. Wilson, 1975). Only a few agents have demonstrated the high risk of teratogenicity which *almost always results* in a dead, deformed, or biochemically affected fetus if exposure takes place during organogenesis (organ formation).

Highly Probable Teratogens   The first category includes highly probable teratogens, or those *definitely related* to fetal injury. For instance, almost 100 percent of the fetuses exposed to thalidomide between days 34 and 50 had some type of deformity or were aborted. Rubella also carries a very high risk in the first 8 weeks. Certain viral diseases (see Table 1-1), syphilis, steroid sex hormones, folic acid antagonists, and heavy metals are proven teratogens. Tetracyclines, antithyroid agents, and coumadins in therapeutic maternal doses will also cause definite, although usually not life-threatening effects.

Suspected Teratogens   Agents with a suspected relationship are those which have a lower incidence of risk and yet those for which a clear relationship has been shown in *some cases*. The agent *does not* always cause problems, however, since many more exposed women have healthy offspring than have affected fetuses. Thus, effects may occur under multiple influences of genetic susceptibility, placental problems, or maternal disease. In this group fall the effects of anticonvulsants, streptomycin, chronic high alcohol intake, certain appetite suppressants, sulfonylurea hypoglycemics, chemotherapeutic and alkylating agents, and therapeutic doses of radiation (over 5 rad). Certain disease states of diabetes and epilepsy, in which the biochemical problems in the mother may intensify drug effect on the infant, must be included here.

Rarely Teratogenic   Under certain multifaceted conditions, some drugs may occasionally be implicated in teratogenesis in humans. In large doses in lab animals, these drugs have demonstrated clear-cut adverse effects. Into this category are placed agents which show clearly adverse reactions in vitro (test tube) and in vivo in lab animals. However, dosage ranges used may be extraordinarily high, and results may only be applied tentatively to pregnancy situations, as cell responsiveness may be different in human beings. High doses of aspirin, certain antibiotics and antituberculosis drugs, quinine, imipramine, and very high insulin levels are included in this group. Many reports have yet to be verified by prospective surveys.

Improbable Teratogens　　Improbable teratogens are agents which are thought to have a *very low* risk but which might, in rare instances, have an adverse effect, given proper conditions or maternal disease. Drugs which have demonstrated some effects in lab animals but which have been thoroughly studied and found to have a very low risk in humans are placed in this category. In usual doses, agents which are *unlikely* to cause adverse effects are diagnostic radiation (under 5 rad) and active immunization with killed agents. (Physical and psychologic trauma are included in this group.) After study, agents formerly thought to have had teratogenic potential but which now seem to be of very low risk have been moved to this classification. Such agents as LSD, sulfonamides, cortisone, antihistamines, and most tranquilizers and antiemetics now are placed in this category.

Proving teratogenicity is not the final goal of study, however. The problem of unknown long-term biochemical and behavioral disturbances still remains. The principle of prescribing the least possible medication as well as being alert to avoid exposure to environmental pollutants must underlie all care for pregnant women.

DEVELOPMENTAL TIMETABLE

In order for nurses to administer drugs intelligently, there must be some awareness of how the environment and fetal target changes during pregnancy. From conception to implantation, the ovum is enroute through the tube, bathed in fluid and susceptible only to the drugs which may pass into that tubal fluid. Any damage during this time would probably be lethal, since tubal fluid consistency would be affected. By days 8 to 10, when implantation has begun, trophoblastic cells begin to break down maternal tissue to form lacunae, the villi, and the placenta. The blastocyst is firmly implanted by days 14 to 17, and placental function is present from day 21. Once placental function begins, the transfer of almost every substance in maternal circulation will take place, usually *at maternal dosage*.

Organogenesis

The main period of organ formation is considered to be from days 15 to 56 after fertilization. In this period, incredibly rapid cell duplication (proliferation) and sorting out into different layers, organs, and functions (differentiation) takes place on a strict schedule. It is clear that any agent toxic to cell growth, even with a single dose, could arrest or distort that growth, and it is sometimes possible to name the week of the insult by the anomaly. In other cases, cause and effect are less clear. However, almost all major structural anomalies are produced within these first 56 days.

Period of Fetal Growth

During the fetal growth period (days 57 to 266), some organogenesis will continue, especially further development of the central nervous system, teeth, eyes, and genitalia (Fig. 1-2). However, the major changes to be noted in these later days of pregnancy are those of growth by duplication of cells and enlargement of the already established cells in organs and tissues. As has been noted, insult during this period will usually take the form of slowing this cell growth, resulting in smaller size of the individual part, or reducing the growth of the whole infant (intrauterine growth retardation). Fortunately, unless it is under extra stress, the brain is usually protected and often will be of normal size when other body organs are smaller.

During this period, drugs begin to affect the fetus in the same biochemical ways that occur in the mother, with a gradual progression to the neonatal level of response to drugs. Fetal pathways of metabolism and excretion begin to function,

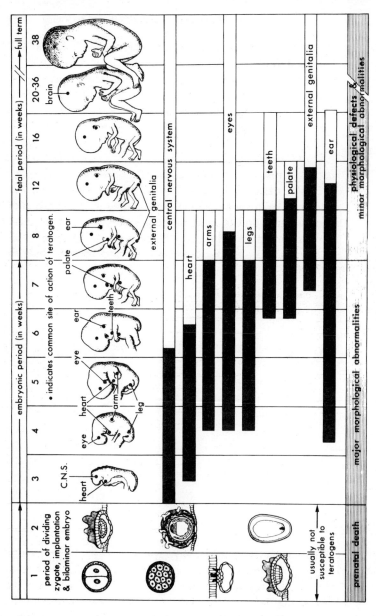

Figure 1-2 Schematic illustration of the sensitive or critical periods in human development. (Shaded areas denote highly sensitive periods.) *(After Keith L. Moore, Before We Are Born, W. B. Saunders, Philadelphia, 1975. Used by permission of author and publisher.)*

although the timing of metabolism and excretion may be much different from a newborn or older infant. Studies of the fetus are discovering some very surprising information about drug metabolism. It appears that drugs are handled very early by the fetus but in unpredictable patterns.

Based on these findings, treatment of the fetus in utero is possible. Sophisticated biochemical studies of amniotic fluid and metabolism in immature infants have demonstrated that the fetus can, in some instances, be treated for diseases such as heart failure or anemia in erythroblastosis fetalis, and drugs can be given to the mother to stimulate maturation of fetal enzymes and to increase lung maturity when preterm birth is imminent (Chez and Fleishman, 1975). More will develop in this field as studies already in progress come to conclusions.

Transitional Period

A highly critical period for the infant is just before, during, and just after delivery. During this transitional period, maternal–fetal equilibrium of a drug can, in most cases, be reached by 40 minutes after oral ingestion and much faster with intravenous administration to the mother. Thus, depending on the timing of administration and the rate of maternal excretion, drug levels in the infant at birth may be near or higher than maternal levels. This major newborn environmental problem is discussed in Chapter 8.

Newborn Period

Once it is on its own, the newborn must route drugs through its own immature liver and kidneys. The results are varied, since each drug has its own pattern of excretion. For some drugs, the delay in excretion is 10 times longer than in the mother, while other drugs are handled with only minor delays.

A factor to consider in the newborn period is that the immaturity of metabolic pathways may sometimes cause incomplete metabolism, leaving partially reduced metabolites in the blood for longer periods than is usual. Some of these metabolites may be more active than the parent drug, thus causing, in some instances, unexpectedly high blood levels of active drug and increased adverse effects.

Brackbill studies the effect of analgesia and anesthesia on the newborn's subsequent learning ability and ability to cope. She discovered marked differences in the baby's ability to adapt to nonsignificant noise (Brackbill, 1975). The nonmedicated baby (2 days old) learned to stop listening to short bursts of "white noise" after 26 episodes. For babies with regional anesthesia it took 58 episodes, and for those born with general anethesia it took 90 or more episodes. A continued adverse effect was noted, as scores were not much different when the same infants were 1 month old! There now needs to be exploration of the possible relationship of early medication to some learning disabilities.

Brackbill states that the infant's performance is disturbed in direct proportion to the dose or potency of the medication. There may be no correlation that can be proved because so many environmental factors impinge on later learning ability, but since in a number of learning disabilities, the child is often unable to stop paying attention to nonmeaningful stimuli in order to concentrate, the parallel must be examined.

Once the variables in the newborn infant's ability to metabolize and excrete specific drugs are clarified, it becomes evident that doses for prematures and term newborns must be carefully calculated, not by rules, but by each drug's potential metabolic pattern in the infant. In general, the younger the infant, the less able it will be to handle drug metabolism, and the more susceptible it will be to delayed excretion and possible resultant overdoses, cumulative effect, or adverse side effects. Hypoglycemia, cold stress, respiratory difficulty, and birth trauma will further complicate the outcome. Factors influencing the infant's ability to utilize drugs are discussed in Chapter 7.

DRUGS DURING LACTATION

Interest in lactation is growing in this country after decades of emphasis on bottle feeding. The interest parallels the growth in women's concerns to know what is happening with their bodies and their infants during pregnancy, labor, and the recovery period. Increasingly, mothers are asking questions about safety of medication. Nurses are being challenged as they distribute routine medications on the unit. It is not enough to state, "The doctor ordered this for you." The mother wishes to know if it is really necessary, and if she is breast-feeding, what the drug's effect will be on the infant. The nurse must know how to answer and have a resource available. Fortunately, the same questions are being asked by researchers in pharmacology, and recent articles do provide some guidance. Drug use during lactation is discussed in detail in Chapter 3.

LEGAL ASPECTS

No woman would deliberately seek to harm a growing fetus. Should she find out that she had inadvertently taken a harmful drug, she would feel terribly guilty and be intensely angry with those who knew better and did not warn her against the drug. Thus, it is important for those involved in preventive care to keep abreast of current research and to continue to interpret new findings. In addition, continuing education about adverse effects of agents on the developing infant must be given to every level of society. Otherwise, exaggerated and incorrect information will be gleaned by parents from newspapers and magazines.

Brent (1976) states that there is an epidemic of legal suits in this area. Many suits are instigated because of uninformed anger, when parents blame agents which are not teratogenic or even blame the doctor for genetic factors. Some of these suits could have been avoided by careful explanation when the drugs were first prescribed. Other suits are well-founded and based on real negligence. As the public becomes more informed, and less acquiescent, those prescribing and administering medications may be held even more responsible for their role in therapy of mother and fetus.

NURSING MEASURES

The expanding role for nursing should include both assessment and teaching aspects related to pharmacology in maternal and newborn care. As a result of understanding the implications of the wider definition of the teratogenic effects of drugs, the nurse must include in her care plan both observation and assessment of drug effects on her patients and teach preventive care. The following steps can be taken to increase awareness and improve assessment.

1. Drug "alerts" and results of new findings should be regularly included in nursing conferences.
2. Lists of nonrecommended drugs during pregnancy and lactation should be posted in each medication room (Table 1-2).
3. The pharmacist should be involved whenever a question arises about the safety or the effect of a drug during pregnancy.
4. Education about drugs should be included in antepartum and postpartum classes, and for every lactating woman.
5. Assist each mother who must take a questionable drug to understand the benefit-to-risk ratio for that drug.
6. Counsel all mothers about nonpharmacologic methods for alleviating minor discomforts of pregnancy and recovery.
7. Encourage women to take childbirth classes to help reduce medication levels during delivery, and then support the educated mother in her attempts to cope with labor and delivery.
8. During interview and assessment of the mother on admission to labor, include a record of any incidental nonprescription or prescription drugs taken prior to labor.

9. Inform nursery nurses of any transitional drugs that might affect newborn during recovery. Inform nursery nurses of timing and level of analgesia and anesthesia.

10. Increase ability to assess the newborn for normal behavioral responses. Records must be more descriptive during the newborn period if long-term behavioral effects of drugs are to be evaluated.
    a. Note iatrogenic factors affecting infant's responses.
    b. Be alert for delayed excretion, cumulative effects, and altered physiologic states whenever noting drug effects in the newborn.
    c. Note and record feeding ability. Check the mother's chart when her infant sucks poorly, falls asleep during feedings consistently, or will not interact with mother.
    d. Make every effort to teach the mother how to feed and handle a sleepy baby and when to expect improvement.
    e. Increase efforts to support the bonding process when the infant is sick and receiving special care or when it is recovering from the effects of delayed excretion of drugs.
    f. Support the breast-feeding woman, providing information to answer questions about drug effects on the infant.

When these steps are taken, it should be possible to provide informed nursing support to any woman during pregnancy or recovery and to discover subtle signs of medication influence on the infant.

Table 1-2   Effects of Drugs on Fetus and Neonate

Agent	Implications
ANALGESICS	
Alphaprodine (Nisentil)	Depressed fetal responses
Acetylsalicylic acid (aspirin; many trade names)	Albumin-binding capacities are lower; may compete with bilirubin, causing possible neonatal bleeding from platelet dysfunction, GI ulceration, kidney malformation; best to avoid during first and third trimesters; may prolong gestation, delaying labor by interfering with prostaglandin syntheses
Codeine	Withdrawal symptoms
Heroin	Addiction; withdrawal symptoms, low birth weight
Indomethacin	May lead to closure of ductus arteriosus in utero. May prolong gestation by inhibiting prostaglandin release
Meperidine hydrochloride (Demerol)	Respiratory depression in the newborn; dose-related response; stimuli response decreased; effects detected up to 30 days
Methadone (Dolophine)	Withdrawal symptoms in newborn; usually later onset of symptoms than morphine-addicted infant
Morphine	Acute: Respiratory depression. Chronic: Dependency, withdrawal symptoms
Propoxyphene (Darvon)	May have withdrawal syndrome; temperature elevation, irritability, aggressive feeding, loose stools, weight loss
ANESTHETICS	
General	Fetal depression, apnea
Local (Paracervical route especially)	Bradycardia, fetal acidosis, decreased fetal neurologic reaction
ANTACIDS	
Magnesium hydroxide	Large, frequent amounts can cause fetal neuromuscular damage or cardiovascular impairment from magnesium poisoning
Magnesium trisilicate	Large, frequent doses can cause fetal kidney damage
Sodium bicarbonate	Large doses can cause metabolic alkalosis

Table 1-2   Effects of Drugs on Fetus and Neonate *(Continued)*

Agent	Implications
ANTICHOLINERGICS	
Scopolamine	Use during labor may mask fetal distress and smooth the beat-to-beat variations as seen on the fetal monitor
ANTICOAGULANTS	
Bishydroxycoumarin (Dicumarol)	May cause fetal hemorrhage and fetal death; avoid in first and third trimester
Heparin	No effect—large molecule does not cross placenta
Warfarin (Coumadin)	Possible fetal hemorrhage; avoid in first and third trimester
ANTICONVULSANTS	
Phenytoin (Dilantin)	Congenital disorders, cleft palate, folic acid deficiencies, hemorrhagic disorders
ANTIDEPRESSANTS	
Imipramine (Tofranil)	Stunted extremities, CNS and craniofacial abnormalities, withdrawal symptoms
ANTIDIABETIC AGENTS	
Chlorpropamide (Diabinese)	Respiratory distress, prolonged hypoglycemia, increased risk of fetal mortality
Insulin	No proven effect; drug of choice for pregnant diabetic patient
Tolbutamide (Orinase)	Reports of multiple congenital defects, neonatal hypoglycemia; fetal deaths three times higher than those whose mothers were on insulin
ANTIEMETICS	
Cyclizine (Marezine), meclizine (Bonine, Antivert)	Both have been known to cause limb deformities, cleft lip and palate in animal studies; not generally recommended for use during pregnancy
ANTIHISTAMINES	
Promethazine hydrochloride (Phenergan)	Depresses infant responses when given during labor

Table 1-2   Effects of Drugs on Fetus and Neonate *(Continued)*

Agent	Implications
ANTIHYPERTENSIVES	
Hexamethonium bromide	Paralytic ileus
Reserpine	Bradycardia, nasal stuffiness and discharge, respiratory distress, hypothermia, hypotonus, vasodilation, anorexia
Magnesium sulfate	Possible temporary myoneural junction paralysis; inhibited muscle tone if given too close to delivery; convulsions
ANTIMALARIALS	
Quinine (quinine contained in tonic water)	Possible congenital anomalies of CNS (including auditory and optic nerve damage), possible anomalies of the extremities, thrombocytopenia, abortifacients
Chloroquine phosphate	Deafness, mental retardation, or thrombocytopenia
ANTIMICROBIALS	
Amphotericin B	Multiple abnormalities, abortion
Cephalexin (Keflex), cephalothin (Keflin)	Coombs' test interfered with; half become false positive
Chloramphenicol	Gray syndrome (newborn) (if given during transition period so that drug is still in newborn's system or if given to newborn)
Cloxacillin, dicloxacillin	Kernicterus, jaundice (if given during transition period so that drug is still in newborn's system or if given to newborn)
Erythomycyin	Possible liver injury
Isoniazid	Possibly retards psychomotor activity
Metronidazole (Flagyl)	Crosses placental barrier easily; manufacturer discourages use during second and third trimesters
Nitrofurantoin	Hemolysis in fetus with glucose 6-phosphate dehydrogenase defect
Novobiocin	Hyperbilirubinemia
Tetracyclines	Tooth discoloration and damage, bone growth inhibition

Table 1-2   Effects of Drugs on Fetus and Neonate *(Continued)*

Agent	Implications
Streptomycin	Hearing loss if given early in pregnancy
Sulfonamides	Kernicterus by displacing protein-bound bilirubin; hemolysis in G6PD patients
ANTITHYROIDS (GOITROGENS)	
Iodides (ingredient in many over-the-counter cough syrups),methimazole (Tapazole), potassium perchlorate, propylthiouracil	All antithyroid agents cross the placenta and can cause neonatal goiters and hypothyroidism
Sodium iodine (^{131}I)	May cause permanent thyroid suppression
CANCER CHEMOTHERAPEUTIC AGENTS	(In general, all should be *avoided*, at least during the first trimester)
Aminopterin	Fetal death, multiple malformations and congenital anomalies, abortion
Chlorambucil (Leukeran)	Growth retardation, genitourinary abnormalities (absence of kidneys and ureters), abortion
Cyclophosphamide (Cytoxan)	Congenital anomalies, fetal death, abortion
Mercaptopurine (Purinethol) alternated with busalfan (Myleran)	Abortifacient, possible structural alterations in fetus (cleft palate, others), hemolytic anemia of newborn
Methotrexate (Amethopterin)	Congenital anomalies, hypertelorism (increased distance between organs or parts), abortion, cleft palate
DIURETICS	
Thiazides, ammonium chloride (found in Aqua-Ban)	Neonatal thrombocytopenia, electrolyte imbalance (especially if given in transitional phase of labor), acidosis, respiratory distress
HORMONES	
Androgens, progestins	Advanced bone age, masculinization of female fetus, labioscrotal fusion prior to twelfth week, phallic enlargement after twelfth week, possible congenital anomalies, possible increased bilirubin

Table 1-2 Effects of Drugs on Fetus and Neonate *(Continued)*

Agent	Implications
Estrogens	
Natural steroidal	Feminization of male fetus
Synthesized nonsteroidal	Masculinization of female fetus
Diethylstilbestrol	Vaginal cancer in female offspring; possible psychosocial difficulties and genitourinary anomalies in male offspring
Corticosteroids	May suppress adrenal activity; cleft palate, small-for-date infants
Dexamethasone (Decadron)	Placental insufficiency syndrome, possible fetal distress during labor
Ovulatory agents	Multiple pregnancy, possible chromosomal defects in abortus, possible anencephaly
LAXATIVES	
Mineral oil	Low maternal absorption of vitamins A,D,E, and K may affect fetus
NARCOTIC ANTAGONIST	(In the absence of narcotic, may cause severe respiratory depression in neonate)
Levallorphine (Lorfan)	In asphyxia neonatorum, irritability and a tendency to increased crying may occur
Nalorphine (Nalline)	Decreases neonatal depression caused by narcotic
Naloxone (Narcan)	No neonatal depression
OXYTOCICS	
Ergonovine maleate (Ergotrate), methylergonovine maleate (Methergine)	Abortions; not to be used during labor or delivery until after placental separation
Oxytocin	May have some effect on bilirubin metabolism
PSYCHOTROPIC DRUGS	
Chlordiazepoxide (Librium)	Possible cleft palate. Large doses: hypotonicity, listlessness, hypothermia, and anorexia

Table 1-2   Effects of Drugs on Fetus and Neonate *(Continued)*

Agent	Implications
Diazepam (Valium)	Hypotonia, poor sucking reflex and fetal response, possible teratogenic effect (cleft palate), low Apgar scores with doses greater than/30 mg before delivery, hypothermia
Lithium compounds	Teratogenic in mice; neonatal serum levels reach adult toxic levels; lethargy, cyanosis in newborn, respiratory distress
Lithium carbonate	May cause neonatal goiter
Phenothiazines	Extrapyrmidal effects in newborn if given in the third trimester, hypotonia, unresponsiveness, hyperactivity (tremors, agitation); may prolong labor; possible effect on eyes; possible chromosomal breakage
SEDATIVES	
Barbiturates	Minimal dose: Fetal depression. Large dose: Apnea, fetal distress, increased drug metabolism; penetrates white matter, causing longer sleeping time than in adult, poor sucking ability, neonatal bleeding, lowers bilirubin level. Chronic use: Neonatal withdrawal (high incidence of seizures)
Bromides, potassium (contained in Alva-Tranquil, Nervine)	Lethargy, hypotonia, high-pitched cry, feeding problems, rash
Paraldehyde	Large dose decreases fetal responsiveness; increased drowsiness in neonate
Thalidomide	Severe congenital limb malformations (phocomelia)
THYROID PREPARATIONS	
Sodium levothyroxine (Letter, Synthroid), sodium liothyronine (Cytomel)	Thyroid preparations cross the placenta but rarely cause problems
VITAMINS	
A	Excessive doses may cause teratogenic effects in fetus: bone and skeletal abnormalities; CNS abnormalities; eye, cleft palate, genitourinary disorders,
C	Possible kidney stones in fetus in excessive doses

Table 1-2   Effects of Drugs on Fetus and Neonate *(Continued)*

Agent	Implications
D	In excessive doses, congenital/cardiac malformations (supravalvular aortic stenosis), peculiar facies and hypercalcemia (calcification of placenta and kidney); mental retardation can occur
K	A dose of 10 mg or more may cause hyperbilirubinemia, kernicterus, hemolysis
Folic acid deficiency	Thought to be teratogenic in humans
OTHER AGENTS	
Alcohol (ethyl alcohol)	"Fetal alcohol syndrome," decreased birth weight, decreased head size, withdrawal symptoms, retarded psychomotor development, CNS agitation or depression, metabolic acidosis
Carbon monoxide	Anoxia which may lead to brain damage; stillbirth
Cholecystographic agents containing iodine, iophenoxic acid (Teridax)	May remain in maternal blood for decades; one recorded case of mother who bore three retarded hypothyroid children several years after Teridax was used; her first three children born before Teridax were normal
Dextroamphetamine sulfate (Dexedrine)	May cause withdrawal symptoms; may cause transposition of great vessels
Edrophonium chloride (Tensilon)	Transient muscle weakness
Food preservative (benzoic acid)	When given concurrently with aspirin, thought to enhance teratogenicity of aspirin
Heavy metals (lead, mercury, arsenic)	Cerebral palsy, mental retardation, abortion, congenital anomalies
LSD	Increased risk of abortion; may cause chromosomal breakage in users, although never substantiated; apparently no effect on sex cell chromosome
Smoking (excessive)	Intrauterine growth retardation, prematurity; newborn's weight averages 300 g below that from nonsmoking mothers
Ionizing radiation	Congenital anomalies, fetal death; linked with juvenile leukemia; avoid during pregnancy, particularly in first trimester

BIBLIOGRAPHY

* Brackbill, Yvonne: "Psychophysical Measures of Pharmacological Toxicity in Infants," in P. L. Morselli (ed.), *Basic and Therapeutic Aspects of Perinatal Pharmacology*, Raven Press, New York, 1975.

Brent, R.L.: "Medicolegal Aspects of Teratology," Second Semmelweiss Seminar, New Jersey College of Medicine, September 1976.

Chez, R.A., and A.R. Fleischman: "Fetal Therapeutics—Challenges and Responsibilities," *Clinical Pharmacology and Therapeutics*, **14**(4) (part 2):754, 1975.

Eriksson, M., Charlotte S. Catz, and Sumner J. Yaffee: "Drugs and Pregnancy," *Clinical Obstetrics and Gynecology*, **16**:1:199, March 1973.

Fofar, J.O., and M.M. Nelson: "Epidemiology of Drugs Taken by Pregnant Women," *Clinical Pharmacology and Therapeutics*, **4**:632, July-August 1973.

* Heinonen, O.P., D. Slone, and S. Shapiro: *Birth Defect and Drugs in Pregnancy*, PSG Publishing, Littleton, Mass., 1977.

Herbst, A.L., et al.: "Prenatal Exposure to Stilbestrol," *New England Journal of Medicine*, **292**:7:334, February 13, 1975.

McCrory, W.W.: Concluding Remarks, in "Symposium on Drugs and the Fetus," *Clinical Pharmacology and Therapeutics*, **14**:700, July-August 1973.

Nishamura, H., and T. Tahashi: *Clinical Aspects of the Teratogenicity of Drugs*, Experta Medica, American Elsevier, New York, 1976.

Overbach, Avrin M.: "Drugs Used with Neonates and During Pregnancy," Parts I, II, III, *RN*, October, November, and December, 1974.

Pomerance, J.J., and S.J. Yaffee: "Maternal Medication and Its Effect on the Fetus," *Current Problems in Pediatrics*, **4**:1–60, 1973.

*Denotes particularly pertinent references.

Sirrat, G.M.: "Prescribing Problems in the Second Half of Pregnancy and During Lactation," *Obstetric and Gynecological Survey*, **31**:1, 1976.

Smithells, R.W.: "Defects and Disabilities of Thalidomide Children," *British Medical Journal*, 1:269, 1973.

Waziri, M., V. Ionasecu, and H. Zellweger: "Teratogenic Effect of Anticonvulsant Drugs," *American Journal of Diseases of Children*, **130**:1022, September 1976.

* Wilson, James G.: "Present Status of Drugs as Teratogens in Man," *Teratology*, **7**:3–16, 1975.

* ———: *Environment and Birth Defects*, Academic Press, New York, 1977.

Wilson, J.T.: "Pragmatic Assessment of Medicines Available for Young Children and Pregnant or Breast-feeding Women," in P.L. Morselli (ed.), *Basic and Therapeutic Aspects of Perinatal Pharmacology*, Raven Press, New York, 1975.

Yaffee, Sumner J.: "A Clinical Look at the Problem of Drugs in Pregnancy and Their Effect on the Fetus," *Canadian Medical Association Journal*, **112**:6:728, 1975.

Yalom, Irvin D., Richard Green, and Norman Fish: "Prenatal Exposure to Female Hormones, Effect on Psychosocial Development in Boys," *Archives of General Psychiatry*, **28**:554, 1973.

2

Drug Utilization in Pregnancy

Elizabeth J. Dickason

Until recent years, drug studies have focused attention on the pathologic and teratogenic effects during the period of organogenesis. Now, however, research is being directed toward the effect of the sum of physiologic differences during pregnancy on drug utilization. Of particular relevance to the pregnant woman and her fetus are mechanisms regulating placental drug transfer and movement of agents across the barrier separating blood and breast milk. Physiologic changes in hormonal levels, body water, fatty tissue, and blood volume during pregnancy are also becoming recognized as influencing drug utilization in pregnancy.

The nine months of pregnancy should be viewed as a period of constantly changing, complex interactions between mother and fetus. During this period, most drugs ingested by the mother will cross the placenta to the fetus, achieving equilibrium and, in some cases, higher concentration in fetal circulation than in maternal circulation. At the same time, the continuum of fetal development is marked by an increasingly sophisticated ability of the fetus to metabolize the drugs passed transplacentally. Research now indicates that the fetus and newborn are unique organisms, varying greatly from the older child and adult in their ability to metabolize and excrete substances within a reference time interval. As a result of this fact, drug ingestion by the mother, especially in the third trimester, must be carefully monitored. Administration of drugs during the transitional period and the newborn period deserves every possible precaution.

ABSORPTION

A drug must be absorbed to reach its site of action. Absorption usually involves penetration through a membrane barrier made of lipid (fat) and protein molecules containing small pores through which water and some water-soluble substances can move, depending on molecular weight. Three major groups of substances are absorbed by different methods of transportation.

1. Fat-soluble (nonionized, undissociated) drugs move rapidly, diffusing across a membrane by *passive diffusion* (without using energy) because they are readily dissolved in and move through the membrane's lipoid substance. The direction of movement depends on the amount of drug on each side of the membrane, since a compound moves from an area of higher concentration to one of lower concentration. After traversing the membrane, the drug moves by way of systemic circulation to its site of action.

2. Water-soluble (ionized, dissociated) drugs can move through the sievelike membrane in relation to the pH, osmotic, and electrochemical differences on each side of the membrane. Water, carrying small molecules with it, moves from the side of higher concentration to that of lower concentration. Drugs with low molecular weights and many of the inorganic ions move in this way, but their movement is generally slower than that of fat-soluble molecules.

3. Lipid-insoluble drugs, which have higher molecular weights and are *ionized* (dissociated, possessing an electrical charge), are not able to pass through body membranes easily. Some of these drugs need to combine with a carrier substance (a protein) to be transported; once the interstitial fluid or plasma has been reached, the drug is released. The rate of transport, in fact, depends upon the availability of protein molecules; if all are "busy" (saturated), absorption is impaired.

The degree of ionization of a drug also influences its ability to be absorbed and excreted. Fat-soluble drugs tend to be nonionized and absorbed easily, while water-soluble drugs tend to be ionized and less readily absorbed. Drugs can be altered to become more or less ionized when in pH environments different from their own. Acidic drugs would become more ionized in an alkaline pH, e.g., small intestine, and alkaline drugs would become more ionized in an acidic pH, e.g., stomach and duodenum. However, "drugs are usually weak acids or bases which may exist in solution as a mixture of ionized and non-ionized forms" (Dipalma, 1976, p. 18). Thus, when the pH of the stomach or intestines is changed by food or medication, drug absorption may also be changed. If a person becomes acidotic (blood pH drops below 7.35–7.45) drug absorption is also influenced; i.e., acidic drugs are absorbed more easily and excreted less readily. In instances where alkalosis occurs, the reverse would be true; basic drugs would be absorbed more easily and excreted less readily.

Oral Medication

The absorption of oral (PO) medication is affected by many factors: gastrointestinal motility (length of time in the stomach), the dosage and form of the drug (i.e., liquid, tablet, enteric coated, or sustained released), the presence of food or other medication in the stomach, and the pH of the stomach, duodenum, and intestine. Food in the stomach may chemically react with the drug or limit absorption by significantly changing the pH of the stomach and upper intestine, carrying the drug past the sites of absorption. This explains why a drug may be ordered 1 hour before meals (ac) or 2 hours after meals (pc). Other foods, such as those with high fat or oil content, may combine with fat-soluble vitamins (A, D, E, and K) or drugs, thus reducing availability for absorption. (Sometimes, drug absorption is enhanced by a fatty meal, e.g., griseofulvin.) Drugs taken concurrently may interact and either reduce or increase the degree of absorption. Absorption from the gastrointestinal (GI) tract is also affected by factors such as state of nutrition (starvation), fluid and electrolyte balance (dehydration), and the presence of diseases affecting GI function (malabsorption syndromes).

During pregnancy the digestive tract changes in a number of ways. There is reduced formation of hydrochloric acid in the stomach and delayed gastric emptying, which are two factors leading to delayed drug absorption of those medications which are usually absorbed in an acid environment or absorbed only in the small intestine. In addition, the absorption rate in the small intestine is slowed, but for some substances, this is balanced by slowed motility of the whole tract.

This slower absorption must be taken into account when evaluating a glucose tolerance test during pregnancy. The normal pregnancy pattern is "delayed, with a lower peak, but with prolonged sustained glucose elevations" resulting from the loading glucose dose remaining in the intestine longer (Greenwald and Kirschbaum, 1975, p. 299).

Parenteral Medication

Drugs administered by injection into skin (intradermal), fatty tissue (SC), muscle (IM), or the vascular system (IV) bypass the membrane barriers of the GI tract and are delivered rapidly to their site of action. Each injection site has properties which limit the type and volume of medication given during pregnancy (see Appendix B).

Drugs injected into the skin and subcutaneous tissue should be highly water-soluble, isotonic, and should not contain precipitates nor be in an oily base. If a very slow rate of absorption is desired, a drug is injected as a suspension of slowly soluble crystals (procaine penicillin) or is implanted as a pellet. Absorption takes place into lymph (large molecules) and capillary vessels (small and lipid-soluble molecules) and thus may bypass the liver, depending on the site of injection. Initially bypassing the liver, where most drug metabolism occurs, may contribute to a slightly prolonged action (eliminating the "first-pass" effect).

During pregnancy, drugs administered into subcutaneous and intradermal tissues may be absorbed more rapidly as a result of peripheral vasodilation, but injections into muscle tissue should not differ in absorption rate. Medication deposited in muscle richly supplied with blood vessels will usually be rapidly absorbed. Irritating, insoluble, or oily substances, as well as those easily absorbed, are injected into muscle tissue. Since the rate of absorption can be changed, drug solvents are selected to retard or speed absorption from muscle tissue.

All injections are thought to cause trauma to muscle tissue, but trauma varies with the injection technique as well as with drug concentration and vasoconstricting (epinephrine) qualities. Thus the injection site must be rotated and observations made about pain, signs of injury, and inflammation. Repeated use of the same site may produce fibrosis and decrease absorption.

The injection of drugs into the venous circulation produces rapid onset of action. Once injected, the drug reaches its site of action as fast as blood travels through the system. Precautions include absolute control over both the amount and rate of drug injected; i.e., always use a slow rate of injection and never inject a bolus. (There are a few exceptions to this rule, e.g., diazoxide with an injection rate within 10 seconds.) Slow injection is important because "rapid injection will saturate binding capacity of protein bound drugs in a limited blood volume with which drug mixes, producing very much higher concentration of free drug available to act at the receptor site" (Koch-Weser and Sellers, 1976, p. 314).

Strict aseptic technique must be exercised when the intravenous route is used. In addition, a drug must be compatible with blood, must not precipitate at blood pH, nor be administered in incompatible or oily liquids. Direct venous injection is often the responsibility of the physician, but the nurse prepares the dose and, in certain settings, administers it.

Control of intravenous infusions containing added drugs is the responsibility of the nurse. Whenever a potent drug is administered, the rate should be controlled by a constant infusion pump, e.g., use of heparin or pitocin. All other medications given intermittently via infusion should be delivered through a "piggyback line" using a controlled volume infusion set (see Appendix B).

Dermatomucosal Medication

The absorption rate of drugs applied to the skin depends on the skin site, epidermal thickness, and the presence of any breaks in the skin. The mechanism of absorption is diffusion, and fat-soluble drugs transfer most readily. The higher the concentration of the drug in contact with the skin and the larger the surface covered, the greater the amount transferred. Thus, if systemic absorption is not desired, caution should be used in drug concentration and the amount of surface area covered.

Mucous membranes can be used to administer either local or systemic drugs. This skin surface contains connective tissues and epithelial cells, some of which secrete mucus. The thickness of the mucous membrane layer and its vascularity determines the rate of absorption. Any drug intended for absorption through the mucous membrane should be placed in contact and left to be slowly dissolved. (If placed in the nose or mouth, it should not be swallowed.) Buccal, nasal, rectal, and vaginal mucosa are common sites for administration. The vagina possesses relatively thick epithelial tissue and is usually used only for local medicinal effect, although increased vascularity during pregnancy may speed absorption.

Lung alveolar membrane has a very rapid rate of absorption because it is thin and has a rich blood supply (which is augmented during pregnancy). Particles of 2 μm will usually deposit in nasal passages or in the trachea. Finer aerosol sprays (smaller particle size) will precipitate in smaller airways. Since absorption is erratic, this route is rarely used when systemic effects are desired. In addition, gaseous anesthetics are used with caution during pregnancy because of the increased induction rate resulting from hyperventilation and the greater circulation to lung tissue (Kennedy, 1974).

Transfer of drugs is slow across the sclera or cornea of the eye. Drops placed in the eye are intended for local effect and should always be directed so that they avoid entering the lacrimal ducts, which lead into more readily absorptive areas.

DISTRIBUTION

Once they are systemically absorbed, drugs encounter alterations in plasma and tissue caused by physiologic changes of pregnancy. Along with peripheral vasodilation and increased interstitial and cellular water, there is a dramatic increase in plasma volume of 30 to 40 percent in early pregnancy (by 8 to 10 weeks), a factor which changes the ratios of blood constituents.

Protein Binding

To become effective, a drug must be free to move to its receptor site. Tissue and protein binding are mechanisms which limit effectiveness by removing a free drug from the circulation. In the circulation, a drug may be dissolved in serum water or bound in many ways; it can be linked loosely with nucleoproteins, blood erythrocytes, globulins, lipoproteins, or albumin, or the drug may be taken up by other body tissues.

Most bound drugs are linked to an albumin molecule by ionic bonds which may easily be reversed.

Unbound drug + albumin = drug–albumin complex

Binding of a drug is limited by the available number of albumin molecules (Koch-Weser and Sellers, 1976, p. 311) and by the specific binding sites available for that drug.

Other factors such as hydrogen or hydrophobic bonding promote the drug–albumin bond. Drugs which are poorly soluble in water (lipophilic, hydrophobic) are often highly protein-bound (Koch-Weser and Sellers, 1976, p. 315). A bound drug is not able to move to its site of action until released to replace the drug at the receptor site once it has completed its action. Thus, protein binding is an important factor to consider in dosage and rate of excretion of a specific drug.

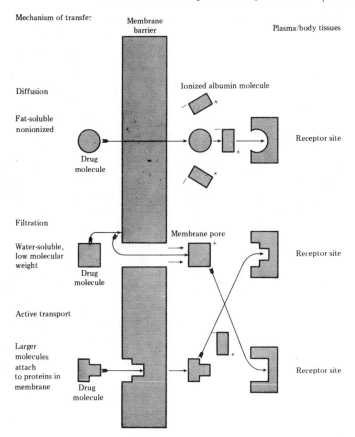

Mechanism of transfer

Membrane barrier

Plasma/body tissues

Diffusion

Fat-soluble nonionized

Ionized albumin molecule

Drug molecule

Receptor site

Filtration

Water-soluble, low molecular weight

Membrane pore

Drug molecule

Receptor site

Active transport

Larger molecules attach to proteins in membrane

Drug molecule

Receptor site

Figure 2-1   Schematic representation of drug absorption across membrane barriers.

When the concentration of the free drug falls, displacement occurs in an attempt to maintain equilibrium (Fig. 2-1). This displacement continues until the free drug reaches equilibrium in the serum and extracellular water. It is this concentration which is important for drug action at specific receptor sites, because only a free drug has the ability to reach the receptor site. For many drugs, only 5 to 20 percent of the drug is left unbound at one time (e.g., chlorothiazide, 95 percent bound; nafcillin, 90 percent bound). In these cases, higher doses may be needed to obtain initial action. In addition, the effect of a highly bound drug will usually be prolonged by slower elimination as drug is released from its reservoir of albumin-binding sites.

Although there is an increase in total albumin in the plasma during pregnancy, it is not proportionate to the increase in water, and the ratio of albumin/water falls approximately 1 g/100 ml (Greenwald and Kirschbaum, 1975, p. 296; Hytten and Leitch, 1971, p. 30). This change in the albumin/water ratio may allow further dilution of the free drug in tissue and plasma and affect the protein-binding capacity, slightly increasing the level of free drug expected from doses considered safe in nonpregnant states.

Competition for Binding Sites Adverse effects may occur when drugs compete for protein-binding sites. Those more highly ionized replace weakly ionized drugs because they have a higher affinity for the binding site. The release of all the formerly bound drug molecules into free circulation may result in a toxic level of free drug in the plasma.

During pregnancy, there appears to be increased competition for binding sites for several reasons. Endogenous estrogen and progesterone are protein-bound and will take up available sites in greater amounts during pregnancy. In addition, metabolic sources of energy are altered to conserve carbohydrates while increasing fatty tissue metabolism, resulting in a rise in free fatty acids, triglycerides, cholesterol, and phospholipids, all of which are carried in the plasma attached to proteins. Through this additional alteration, sites for protein binding may be further reduced. If such sites are not as readily available for binding drugs during pregnancy, a larger percent of the drug will be free to move to receptor sites or to cross membrane barriers such as the placenta. In an illustration of this effect, some women comment on their increased sensitivity to particular drugs which they had taken regularly before pregnancy (higher concentration of free drug = greater effect of the drug).

Tissue Binding

Some drugs have an affinity for tissues other than plasma proteins and may be deposited at these sites instead of at the proper receptor. Drugs may deposit first in bone or teeth (tetracycline) or in hair, nails, cell nuclei, adipose tissue, or in other tissues. Tissue binding may lead to storage of large amounts of drug, and saturation may have to be reached in specific tissue sites before there is sufficient free drug to be effective at the receptor site (e.g., thiopental's attraction for fat and muscle draws it away from the brain and gives it a very short duration of action at its receptor). When the drug is discontinued, tissue deposits give up their share slowly, causing a persistence of drug effect. For example, many lipid-soluble substances are stored in fatty tissue. Thus, in pregnancy, the increase in adipose tissue may slightly reduce the specific amount of a highly lipid-soluble drug in circulation (e.g., sedatives and hypnotics that leave a "hangover" because of slow release).

MEMBRANE BARRIERS TO DRUG TRANSPORT

Once absorbed, the drug will have to cross the body membranes which enclose each fluid reservoir and surround each organ, cell, and cell nucleus. Major membranes affecting drug responses in pregnancy are the placental barrier, the blood-brain barrier, and after delivery, the blood-milk barrier. Transport across these membranes influences which drugs will affect the fetus by entering its central nervous system or being excreted into its urine. Later, membrane transfer governs the degree to which drugs will pass into breast milk.

Placental Barrier

The placenta, a unique biologic membrane, possesses some similarities to, yet has some unique differences from, other body membranes. The placental membrane at the embryonic stage is composed of several cell layers of tissue separating the mother's blood from that of the embryo. This barrier is the layer of chorionic cells that makes up the lining of the villi in each placental cotyledon. The thickness of this layer diminishes from 25 μm to 2 μm in the course of pregnancy (Mirkin, 1975), suggesting that its permeability changes to facilitate the passage of substances as pregnancy proceeds. In fact, it has been shown that even early in pregnancy, most drugs, except some of high molecular weight (1000+), pass this lipoid membrane. In the later stages of gestation, large molecules, notably antibodies, may in some cases traverse the membrane.

The placental membrane is composed of lipoprotein and permits passive or active transport of free non-protein-bound drugs to the fetal circulation. Usually within 40 minutes of oral drug intake by the mother, drug equilibrium will be reached with the fetal circulation by the following mechanisms: (1) passive diffusion—from higher to lower concentrations, (2) active transport—using a carrier system and moving against a concentration gradient (e.g., Na^+, K^+, amino acids, or using facilitated diffusion), not against a concentration gradient (e.g., glucose, pyrimidines), and (3) placental metabolic conversion (Eriksson et al., 1973).

Variations in placental blood flow will influence the transfer of materials. The condition of intrauterine growth retardation, when secondary to placental dysfunction, will often be associated with diminution of nutrient and waste transfer. Either maternal hypotension or hypertension (the latter causing placental ischemic areas as a result of vasoconstriction) would diminish blood flow to the membrane and change transfer rates because of pressure (gradient) differences.

Differences in maternal and fetal pH will also promote or hinder transfer and reabsorption of drugs. This pH *gradient* influences membrane transfer at every site but is especially important in terms of placental function in cases of fetal hypoxia and acidosis during fetal distress. The pH of cord blood is normally 0.10–0.15 pH units lower than maternal blood pH (Mirkin and Singh, 1976, p. 26). Changes in this pH relationship may result in drug redistribution secondary to impairment of membrane transport.

Blood-Brain Barrier (BBB)

Another significant biologic membrane, the blood-brain barrier, acts selectively to prevent certain substances from entering into brain tissue. This membrane, consisting of capillary walls and the glial membranes which separate plasma from the extracellular fluid (ECF) of the brain, develops toward the end of pregnancy. It has no pores, and since the capillaries are covered with a tight lipoid sheath, lipid-soluble, non-protein-bound drugs have the greatest possibility of entering the brain ECF. Most others are excluded, unless the patient is in a state of respiratory acidosis or alkalosis severe enough to change the ECF pH. Anoxia, trauma, or inflammation of the brain (meningitis) will also alter the permeability of the blood-brain barrier to drugs.

Blood-Milk Barrier

The membrane barrier between maternal plasma and breast milk consists of an epithelial layer lining the mammary alveolar ducts. Transfer is mainly by diffusion of lipid-soluble substances. The pH of milk is 0.4–0.7 pH units below plasma; therefore, basic drugs are favored in transfer and may be found to concentrate in larger amounts in milk than in plasma, while acidic drugs would be less readily transferred, and neutral substances would be evenly divided (Vorherr, 1974). Highly protein-bound substances and drugs of high molecular weights are less readily transferred.

Determination of which drugs will affect the infant has been difficult because of the complex process of milk production, the variation within each 24 hours in the constituents of milk, and the difficulty in predicting whether the free drug or an inactive metabolite will be transferred. In addition, once a drug is solubilized in breast milk, it may be broken down by the enzymes and flora in the newborn GI tract or passed through rapidly producing incomplete absorption. Thus the effect of drugs on the nursing infant has been largely determined by empirical studies, with all the attending problems of measurement. Lists of approved and nonrecommended drugs during lactation are given in Chapter 3.

BIOTRANSFORMATION

Drugs produce their effects by combining with enzymes or cell components. This drug-cell interaction produces an alteration of membrane structure and cellular function which results in a chain of biochemical and physiologic changes specific for a given drug. The initial result of the drug–cell interaction is termed the *action*, while the resultant occurrences are the *effects*. Drug action precedes and produces the effect. Although most drugs act at specific body sites, the ultimate effect of a drug might take place far from its locus of action. Many drugs exert multiple actions, and these actions tend to be related.

Drugs can be used to replace a missing substance (L-dopa), counteract an already present drug (protamine and heparin), correct a chemical imbalance, or change body function by their general presence in the body. Some drugs are termed *mimetic agents* because they mimic or duplicate the action of a normal body chemical transmitter. Other drugs act by inhibiting enzyme function or steps in metabolism (allopurinol, MAO inhibitors). Antibiotics (sulfamethoxazole) act on microorganisms in this way, thereby blocking the organism's growth or ability to function.

It has been hypothesized that most drugs act by combining with cellular components which have an affinity or attraction for the drug. This intracellular component is termed a *receptor*. (Drug-cell interactions which do not produce drug action are thought to involve silent receptors.) Adherents of the receptor theory define *agonists* as drugs which combine with receptors to produce a sequence of effects and *antagonists* as drugs which interact with a receptor to inhibit action of an agonist. Receptors are classified according to effects of agonists and lack of effects of antagonists.

Drug action is usually terminated by metabolism and excretion or by redistribution from the site of action into other tissues. Some drugs are inactivated on the first pass through the liver, while others are metabolized much more slowly because of high levels of protein and tissue binding. Regardless of the rate, the metabolic process will continue until the drug is completely altered, either into an active metabolite form or, after being metabolized, into an inactive product. The process works toward making a drug less fat-soluble and weakly ionized and thus less able to bind to protein, to cross membranes, or to be reabsorbed by the kidney.

These biotransformations are either nonsynthetic or synthetic. In phase I (nonsynthetic) reactions, a single drug may be changed to a number of different metabolic products, some of which are inactive, some of which are active, and a few of which may be more active than the parent drug. Nonsynthetic reactions result from oxidation, reduction, or hydrolysis and change a parent drug to metabolic products which are weakly ionized and less fat-soluble. These metabolic processes take place primarily in the microsomal fraction of the liver, although some reactions may also occur in the plasma, the kidneys, and the GI tract.

If it is not rendered inactive by phase I reactions, a drug will undergo phase II (synthetic) reactions before excretion. Synthetic reactions generally convert nonionized drugs by mechanisms of conjugation to the ionized form, which can be excreted in the bile or the urine.

The microsomal portion of the liver produces many of the enzymes which are active in drug metabolism. These hepatic microsomal enzymes can be induced (barbiturates, phenytoin, alcohol) or inhibited (MAO inhibitors) by pharmacotherapeutic agents and depend as well on environmental influences, genetic factors, and patient age. Agents known as *enzyme inducers* stimulate increased enzyme production by increasing the size and content of the endoplasmic reticulum, resulting in faster drug metabolism than might otherwise be expected. Both the inducers themselves and the results of induction may be helpful or harmful. *Enzyme inhibitors* inhibit metabolism and can delay excretion of a drug. A cumulative effect may result, which can be dramatically illustrated when an anticoagulant is administered with an enzyme inhibitor and bleeding results as drug doses are continued while the drug is not being metabolized in usual amounts.

The liver excretes many of its metabolic products into the biliary tree, which drains into the small intestine. There, partially metabolized substances may be further altered, reabsorbed into the circulation, and later presented to the liver for conjugation and excretion. This *enterohepatic cycle* appears to be quite prominent in the newborn, who as a result, may experience many hours or days of delay in final clearance of a drug. Ampicillin and all tetracyclines are involved in this cycle to some extent. Diazepam and chlorpromazine also undergo recycling.

Certain functions of the microsomal portion of the liver are slowed during pregnancy, which delays metabolism of some drugs. In addition, the gallbladder becomes hypotonic in response to the vasodilating effect of estrogens, and there is delayed excretion of bile (with an increased possibility of the formation of gallstones.) Thus, in another way the enterohepatic cycle may be slowed, allowing drug action to be sustained.

Metabolism by the Placenta

There are a number of unresolved questions about the metabolic role of the placenta. It is recognized that one of its primary activities is to metabolize endogenous hormones, e.g., androgen to estrogen; maternal cholesterol to pregnenolone and then to progesterone. The fetal–placental unit demonstrates its integrated function by placental metabolism to estriols of *dehydroepiandrosterone*, which has been formed in fetal adrenals. Drugs which compete at the placental level for this enzymatic activity may alter steroid production significantly and thus interrupt the function of those hormones controlling fetal development.

Cigarette smoking has been shown to increase some placental metabolic function. In doing so, metabolism of hormones or drugs may be speeded. The result of this effect is not yet clear.

Half-life

Half-life $(T_{1/2})$ has been described in many ways but can be generally considered as the time period in which half the absorbed dose is metabolized (Martin, 1969, p. 120). Knowl-

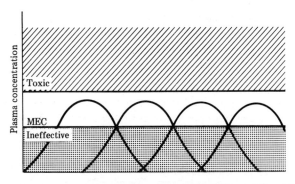

Figure 2-2   Minimum effective concentration (MEC) is achieved by administering a drug at intervals determined by its rate of metabolism.

edge of a drug's half-life, including modification of absorption, biotransformation, and excretion, may especially modify dosage regimens in the transitional and newborn periods.

Minimum Effective Concentration

Another useful measurement of drug absorption, distribution, and metabolic rate is the level of *minimum effective concentration* (MEC) achieved in the blood. Drug doses should be given at intervals close enough to maintain the correct MEC. The ideal dosage regimen is to space drug intake in such a manner as to keep plasma levels above the MEC and below the toxic level (Fig. 2-2). Drugs which are rapidly metabolized must be given at more frequent intervals or by continuous infusion (heparin, nitroprusside). Drugs which are highly protein- or tissue-bound may take several days to reach their MEC, and once discontinued the drug may require additional time to be completely metabolized and eliminated. Measurement of drug blood levels is a valuable aid in understanding drug metabolism, but such determination must never replace a nurse's close observation of signs and symptoms suggestive of cumulative, toxic, or poor drug effect. Information pamphlets provide general data on rates of metabolism, but wide variation in individuals' ability to metabolize drugs means that a "safe" dose for one patient may be inadequate or toxic for another.

EXCRETION

Drugs can be eliminated through feces, saliva, respired air, sweat, bile, or urine, but the major route is through urine, that which is formed by filtration by renal glomeruli, dependent mainly on diffusion, and by tubular secretion utilizing active transport. The renal glomerular membrane acts like other membrane "barriers" in the body but contains many more large pores through which water can move, carrying with it dissolved metabolites. This process of filtration carries the bulk of solutes from plasma into urine. The more water-soluble substances would be more readily excreted without reabsorption, while fat-soluble substances are, in large measure, reabsorbed across the tubular membrane and recirculated for a prolonged drug effect. Reabsorption of very large amounts of water and electrolytes, as well as other substances in plasma, is the key process in maintaining fluid and electrolyte balance.

A 50 percent increase in renal plasma flow is maintained through the second and third trimesters. This rate is altered by body position, for when the woman is lying supine the compression of vessels to the kidney will reduce blood flow.

The glomerular filtration rate is increased even more during pregnancy, a factor which, with a sodium-preserving factor, appears to allow increased excretion of waste products without significantly changing urine volume. Because of the increased circulation of blood to kidney, those drugs easily excreted may be metabolized more quickly than in the nonpregnant state.

Reabsorption may be hindered or speeded up by changing the pH of the urine. Bases are excreted more rapidly into acidic urine (meperidine), and acid substances (phenobarbital, salicylic acid) are excreted more rapidly into alkaline urine. The pH of urine can be changed by administration of large doses of substances, such as vitamin C or cranberry juice toward acidic levels and sodium bicarbonate toward alkaline levels. Active transport can also be altered by concurrent administration of specialized drugs. Probenecid may be given with penicillin to reduce or inhibit the rapid excretion of this antibiotic. Since such a drug may affect other medications as well, it must be considered in dosage regimens for that medication.

Only free drug molecules can be eliminated from glomeruli and tubules. Some drugs are excreted as free and unmetabolized, e.g., gentamycin, 92 to 98 percent unmetabolized.

As active transport eliminates a free drug, release of a protein-bound drug occurs, maintaining equilibrium. In this manner, depending on drug amount and transport availability, the entity is gradually or rapidly excreted. Other drugs bound to albumin or tissues are not excreted until released and metabolized. Some highly bound drugs therefore have prolonged elimination times and are excreted very slowly in decreasing amounts for days or weeks.

BIBLIOGRAPHY

DiPalma, Joseph R.: *Basic Pharmacology in Medicine*, McGraw-Hill, New York, 1976.

Eriksson, M., C. S. Catz, and S. J. Yaffee: "Drugs and Pregnancy," *Clinical Obstetrics and Gynecology*, **16**(1):201, March 1973.

Greenwald, E.F., and T. H. Kirschbaum: "Changes in the Status of Women During Pregnancy," in S.L. Romney, (ed.), *The Health Care of Women*, McGraw-Hill, New York, 1975, chap. 22.

Hytten, F. E., and I. Leitch: *The Physiology of Human Pregnancy*, Blackwell Scientific Publications, Oxford, 1971.

Kennedy, R. L.: "General Analgesia and Anesthesia in Obstetrics," *Clinical Obstetrics and Gynecology*, **17**(2):230, June 1974.

Koch-Weser J., and E. M. Sellers: "Binding of Drugs to Serum Albumin," *New England Journal of Medicine*, **294**(6):311, 1976.

Martin, E. W.: *Hazards of Medication*, J. B. Lyppincott, Philadelphia, 1969.

Mirkin, Bernard L.: "Maternal and Fetal Distribution of Drugs in Pregnancy," *Clinical Pharmacology and Therapeutics*, 14(4):645, 1975.

————, and S. Singh: *Perinatal Pharmacology and Therapeutics*, Academic Press, New York, 1976.

Vorherr, H.: "Drug Excretion and Breast Milk," *Postgraduate Medicine*, **566**:97, 1974.

3

Drugs Used in Normal Pregnancy and Lactation

Martha Olsen Schult

This chapter discusses those drugs prescribed during pregnancy which have been shown to have no harmful effect on the fetus or neonate (at this time). Drugs which may have a harmful effect are listed in several of the following tables. In such a rapidly changing field, many statements must of necessity remain tentative until conclusive proof is obtained.

ANTACIDS During pregnancy the motility of the stomach is slowed, and early in pregnancy, gastric acidity is reduced. Therefore, an antacid is rarely necessary. Later, however, the cardiac sphincter becomes slightly relaxed, and the pressure of the enlarging uterus causes slight regurgitation of stomach acid through the sphincter into the esophagus. The acid reflux irritates the mucosa, causing a burning sensation. In addition to this discomfort of *heartburn*, increased movement of the diaphragm and the flaring rib cage may create a temporary *hiatus hernia*.

Nonpharmacologic remedies for these problems should be advised before drug therapy is begun. Such remedies include (1) drinking milk between meals, (2) eating small, frequent meals, (3) avoiding gas-producing and fatty foods, and (4) alternating dry and liquid meals.

Any antacid should be prescribed by the physician, and the patient should be advised against taking extra doses.

Large quantities of calcium carbonate can cause "milk-alkali syndrome" or acid rebound, inducing the stomach to secrete *more* acid. Schenkel and Vorherr (1974) report that large doses of magnesium trisilicate may damage fetal kidneys, and fetal neurologic and neuromuscular systems can be damaged by magnesium hydroxide. Sodium bicarbonate should probably be avoided completely during pregnancy because of its high sodium content, its systemic absorption, and the gaseous carbon dioxide produced by it in the stomach. Whenever antacids are necessary, they should be used judiciously and avoided in the first trimester whenever possible. Table 3-1 lists the ingredients of various over-the-counter antacids.

Antacids During Labor

During labor, many physicians will order either an immediate (stat) dose or q 2 h doses of an antacid to neutralize stomach acidity. A dosage regimen of 15 ml of magnesium trisilicate q 2 h to raise the gastric pH to above 2.5 is recommended to reduce pulmonary complications should the patient vomit and aspirate during the labor or delivery.

Nursing Implications

1. Instruct the patient to take the least amount of medication for the shortest time possible to control the symptoms and to follow physician's directions.

2. Magnesium products have a laxative tendency, and aluminum and calcium have a constipating effect, but combinations of aluminum–magnesium seem to have few untoward effects.

3. If a choice of medication is available, a liquid is generally more desirable in terms of effectiveness. If the tablet or wafer form is given, be sure it is chewed thoroughly and followed with liquid (at least 60 to 90 ml); otherwise the antacid may be ineffective or remain undissolved in the stomach.

4. Check the medication for sodium content for patients on salt-restricted diets.

Table 3-1 Ingredients of Over-the-Counter Antacids

Trade Name	Aluminum Hydroxide (gel)	Magnesium Carbonate, Hydroxide, Peroxide, or Trisilicate	Calcium Carbonate	Acetylsalicylic Acid (Aspirin)	Sodium or Sodium Bicarbonate
AlCaroid	x	x			
Alka Seltzer			x*	x	1901 mg
Alkets		x	x		
Amphojel	x				
A-M-T	x	x			25.5 mg/15 ml
Bisodol		x	x		
Camalox	x	x	x		1.5 mg/tablet; 2.5 mg/5 ml
Creamlin	x	x			9 mg/15 ml; 41 mg/tablet
Chooz		x	x		
Citrocarbonate		x	x		2100 mg/15 ml
Di-Gel	x	x			25.5 mg/15 ml; 10.6 mg/tablet
Ducon	x	x	x		45 mg/15 ml
Fizrin				x	1820 mg
Gaviscon	x	x			70 mg
Gelusil	x	x			9 mg/tablet; 8 mg/5 ml
Gelusil-Lac	x	x			7.5 mg
Kolantyl	x	x			10 mg/wafer; 20 mg/tablet
Kudrox	x	x			

*Calcium phosphate.

Table 3-1 **Ingredients of Over-the-Counter Antacids (*Continued*)**

Trade Name	Alumi-umi-Hydrox-ide (gel)	Magnesium Carbonate, Hydroxide, Peroxide, or Trisilicate	Calcium Carbo-nate	Acetyl-salicylic Acid (Aspirin)	Sodium or Sodium Bicarbonate
Krem		x	x		
Maalox	x	x†			7.5 mg/15 ml
Maalox #1	x	x†			1 mg/tablet
Maalox #2	x	x†			2 mg/tablet
Magnatri	x	x			
Magnesium-Alum HydroxideGel	x	x			25.2 mg/15 ml
Malcogel	x	x			
Mucotin	x	x			
Mylicon		‡			
Mylanta	x	x†			11.7 mg/15 ml; 0.79 mg/tablet
Mylanta II	x	x†			1.6 mg/tablet; 4–10 mg/5 ml
Ratio		x	x		0.6–0.8 mg
Riopan	x	x			0.7 mg/tablet; 2.1 mg/15 ml
Silain-Gel	x	x†			
Sippyplex	x	x			
SodaMint					324 mg (sodium bicarbonate); 87.4 mg (sodium)
Syntrogal	x	x	x		
Tricreamalate	x	x			123 mg/15 ml

†Plus simethicone.
‡Simethicone only.

Table 3-1   Ingredients of Over-the-Counter Antacids (*Continued*)

Trade Name	Aluminum Hydroxide (gel)	Magnesium Carbonate, Hydroxide, Peroxide, or Trisilicate	Calcium Carbonate	Acetylsalicylic Acid (Aspirin)	Sodium or Sodium Bicarbonate
Trisogel	x	x			48 mg/15 ml
Trisomin		x			
Tums		x	x		2.7 mg
WinGel	x	x			7.5 mg/15 ml; 2.5 mg/tablet
Zylase		x	x		

5. Nonsystemic antacids are preferable to systemic ones that may cross placental barrier.

6. Antacids inhibit the absorption of anticholingerics and barbiturates. Aluminum, magnesium, iron, and calcium—all heavy metal ions—inhibit tetracycline absorption.

ANTIEMETICS

Nausea is one of the most common complaints of the first trimester for about 50 percent of all pregnant women. Although psychologic factors, such as ambivalence toward the pregnancy, may be involved, there is a physiologic basis for nausea in the marked gastrointestinal changes and in elevated human chorionic gonadotropin (HCG) levels. Fortunately, by the thirteenth week, most women are free of "morning sickness."

Before any antiemetic is prescribed, other avenues of relief should be explored. Women are often advised to eat a few dry crackers or toast before arising from bed in the morning. Dry, easily digested carbohydrate food in the stomach may prevent symptoms, and frequent, small meals may provide more relief than large ones. Since fat slows down peristalsis, low-fat meals will not aggravate the already slowed motility that underlies these symptoms. Liquids should be consumed between meals to prevent dehydration. If vomiting persists or is severe, the physician should be notified for treatment. Medications to stop nausea and vomiting must be by prescription, not an over-the-counter purchase. If an antiemetic is needed, it should be used judiciously during the first 5 to 8 weeks, since conclusions on adverse effects on organogenesis are not complete.

Benzquinamide Hydrochloride (Emete-Con)

Emete-Con is thought to exert a depressant effect on the chemoreceptor trigger zone (CTZ), thereby suppressing nausea. It is used only in severe vomiting.

Adverse Effects   Drowsiness, headache, dry mouth, restlessness, nervousness, flushing, blurred vision, excitement, insomnia, shivering, sweating, and salivation. After intravenous injection, cardiovascular effects may be noted.

Dosage   A dose of 50 mg IM may be repeated in 1 h, then q 3 to 4 h as needed (prn); 25 mg IV, single dose only.

Nursing Implications
1. Use sparingly since teratogenicity has not been established.

2. Intravenous medication must be given slowly.

Dicyclomine Hydrochloride, Doxylamine Succinate, and Pyridoxine Hydrochloride (Bendectin)

The antiemetic action of Bendectin is related to the antispasmodic and antihistaminic action of its ingredients. Delayed action coating promotes action in early morning.

Adverse Effects   Atropinelike effects (dry mouth, blurred vision, thirst, dizziness), rash, fatigue, sedation, constipation, anorexia, nausea, vomiting, headache, dysuria, nervousness, epigastric pain, palpation, diarrhea, disorientation, and irritability.

Dosage Two tablets at bedtime (hs). If necessary, 1 additional tablet in the morning.

Nursing Implications
1. Because of the antihistaminic component of the drug, patients should be cautioned about accompanying drowsiness.
2. Bendectin is specific for nausea and vomiting of pregnancy and is a researched drug.

Levulose, Dextrose, and Orthophosphoric Acid (Emetrol)

Emetrol acts locally on the walls of the GI tract to reduce smooth muscle contraction in direct proportion to the amount taken. It acts quickly to alleviate nausea and vomiting. There are no reported adverse effects.

Dosage For nausea of pregnancy, 1 or 2 tbsp (5 to 10 ml) on arising; may be repeated q 3 h prn. Do not dilute the medication; instruct patient not to drink fluids before or until 15 min after the dose is taken.

Trimethobenzamide Hydrochloride (Tigan)

The antiemetic action of Tigan is directed toward the CTZ in the medulla oblongata through which emetic impulses travel.

Adverse Effects Drowsiness, occasionally Parkinsonlike symptoms, skin reactions. Rarely, blurred vision, coma, depression, convulsions, diarrhea, dizziness, headache, jaundice, muscle cramps, and opisthotonos.

Dosage 250 mg PO (capsule) tid or qid; 200 mg rectally (suppository) tid or qid; or 200 mg (2 ml) IM tid or qid.

Nursing Implications
1. Do not give suppository to benzocaine-sensitive individuals.

2. Although side effects are rare, they do occur, and skin reactions are the first sign of hypersensitivity. Drowsiness may occur.

3. Tigan is well tolerated and researched. Although all studies are not complete, it has not been proven harmful to mother or fetus.

Antiemetics Best Avoided During Pregnancy

Buclizine, cyclizine, and meclizine are antihistamines not presently used in view of the teratogenic effects of these piperazines in animal studies. Nor is Compazine to be used during pregnancy.

LAXATIVES With the slowing of peristalsis during pregnancy, more vitamins, minerals, and other nutrients are extracted from foods eaten. In the process, however, water is also extracted. Adequate exercise, increased fluid intake, and foods containing roughage will help to alleviate constipation, but the physician may also have to order a laxative or stool softener. Tables 3-2 and 3-3 list, respectively, laxatives to avoid during pregnancy and laxatives used during pregnancy.

Table 3-2 Laxatives to Avoid During Pregnancy

Drug	Caution
Liquid petrolatum (Kondremul, mineral oil, retention enema)	Blocks absorption of fat-soluble vitamins A, D, E and K. During pregnancy, blocked absorption of vitamin K can lead to hypoprothrombinemia in the newborn.
Danthron	Systemic absorption; thus contraindicated.
Castor oil	Causes too severe catharsis.
Disacodyl tannex enema (Clysodrast)	Tannic acid may be hepatotoxic if absorbed.
Casanthrol	Ten times as potent as cascara and too severe for pregnancy.

Table 3-3 Laxatives Used During Pregnancy

Drug	Dosage	Comments
Dioctyl calcium sulfosuccinate (Bu-lax,	Pink: 1 to 3 capsules (50 mg) daily Red: 1 capsule (250 mg) daily	Stool softener. Wetting agent with no peristaltic action. Nonsystemic. Does not alter physiology or interfere with vitamin absorption. Non-habit-forming. Causes occasional, mild cramps. Do not give in presence of nausea, vomiting, intestinal obstruction, or abdominal pain.
Dioctyl sodium sulfosuccinate (Bu-lax, Colace, Disonate, DioMeodicone, Doxinate, Ilozoft)	1 or 2 capsules (100 mg) daily. Liquid syrup available.	Wetting agent and stool softener. Not a laxative. May promote mineral oil absorption. Occasionally causes nausea, vomiting, abdominal pain, and intestinal obstruction. Mix liquid form with ½ glass of milk or juice to mask taste.
Dioctyl sodium sulfosuccinate with casanthranol (Di-Sosul, Pericolace, Stimulax, Comfolax-plus, Forte tablets)	1 to 2 capsules hs or 1 to 3 tablets qd	Mild laxative with peristaltic stimulation. Occasional nausea, griping loose stools, or constipation rebound. Given postpartum. Prolonged use may cause dependence.
Dioctyl sodium sulfosuccinate with psyllium mucilloid (Sof-cil)	1 rounded tsp stirred into glass of fruit juice bid or tid	Two agents. Controlled bulk and wetting agent. No adverse effects. Stir in liquid quickly. Do not allow to stand.
Dioctyl sodium sulfosuccinate with senna concentrate (Senokap Dss Capsules)	1 to 2 capsules hs	Stool softener; stimulates peristaltic action in 8 to 10 h; ½ dose during pregnancy.
Malt soup extract (Maltsupex)	2 tbsp bid or hs mixed with 1 full glass of liquid	Mild, effective laxative with no adverse effects. Allow for CHO content if patient diabetic (14 g/tbsp, liquid).
Methylcellulose (Cellothyl, Cologel, Methocel, Hydrolose, Syncelose)	1–5 g up to qid	Increases bulk by swelling, forming mass and thus stimulates peristalsis. May cause diarrhea, nausea/vomiting. Patient must *not* chew tablets. Drink at least 2 glasses water. Not for chronic use or when GI pain, obstruction, or diarrhea are present.

Table 3-3   Laxatives Used During Pregnancy (*Continued*)

Drug	Dosage	Comments
Psyllium hydrophilic mucilloid (Betajel, Konsyl, Metamucil, Mucilose)	1 rounded tsp (7 g) stirred into glass of liquid once daily, bid, or tid	Soft celloidal bulk does not interfere with absorption of vitamins. Causes physiologic peristalsis. Must be taken with adequate fluid (1 to 2 glasses of water), otherwise, could cause impaction. Do not let stand after mixing.

NONNARCOTIC ANALGESICS

Pain, other than an occasional discomfort, is abnormal during pregnancy, and its cause should be assessed before any pregnant woman is given an analgesic. When a pregnant woman does experience discomfort during pregnancy, it is usually due to lower back pain, sciatic pain, headache, or muscle cramps. If the pain is caused by tension, poor posture, pressure symptoms from uterine enlargement, or by other physiologic changes of pregnancy, measures other than drug therapy may be utilized.

Muscle cramps may be a result of calcium–phosphorus imbalance or may be due to unusual or excessive exercise. To relieve the pain of muscle cramps, standing on a cold floor or pressure on the knee while dorsiflexing the foot may be helpful.

Analgesics are to be used sparingly in pregnancy. It has been shown that aspirin, which has been commonly used, can cause problems in the neonate. Schenkel and Vorherr (1974) report that studies indicate that 3 g of aspirin (or 9 tablets) taken daily for 3 to 6 days could cause fecal blood loss of about 5.0 ml per day, and even 2 aspirin tablets a day can increase the bleeding time significantly. They further report that aspirin taken as long as 2 weeks prior to delivery resulted in infants with a 10 percent higher risk of developing cephalohematoma, purpura, and a transient melena. Potential hazards of salicylates to developing infants include teratogenic effects on the central nervous system (CNS) through-out pregnancy and upon the kidneys during second to fifth month, GI tract bleeding with possibility or hemorrhage at delivery, and salicylate poisoning of the newborn.

Para-aminopheral derivatives (acetonalid, acetaminophen, and phenacetin) also have the potential for causing teratogenic effects, particularly when given in large doses and in com-bination with other drugs, as in headache mixtures (Schenkel and Vorherr, 1974). In light of these findings, it is probably best for the infant if the mother refrains from taking *any* analgesics containing these substances during the first 8 weeks of her pregnancy and within 2 weeks of her EDC.

Postpartum patients do not have to take the same pre-cautions because the neonate can no longer be affected by medication unless the baby is being breast-fed.

Most primaparas do not experience strong "after-pains," but multiparas and nursing mothers do. Local anesthetic sprays, compresses, sitz baths, and/or ice packs are usually sufficient to alleviate the pain from the episiotomy site. In addition, Kegel exercises are also helpful for perineal discom-fort. The analgesics listed below will usually suffice to relieve postpartum discomfort, but narcotic analgesics may be neces-sary to relieve the more severe pain caused by cesarean section.

Acetaminophen (Apamide, Capital, Datril, Lyteca, Tapat, Tempo, Tempra, Tylenol, and Many Others)

An analgesic and an antipyretic, acetaminophen is generally free of untoward effects unless taken in large, frequent doses, in which case liver damage can result. If a rare sensitivity occurs, drug should be stopped.

Dosage   325 mg, 1 or 2 tablets, tid or qid.

Nursing Implications   Caution patient about ingesting large doses of this or any other medication, as hepatotoxicity and other toxic reactions may result.

Table 3-4   Common Medications Containing Nonrecommended Ingredients

SALICYLATES

Alka Seltzer	Bayer Aspirin*	Excedrin	Pyra-Gesic
Anacin	Bufferin	Femicin	Salicorbate
APC	Comeback	Liquiprin*	St. Joseph*
ASA Compound	Cope	Measurin*	Trigesic
Ascriptin	Ecotrin*	Midol	Vanquish
Aspergum*	Empirin Compound	Pamprin	

PARA-AMINOPHENOL DERIVATIVES: PHENACETIN, ACETONALID, ACETAMINOPHEN

APC

ASA Compound	Datril*	Monthly Ets*	Pyra-Gesic
Bromo-Seltzer	Empirin Compound	Nebs*	Tempra*
Comback	Excedrin	Nilprin 7½*	Trendar
Contramal	Febrinol Tablets*	PAC	Trigesic
Compound	Femicin	Pamprin	Tylenol*
Counterpain	Medache	Percogesic	Vanquish

CNS STIMULANTS: XANTHINES

Anacin	Comback	Excedrin	Pyra-Gesic
APC	Cope	Femicin	Trigesic
ASA Compound	Easy-Mens	Midol	Vanquish
Bromo-Seltzer	Empirin Compound	Pre-Mens	

*Drug contains one ingredient.

Acetylsalicylic Acid (Aspirin)

Acetylsalicylic acid is an analgesic with antipyretic and anti-inflammatory action having a depressant effect on both the CNS and peripheral pain receptors.

Adverse Reactions   Affects clotting time; causes ringing in the ears, gastric irritation (fetal and maternal), sweating, drowsiness, thirst, and headache. Potential fetal hazards include teratogenic effects, GI bleeding, possible hemorrhage at birth, and salicylate poisoning of the newborn.

Dosage   325 mg, 1 or 2 tablets, q 4 h prn.

Nursing Implications

1. Check the patient's history for sensitivity to this or other salicylates.

2. Avoid during organogenesis and the third trimester (within 2 weeks of delivery) in order to prevent hemorrhagic disorders at delivery.

3. Do not give aspirin if the patient is taking ferrous gluconate or the food preservative benzoic acid, as these are suspected of enhancing the teratogenic aspect of aspirin (Kimmel and Schmacher, 1971).

4. Give the medication with milk to help reduce its irritating effect on the intestinal mucosa.

Propoxyphene Hydrochloride (Darvon, Dolene, Doloxene, Dolocap, Harmar, Propox, Progesic-65, Propoxychel, and Others)

Propoxyphene HCl is an analgesic for relief of mild to moderate pain.

Adverse Reactions   Dizziness, nausea and vomiting, skin rashes; may temporarily impair physical and mental abilities. Interactions occur, and manufacturer's included descriptions must be checked.

Dosage   65 mg, 1 capsule tid, qid, or q 4 h prn

Nursing Implications

1. Advise patient that she may become drowsy, and caution her if she plans on driving or operating any machinery.

2. Best avoided during the latter part of pregnancy, particularly near delivery, as additive effects occur when taken with narcotics.

3. Since safe use in pregnancy is not established, the benefits should outweigh the risks.

4. It is particularly useful for postpartum pain from episiotomy, laceration, after-pains, etc. Not sufficient for pain immediately following cesarean section.

5. Caution patient that abuse can lead to addiction or habituation, since it is structurally related to methadone.

6. Propoxyphene HCl is now a controlled drug in many states and must be counted and recorded.

SEDATIVES

Restlessness and inability to sleep during the last trimester as a result of the pressure symptoms of pregnancy may lead women to seek medication. While discussing sleeping habits with the patient, the nurse should discover specifically why the patient is having difficulty. If she is experiencing dyspnea, assuming a semi-Fowler's and a side-lying position may help. Eliminating external stimuli, such as distracting noises or odors, and talking with the patient and allowing her to express her feelings or problems may help reduce wakefulness. If the patient is still unable to find comfort and rest, her physician may order medication to assist her to sleep and rest.

Adverse Effects

Patients should be especially cautioned against taking over-the-counter sleeping aids without their physicians' knowledge, for many of the ingredients could prove harmful to the infant.

Whenever hypnotics or sedatives are ordered (barbiturates and nonbarbiturates) effects should be noted on the newborn infant. Barbiturates taken near delivery can cause decreased responsiveness, poor suckling ability, depression, apnea in the neonate, and bleeding due to liver damage (Schenkel and Vorherr, 1974). Analgesics and anesthetics may be potentiated by already ingested sedatives. Nurses should ask patients on admission to labor whether they have recently ingested any such drugs.

Table 3-5   Over-the-Counter Sedatives and Antianxiety Agents

Name	Anticholinergics	Antihistamines	CNS Stimulants	Salicylates
AlvaTranquil		x		x
Compoz	x	x		
Cope		x	x	x
Devarex	x	x		x
Dramamine		x		
Lullamin		x		
Neo-Nyte	x	x		
Miles Nervine		x		
Nytol		x		
Rest-On		x		
Quiet World	x	x		x
San-Man	x	x		
Sleep-Eze	x	x		
Sleepwell		x		
Sominex	x	x		x
StaKalm	x	x		
Sure-Sleep	x	x		x
Tranquim		x		

Table 3-5 lists the ingredients of over-the-counter sedatives and antianxiety agents. The following drugs are most commonly prescribed for the pregnant patient who cannot sleep well.

Chloral Hydrate (Aquachoral, Noctec, Somnos, and Others)

Chloral hydrate is a mild CNS depressant which, in therapeutic doses, only slightly depresses the respiratory and cardiovascular systems. Interactions with other drugs include an additive effect with alcohol, an increased effect of anticoagulants such as Coumadin and related compounds, and an increased effect of chloral hydrate by MAO inhibitors.

Adverse Effects   Occasional gastric irritation or skin reaction; rarely, excitement and delirium.

Dosage   Hypnotic dose: 0.5–1 g hs; sedative dose: 250 mg pc tid.

Nursing Implications
1. Administer capsule with a full glass of liquid; syrup in half a glass of liquid,

2. May be habit-forming.

Chloral Betaine (Beta-Chlor)

Dosage   0.44–0.87 g (equivalent to 0.25–0.5 g chloral hydrate), 1 to 2 tablets hs.

VITAMINS AND MINERALS

Poor nutrition may underlie many problems during pregnancy and jeopardize fetal well-being. One of the major responsibilities of nurses is the assessment of and instruction about nutrition for the pregnant woman. Because diet is so intrinsically bound up with life-style, many patients will not change eating habits nor get their necessary daily vitamins and minerals. In many clinics, therefore, vitamin/mineral supplements are given routinely. However, the patient should be instructed to take no other vitamins and minerals without the direction of the physician. Without this precaution, women who have been on fad diets may take "therapeutic" doses that are 10 times more potent than prenatal doses. Patients should be warned not to ingest high doses of the fat-soluble vitamins, since A and D have been linked to fetal anomalies. Also, the ingestion of folic acid without the direction of the physician may mask symptoms of pernicious anemia. Tables 3-6 and 3-7 list, respectively, the vitamin content and mineral content of prenatal tablets.

Calcium   The daily calcium requirement in pregnancy is 1200 mg. Since fetal bone formation requires extra calcium, every pregnant woman should drink at least one quart of milk every day. Unfortunately, many pregnant women do not like milk or do not drink the required amount of milk. For this reason, physicians sometimes prescribe calcium as a nutritional supplement.

Calcium is also prescribed for women who are experiencing muscle cramps from a calcium–phosphorus imbalance. Milk intake should be curbed, since milk contains phosphorus as well as calcium. Calcium is unevenly distributed in food, the largest amount being found in milk and milk products (excluding ice cream), with small amounts found in dark green, leafy vegetables. The calcium content contained in many of the prenatal vitamin and mineral supplements is listed in Table 3-7. Calcium is available either in tablets or in powder form, which can be sprinkled on food. There is some concern that the calcium carbonate preparation may cause milk-alkali syndrome in the patient (see section on Antacids).

Iron

Before pregnancy the average woman absorbs approximately 10 percent of her dietary iron intake. The additional needs of the increased maternal blood volume and fetal stores are partially compensated for by the absence of menstruation and by the increased iron absorption by the body; for example, during the third trimester, about three times the usual amount of iron can be absorbed. At the same time, the fetus needs iron to produce red blood cells and to store for use during its first 3 to 6 months of extrauterine life. Since it is difficult to get the necessary 18+ mg of iron daily from a normal diet, many physicians prescribe an iron supplement.

Iron deficiency anemia is common in women whose diets are deficient in protein, leafy green vegetables, dried peas, beans, apricots, and enriched breads and cereals. Teenagers often have iron deficiency anemia because of their poor eating habits and may need extensive assistance during pregnancy with their nutritional intake. Where a clinic population has a history of poor nutrition, iron is routinely prescribed.

Table 3-6   Vitamin Content of Prenatal Tablets*

MDR:	Vit. A 4000–5000 U	Vit. B$_1$ 1–1.5 mg	Vit. B$_2$ 1.2–1.7 mg	Vit. B$_6$ 2 mg	Vit. B$_{12}$ 2 mg
Calinate	x	x	x	x	x
Calinate-FA	x	x	x	x	x
Chenatal	x	x	x	x	x
En-Cebrin	x	x	x	x	x
En-Cebrin F	x	x	x	x	x
Engran	x	x	x	x	x
Engran-HP	x	x	x	x	x
Feosol Plus		x	x	x	x
Filibon	x	x	x	x	x
Filibon F.A.	x	x	x	x	x
Filibon Forte	x	x	x	x	x
Eivitamin	x	x	x	x	x
Fosfree	x	x	x	x	x
Mission Prenatal	x	x	x	x	x
Mission F.A. or HP	x	x	x	x	x
Natabec Kapseals	x	x	x	x	x
Natabec R	x	x	x	x	x
Natalins	x	x	x	x	x
Natalins R	x	x	x	x	x
Stuart Prenatal	x	x	x	x	x
Stuart Prenatal w/Folic Acid	x	x	x	x	x
"Ulvical Plus"	x	x	x	x	x

*The minimum daily requirement (MDR) for vitamins K and P has not been established.

Pantothenic Acid (Calcium Pantothenate) 10 mg	Nicotinic Acid (Niacin Niacinamide) 20 mg	Biotin 300 g	Folic Acid 0.4 mg	Vit. C 60 mg	Vit. D 400 IU	Vit. E 15 IU
X				X	X	
X	X		X	X	X	
X	X			X	X	X
X	X			X	X	
X	X		X	X	X	
X	X			X	X	
X	X		X	X	X	
X	X		X	X		
	X			X	X	
	X		X	X	X	
X	X		X	X	X	X
X	X		X	X	X	
X	X			X	X	
X	X			X	X	
X	X		X	X	X	
	X		X	X	X	
	X		X	X	X	
	X		X	X	X	X
X	X	X	X	X	X	X
X	X			X	X	
X	X		X	X	X	
X	X		X	X	X	X

Table 3-7   Mineral Content of Prenatal Tablets

Name	Other	Calcium Carbonate	Calcium Gluconate	Calcium Lactate	Potas-sium	Ferrous Fumarate	Ferrous Gluconate
Calinate		x				x	
Calcium gluconate			x				
Calcium lactate				x			
Chenatal	x*					x	x
Cerevon							
Chel-iron	x†						
En-Cebrin		x				x	
Engran	x‡	x					
Feosol							
Feostat						x	
Fergon							x
Ferro-Gradumet							
Filibon		x			x	x	
Filibon Forte		x				x	
Fosfree		x	x	x			x
Ircon*						x	
Livitamin		x				x	
Mission Prenatal		x	x	x			x
Mission F.A./HP		x	x	x			x
Natabec Kapseals		x					
Natalins		x				x	
Natalins R		x				x	
Nionate							x
Stuart Prenatal	x§					x	
"Ulvical Plus"		x				x	
Vitron-C							

*Dicalcium phosphate.
†Ferrocholinate.
‡Ferrous carbonate.
§Calcium sulfate, anhydrous.

Ferrous Succinate	Ferrous Sulfate	Manga- nese	Iodine	Magne- sium	Copper	Zinc	Phos- phorus
		x	x	x	x	x	
x		x	x	x	x	x	x
		x	x	x	x	x	x
	x	x	x		x	x	
	x	x					
			x	x	x	x	
			x				
	x						
			x	x			
			x	x	x	x	

Intramuscular Iron   Intramuscular injections of elemental iron are only given when the patient does not respond to or cannot tolerate oral preparations. Whenever iron is given intramuscularly, it must be injected deeply in the muscle by "Z-track" technique. Improperly injected, iron can stain the tissues for 6 to 12 months; 30 percent remains at the injection site for more than 30 days.

    Since deaths as a result of anaphylactic shock have been reported from the use of iron injections, test doses must always be used before the first IM or IV dose; 0.1 ml can be administered. Urticaria, fever, and headache should be regarded as adverse reactions.

DOSAGE   Calculated by patient's weight and extent of anemia. IM dose (50 mg per 2 ml), up to 250 mg qd for person weighing more than 50 kg; for a person weighing less than 50 kg, dose is no more than 100 mg qd. IV dose (50 mg per 5 or 10 ml) must be fractionated for 3 days; then full dose as above. Give no faster than 1 ml/min. Have patient rest 30 min. Dilute dose in 500 ml dextrose and water and infuse over 12 h as a safer method (*AMA Drug Evaluations*).

Nursing Implications
1. It is generally better if a low dose is started and then gradually increased. Do not give with milk. Give with citrus juice on an empty stomach if tolerated; otherwise, just after meals (pc).

2. Spansules and coated tablets are generally tolerated better than other tablets.

3. Instruct patient that stools may be dark green and diarrhea/constipation may occur.

4. Do not administer oral and parenteral iron simultaneously. This is generally considered unwise, with patients complaining of more side effects.

5. The ferrous form of iron (rather than the ferric form) is used more commonly, since it is more readily absorbed and generally causes less irritation.

6. Ferrous fumarate is a well-tolerated form of iron with little or no gastric side effects.

7. Ferrous gluconate is generally better tolerated than ferrous sulfate with less GI disturbances.

8. Ferrous sulfate is the most efficiently utilized oral form of iron and generally the least expensive.

9. Avoid giving aspirin and ferrous gluconate simultaneously, as Kimmel and Schmacher (1971) report that ferrous gluconate and benzoic acid (the food preserver) may enhance the teratogenic activity of aspirin.

10. Store in tightly sealed containers to prevent oxidation of the ferrous form to the ferric form.

LACTATION

Breast milk is a very unique and complex substance, a composite of more than 100 ingredients containing living cells and enzymes. It is a "living fluid" fluctuating in composition from day to day, from breast to breast, and from "fore" milk to "hind" milk (Catz and Giacoia, 1972). Besides proteins, fats, and carbohydrates (particularly lactose), breast milk contains immunoglobulins which assist the infant in fighting infections. The low pH of breast milk also helps to protect the infant, as organisms generally do not thrive in solutions of low pH, i.e., high acidity. These resistance factors may help to explain why breast-fed babies have fewer upper respiratory infections, gastrointestinal illnessses, septicemia, and allergic reactions.

As a general rule, breast milk, which is more acidic than plasma, will concentrate weak bases more than acids and in concentrations at or greater than the level in the plasma. Smaller, water-soluble particles will diffuse through the capillaries and into the alveolar cells in amounts equal to the level in the plasma. Just as a drug can enter the breast milk, it can also traverse back into maternal circulation when the plasma level falls. Drugs will transfer into breast milk in amounts dependent upon their plasma protein binding, lipid solubility, degree of ionization, ease of dissociation (pK_a), and the pH and fat content of the milk at that particular time.

Colostrom is low in fat content, and thus lipid-soluble drugs may be less concentrated there. Breast milk varies in fat content from 2 to 7 percent depending on the time of day and whether it is the beginning or the end of the feeding. There is generally a higher concentration of fat in the milk at midmorning and less in the early morning. "Hind" milk has a greater concentration of fat than the first part of the feeding ("fore" milk). Therefore, drugs with greater lipid solubility (such as the barbiturates) would be found in greater concentration in the "hind" milk.

Other factors which influence the passage of drugs into breast milk include the concentration of the drug in the maternal circulation and the breast milk and the duration of drug intake.

If the mother is in poor health because of either liver or kidney dysfunction, drugs may not be metabolized or excreted normally, and the breast may become an organ of excretion, with excessive amounts of the drug entering the breast milk. Thus, breast-feeding is contraindicated in these cases.

If drugs must be prescribed for the breast-feeding mother, several guidelines may be employed to decrease ingestion by the infant. Have the mother take medications just *after* feeding her infant rather than before. If the drug is given only once a day, it may be prudent to take the drug after the evening feeding and substitute a bottle for the next feeding. If the medication can be delayed until the infant is a few days older and enzymatic functioning is better established, adverse effects on the infant may be lessened. And, of course, the drug that has been shown to have the least side effects in the infant and mother should be employed (see Table 3-8).

Table 3-8   Drug Excretion in Breast Milk and Effect on the Infant

Drug	Excreted	Implications
ANALGESICS		
Acetaminophen (Datril, Tylenol)	Yes	No significant effect on infant from therapeutic doses
Acetyl salicylic acid (aspirin)*	Yes	Tendency toward bleeding noted; if given to nursing mother, should be given after nursing; check infant for adequate sources of vitamin K
Codeine	Yes	No significant effect on infant reported from therapeutic doses
Heroin†	Yes	Controversial reports as to the long-term effect on infant; usually goes through withdrawal depending on maternal dose
Meperidine hydrochloride (Demerol)	Yes	No significant effect on infant from therapeutic doses
Methadone*	Yes	Controversial as to whether user should breast-feed; if she does, the daily dose should be given after the feeding, and the next feeding should be by bottle
Morphine	Yes	No significant effects on infant from therapeutic doses
Pentazocine (Talwin)	No	
Phenylbutazone* (Azolid, Butazolidin)	Yes	Drug should be used judiciously; manufacturer states that it is excreted in cord blood and breast milk; infant should be monitored; may increase kernicterus—highly protein bound
Propoxyphene hydrochloride (Darvon)	Yes	No significant effect on infant from therapeutic doses
ANTICOAGULANTS		Differing opinions as to whether mother on anticoagulants should nurse; all agree that if she does, infant should be monitored with the mother

*Use with caution in nursing mother.
†Avoid drug whenever possible.

Table 3-8   Drug Excretion in Breast Milk and Effect on the Infant (*Continued*)

Drug	Excreted	Implications
Bishydroxycoumarin* (Dicumarol)	Yes	May cause hypoprothrombinemia in infant; monitor infant
Ethyl biscoumacetate* (Pelentan, Tromexan)	Yes	No significant effect on infant from therapeutic doses, but monitor infant; do not use if infant suffered any birth injury such as cephalhematoma, or forceps damage resulting in vascular injury
Heparin	No	
Phenindione† (Dindevan, Hedulin)	Yes	May cause hypoprothrombinemia; one incident of massive hematoma in infant whose mother received it
Warfarin sodium* (Coumadin)	Yes	May cause hypoprothrombinemia; monitor infant
ANTICONVULSANTS		
Phenytoin* (Dilantin)	Yes	Methemoglobinemia in breast-fed infant; enzyme induction may occur
Primidone† (Mysoline)	Yes	Manufacturer recommends breast-feeding be avoided, since substantial amounts found in breast milk; drowsiness may occur in newborn
ANTIDIABETICS		
Chlorpropamide (Diabinese)	Yes	No significant effect on infant from therapeutic doses
Insulin	Yes	Destroyed in the infant's GI tract
Tolbutamide (Dolipol, Mobenol, Orinase, Tolbutol)	Yes	No significant effects on infant from therapeutic doses
Tolazamide (Tolinase)	?	Has not been completely evaluated; 6.7 times more potent than tolbutamide
ANTIHISTAMINES		
Chlorpheniramine maleate (Chlor-Trimeton)	Yes	May cause drowsiness in the infant
Diphenhydramine (Benadryl, Benhydril)	Yes	No adverse effects on infant from therapeutic doses

Table 3-8   Drug Excretion in Breast Milk and Effect on the Infant (*Continued*)

Drug	Excreted	Implications
Promethazine hydrochloride (Phenergan)	Yes	No significant effects on infant from therapeutic doses
Trimeprazine tartrate (Temaril)	Yes	No significant effects on infant from therapeutic doses
ANTICHOLINERGICS		
Atropine sulfate†	Yes	May inhibit lactation and may cause atropine intoxication in infant; although documentation scarce, best avoided until further research available
Scopolamine	Yes	No significant effects on infant from therapeutic doses
ANTIHYPERTENSIVES–DIURETICS		
Acetazolamide* (Diamox)	Yes	Infant may develop idiosyncratic reaction to this sulfonamide diuretic
Furosemide (Lasix)	No	Women ill enough to receive lasix should not breast-feed
Hexamethonium	Yes	Rarely used drug; very toxic
Reserpine† (Serpasil)	Yes	May cause nasal stuffiness, drowsiness, and diarrhea in infant, galactorrhea in mother
Spironolactone (Aldactone)	No	Watch for potassium deficiency and dehydration in mother
Thiazides†	Yes	Manufacturer suggests avoiding; watch fluid, electrolyte balance
ANTI-INFECTIVES		With all anti-infectives that cross into breast milk, the possibility of sensitization of the infant must be considered
Amantadine hydrochloride† (Symmetrel)	Yes	May cause skin rash and vomiting; manufacturer suggests avoiding
Aminoglycosides*	Yes	Should be reserved for severe infection; avoid in high G6PD-deficient populations, as hemolysis may occur

Table 3-8   Drug Excretion in Breast Milk and Effect on the Infant (*Continued*)

Drug	Excreted	Implications
Ampicillin	Yes	No significant effects on infant from therapeutic doses
Chloramphenicol* (Chloromycetin)	Yes	May effect infant's bone marrow; avoid use, particularly during the first 2 weeks of life
Erythromycin* (E-mycin, Erythrocin, Ilosone, Ilotycin)	Yes	Appears in breast milk in concentrations higher than that of maternal plasma; sensitization possible; estolate form (Ilosone) may cause jaundice
Isoniazid†	Yes	If possible, avoid use during lactation; if given, infant must be monitored for toxicity
Mandelic acid†	Yes	Probably best avoided during lactation; for this urinary antiseptic to be effective, urine must be strongly acid and fluids must be limited
Metronidazole† (Flagyl)	Yes	No adverse oral or GI effects noted in infants, but some authors feel that because of possible carcinogenicity it would be best to avoid, as long-term effects are not known
Nalidixic acid† (Neg Gram)	Yes	Hemolytic anemia, especially in G6PD populations
Nouobiocin†	Yes	May cause kernicterus in large doses
Penicillin	Yes	Possibility of sensitization; may alter intestinal flora of infant
Quinine	Not in clinically significant amounts	In very high maternal doses, thrombocytopenia in infants
Sulfonamides*	Yes	Avoid in high G6PD populations; high doses for long-term use is questionable; may cause kernicterus; avoid in the first 2 weeks of life
Tetracyclines†	Yes	Slows bone growth and deposits in bones and teeth

Table 3-8   Drug Excretion in Breast Milk and Effect on the Infant (*Continued*)

Drug	Excreted	Implications
CANCER-CHEMOTHERAPEUTIC AGENTS†		Breast-feeding is generally considered ill-advised in patients receiving chemotherapy
HORMONES		
Estrogen, progestogen, androgens†	Yes	Breast-feeding not indicated if mother is on oral contraceptives; may alter the composition of breast milk (decreasing the amounts of protein, fats and minerals); long-term effects on infants have not been adequately determined.
Corticosteroids†	Yes	Should be avoided by the nursing mother, as they may interfere with normal function and cause growth suppression
LAXATIVES		
Aloe*	Yes	Conflicting evidence regarding catharsis in infants; avoid in high doses
Cascara†	Yes	Thought to cause diarrhea in infants
Danthron† (Dorbane, Dorbantyl, Doxan, Doxidan)	Yes	Conflicting reports regarding the cathartic effect of these drugs; probably best avoided
Dioctyl sodium sulfosuccinate (Colace)		No reports of having caused any problems in the infant
Milk of magnesia	No	No adverse reactions noted
Phenolphthalein (Evacu-lax, Ex-lax, other nonprescription drugs)	Yes	No significant effects noted in usual doses
Psyllium hydrophilic mucileoid (Metamucil)	Yes	No adverse reactions noted
Senna compounds*	Yes	Controversial reports with moderate doses; high doses may cause diarrhea in infants

Table 3-8   Drug Excretion in Breast Milk and Effect on the Infant (*Continued*)

Drug	Excreted	Implications
MUSCLE RELAXANTS		
Carisoprodol† (Rela, Soma)	Yes	According to manufacturer, two to four times more concentrated in breast milk than in maternal blood plasma; infant may experience CNS depression and GI upset
Methocarbamol (Robaxin)	Yes	No significant effects on infant from therapeutic doses
OXYTOCICS		
Ergot preparations†	Yes	May suppress lactation by blocking the release of prolactin; symptoms in the infant may include vomiting, diarrhea, cardiovascular changes
Oxytocin	Yes	Oxytocin nasal spray used prior to breast-feeding appears to increase the volume of milk produced; may be used for hemorrhaging mother; very short half-life
PSYCHOTROPICS–PSYCHOTHERAPEUTICS		
Butyrophenones, Haloperidol* (Haldol)		Manufacturer recommends that benefits must outweigh risks in the use of these drugs, since their safe use in pregnancy and lactation has not been established
Chlordiazepoxide* (Librium)	Yes	No significant effects on infants from therapeutic doses; some authors suggest using caution
Diazepam* (Valium)	Yes	May cause weight loss, lethargy, jaundice in the infant; some authors feel that breast-feeding should be discontinued if high doses are given to mother
Imipramine* (Tofranil)	Yes	Safe use during lactation has not been established
Lithium carbonate† (Lithonate, Lithane)	Yes	May alter electrolyte balance; most authors state that indications for its use should be unequivocal; long-term effect on infant unknown; best avoided until further evidence available

Table 3–8   Drug Excretion in Breast Milk and Effect on the Infant (*Continued*)

Drug	Excreted	Implications
Phenothiazines* (Compazine, Thorazine, etc.)	Yes	All phenothiazines are excreted in breast milk, and except for reported jaundice in the infant and galactorrhea, no other effects are known at this time

SEDATIVES-HYPNOTICS

Barbiturates†	Yes	May increase the activity of hepatic drug metabolizing enzymes; high single dose may cause more drowsiness than small, multiple doses
Bromides† (ingredient in many nonprescription sleeping medications)	Yes	May cause rash and drowsiness in infant; difficulty in feeding, lethargy, hypotonia or hypertonia
Chloral hydrate (Noctec, Somnos)	Yes	Drowsiness in infant
Chloroform†	Yes	Anesthetic effect in infant
Glutethimide* (Doriden)	Yes	May cause drowsiness in infant; one author suggests avoiding during lactation; manufacturer suggests caution during lactation
Meprobamate† (Equanil, Miltown)	Yes	Very high level in milk (two to four times maternal plasma); alternate drug advised; if given, infant should be monitored for signs of meprobamate toxication

THYROID AND ANTITHYROID PREPARATIONS

Carbimazole† (Neo-Mercazole)	Yes	May cause goiter in infant
Methimazole† (Tapazole)	Yes	Manufacturer recommends that user not breast-feed
Thiouracil† (+ derivatives)	Yes	Excreted in high levels (3 to 12 times maternal plasma levels); may cause goiter or agranulocytosis
Thyroid	Yes	No significant effects on infant with therapeutic doses
Thyroxine sodium† (Choloxin)	Yes	Manufacturer states that use in pregnancy and lactation is contraindicated

Table 3-8   Drug Excretion in Breast Milk and Effect on the Infant (*Continued*)

Drug	Excreted	Implications
IODIDES		
^{131}I† (radioactive)	Yes	All radioactive agents should be avoided in the breast-feeding mother
Iodides† (contained in many nonprescription cough preparations)	Yes	Infant's thyroid functioning may be affected; avoid taking large or frequent doses of iodide-containing cough preparations; may have thyrotropic effect on infant or cause rash
VITAMINS, MINERALS, FOOD PRODUCTS		
Vitamins		
B₁ (thiamine)	Yes	Mothers with severe deficiency (beriberi) should not nurse because of excretion of toxic substances, sodium pyruvate and methylglyoxal, which have caused infant death
B₆ (pyridoxine)	Yes	Some authors report that it successfully suppressed lactation in doses of 150–200 mg po tid
B₁₂ (cyanocobalamin)	Yes	No effect with therapeutic doses
D (Calciferol)	Yes	High doses may cause hypercalcemia in infant
K	Yes	No significant effects on infant with therapeutic doses
Caffeine* (many nonprescription drugs contain caffeine: Awake, 100 mg; NoDoz, 100 mg; Sta-Alert, 100 mg; Vivarin, 200 mg, and coffee and tea, 100–150 mg per cup)	Yes	Unless large amount ingested, no significant effect on infant; ingestion of large quantities of tea or coffee can cause irritability and poor sleeping patterns in infants
Carrots	Yes	In large quantity, may cause yellow discoloration of skin
Egg protein	Yes	Allergic sensitization possible

Table 3-8   Drug Excretion in Breast Milk and Effect on the Infant (*Continued*)

Drug	Excreted	Implications
Fava bean	Yes	In G6PD-deficient infants, hemolysis has occurred
Fluoride (toothpaste, water supply, tablets)	Yes	Not significant in usual quantities; excess may affect tooth enamel; Laleche League advises either *not* breast-feeding or to stop taking fluoride tablets; may cause GI upsets, rash in infants
VACCINES–IMMUNOSUPPRESSIVE		
DPT	Yes	Probably no immunity transfer to baby
Poliovirus	Yes	If infant is immunized after 6 weeks, probably negligible effect on antibody titer
Rh$_o$ (D) immune globulin (human) (Gamulin Rh, RhoGAM)	No	
Rubella	No	Probably no transfer of live virus to infant
OTHER		
Alcohol (ethyl alcohol)	Yes	No significant effect in moderate amount; prolonged ingestion of large amounts may intoxicate infant; large doses may also inhibit the milk ejection reflex, whereas small amount of alcohol prior to nursing may enhance the milk "let down"
Clomiphene citrate (Clomid)		May suppress lactation
Dihydrotachsterol* (DHT)	Yes	May cause hypercalcemia in infant (osteoporosis, bone dysgenesis)
L-dopa		May suppress lactation by inhibiting prolactin secretion
Lead†		Caution against the use of lead acetate ointment in breast creams, as it may lead to encephalitis
Marijuana†	Yes	May interfere with DNA and RNA formation

Table 3-8   Drug Excretion in Breast Milk and Effect on the Infant (*Continued*)

Drug	Excreted	Implications
Mercury†	Yes	In cases of mercury contamination in the environment, watch infant for CNS symptoms and mercury intoxication
Nicotine*	Yes	Probably very little effect on infant with moderate use (20 cigarettes per day or less); may decrease milk production; one recorded case of nicotine intoxication in infant (restlessness, vomiting, diarrhea, insomnia, circulatory disruptions)—mother smoked 20 cigarettes per day; infants of smoking mothers absorb smoke through GI tract, respiratory tract, and skin as well

BIBLIOGRAPHY

Anagnostakis, D., and N. Matfaniotis: "Neonatal Cold Injury and Maternal Reserpine Administration," *Lancet*, **2**:471, August 24, 1974.

*Anderson, Philip O.: "Drugs and Breast Feeding—A Review," *Drug Intelligence and Clinical Pharmacology*, **2**:208-223, April 1977.

Applebaum R.M.: "The Obstetricians' Approach to the Breasts and Breastfeeding," *The Journal of Reproductive Medicine*, **14**: (3):98-116, March 1975.

Berry, D.J., et al.: "Transplacental Passage of Chlordiazepoxide," *British Medical Journal*, **2**:729, June 24, 1974.

Bleyer, W.A.: "Maternally Ingested Salicylate as a Cause of Neonatal Hemorrhage," *Journal of Pediatrics*, **85**(5): 736–737, November 1974.

*Bowes, W.R., E. Conway, Y. Brackbill, and A. Steinchneider: "Effects of Obstetrical Medication on Fetus and Infant," *Society for Research in Child Development*, **35**:137, June 1970.

*Denotes particularly pertinent references.

Burgess, G. E. III: "Antacids for Obstetric Patients," *American Journal of Obstetrics and Gynecology*, **123**(7): 334, February 1975.

Canales, E.S., J.T. Facog, A. Zarate, M. Mason, and J. Soria: "Effect of Ergonovine on Prolactin Secretion and Milk Let-Down," *Obstetrics and Gynecology*, **48**(2):228–229, August 1976.

*Catz, C.S., and G.P. Giacoia: "Drugs and Breast Milk," *Symposium on Pediatric Pharmacology*, **19**:151–166, February 1972.

Chopra, J.G.: "Effect of Steroid Contraception on Lactation," *American Journal Clinical Nutrition*, **25**:1202–1214, 1972.

Chudzik, G.M., and S.J. Yaffe: "Drug Interaction," *Symposium on Pediatric Pharmacology*, **19**:131–139, February 1972.

Cobo, E.: "Effect of Different Doses of Ethanol on the Milk-Ejecting Reflex in Lactating Women," *American Journal of Obstetrics and Gynecology*, **115**:817–821, March 1973.

*Cohen, S., and S. Ganapathy: "Drugs in the Fetus and Newborn Infant," *Clinics in Endocrinology and Metabolism*, **5**:175–190, March 1976.

Cole, P.V., L.H. Hawkins, and D. Robers: "Smoking During Pregnancy and Its Effects on the Fetus," *Journal of Obstetrics and Gynecology of the British Commonwealth*, **79**:782, 1972.

Ditts, T.V.: "Pharmacology in Labor and Delivery," *Contemporary OB/Gyn*, **5**:72, April 1975.

"Drugs in the Fetal Ecosphere," *Hospital Practice*, pp. 21–28, June 1973.

Eriksson, M., A.S. Catz, and S.J. Yaffe: "Drugs and Pregnancy," *Clinical Obstetrics and Gynecology*, **16**(1):199, March 1973.

Erkkolar, E. et al.: "Perinatal Metabolism of Diazepam," *British Medical Journal*, **3** (5928):472, August 17, 1974.

Fofar, J.O., and M.M. Nelson: "Epidemiology of Drugs Taken by Pregnant Woman," *Clinical Pharmacology and Therapeutics*, **14**:632, July-August 1973.

Gerrard, J.W.: "Breast-feeding: Second Thoughts," *Pediatrics*, **54**757–764, December 1974.

Griffenhagen, G.B., and L.L. Hawkins (eds.): *Handbook of Non-Prescription Drugs*, American Pharmaceutical Assn., Washington, D.C., 1973.

Hanson, J.W., K.L. Jones, and D.W. Smith: "Fetal Alcohol Syndrome Experience With 41 Patients," *Journal of American Medical Association*, **235**:1458, 1976.

Hill, R,M.: "Drugs Ingested by Pregnant Women," *Clinical Pharmacology and Therapeutics*, **14**:654, 1973.

*———, J.P. Craig, M.D. Chaney, L.M. Tennyson, and L.B. McCulley: "Utilization of Over-The-Counter Drugs During Pregnancy," *Clinical Obstetrics and Gynecology*, **20**(2):381–394, June 1977.

Hoag, R.W.: "Perinatal Pharmacology," *Birth and the Family Journal*, **1**(3):5–15, 1974.

Jelliffe, D.B.: "Unique Properties of Human Milk," *Journal of Reproductive Medicine*, **14**(4):133–137, April 1975.

Kesaniemi, Y.A.: "Ethanol and Acetaldehyde in the Milk and Peripheral Blood of Lactating Women after Ethanol Administration," *Journal of Obstetrics Gynecology of the British Commonwealth*, **81**:84–88, January, 1974.

Kimmel, C.A., and H.J. Schmacher: "Interrelationships Between Nutrients and Salicylate Teratogenicity," *Teratology*, **4**:233, 1971.

*Knowles, J.A.: "Excretion of Drugs in Milk—A Review," *Journal of Pediatrics*, **66**:1068–1082, June 1965 (comprehensive review).

———: "Breast Milk: A Source of More than Nutrition for the Neonate," *Clinical Toxicology*, **7**(1):69–82, 1974.

McDonald, J.S.: "Preanesthetic and Intrapartal Medications," *Clinical Obstetrics and Gynecology*, **20**(2):447–459, June 1977.

Nymand, G.: "Maternal Smoking and Neonatal Hyperbilirubinemia," *Lancet*, **2**:173, July 20, 1974.

*O'Brien, T.E.: "Excretion of Drugs in Human Milk," *American Journal Hospital Pharmacology*, **31**:844–854, September 1974 (excellent review).

Overbach, A.M., and M.J. Rodman: *Drugs Used with Neonates and During Pregnancy*, Medical Economics Company, Oradell, N.J., 1975.

Palmisano, P.A., and R.B. Polhill: "Fetal Pharmacology," *Pedriatric Clinics of North America*, 19:3–19, 1972.

Rane, A. and F. Sjoquist: "Drug Metabolism in the Human Fetus and Newborn Infant," *Pediatric Clinics of North America*, 19(1):37–49, February 1972.

*Rothermel, P.C. and M.M. Farber: "Drugs in Breastmilk—A Consumer's Guide," *Birth and the Family Journal*, 2(3): 76–88, 1975.

Schenkel, B., and H. Vorherr: "Non-Prescription Drugs During Pregnancy: Potential Teratogenic and Toxic Effects Upon Embryo and Fetus," *Journal of Reproductive Medicine*, 12(1):27–45, January 1974.

Spellacy, W.N.: "Oral Contraceptives Contraindicated for Nursing Mother," *Journal of the American Medical Association*, 221:1415, September 18, 1972.

Stirrat, G.M.: "Prescribing Problems in the Second Half of Pregnancy and During Lactation," *Obstetric and Gynecological Survey*, 31:1–7, 1976.

Sutherland, J.M., and I.J. Light: "The Effect of Drugs Upon the Developing Fetus," *Pediatric Clinics of North America*, 12(3):781–806, August 1965 (excellent bibliography).

Tyson, H.K.: "Neonatal Withdrawal Symptoms Associated with Maternal Use of Propoxyphene Hydrochloride (Darvon)," *Journal of Pediatrics*, 85(5):684–685, November 1974.

*White, M.K.: "Medications for the Nursing Mother," Info. Sheet No. 21, LaLeche League International, Inc., June 1976.

Wyss, R.H., R. Korsznia, W.L. Heinrichs, and W.L. Herman: "Inhibition of Uterine Receptor Binding of Estradiol by Anti-Estrogens (Clomiphene and C.L.-868)," *Journal of Clinical Endocrinology and Metabolism*, 28:1824, 1968.

Yaffe, S.J.: "A Clinical Look at the Problem of Drugs in Pregnancy and Their Effect on the Fetus," *Canadian Medical Association Journal*, 112(6):728, 1975.

Yalom, I.D., R. Green, and N. Fish: "Prenatal Exposure to Female Hormones, Effects on Psychosexual Development in Boys," *Archives of General Psychiatry*, 28:554, 1973.

Zuckerman, H., and S. Carmel: "The Inhibition of Lactation by Clomiphene," *Journal Obstetrics Gynecology of the British Commonwealth*, **80**:822–823, 1973.

4

Drugs Used in Family Planning

Martha Olsen Schult

INFERTILITY

Approximately 15 percent of couples of childbearing age are involuntarily infertile (Garcia and Rosenfeld, 1977). As information is disseminated about rates of success in treatment (35 to 50 percent), more couples are seeking professional help. After extensive and time-consuming procedures to determine the cause of infertility, some couples are treated pharmacologically.

Major factors contributing to female infertility that can be treated with drug therapy are endometriosis, "postpill ammenorrhea," anovulatory cycles, malnutrition (fat, mineral or vitamin deficiency), and infection of the genital tract. In addition, diseases and disorders such as thyroid problems, adrenal, hypothalamic, or pituitary dysfunction, and diabetes may also disturb fertility function. Improvement of chronic disease often returns the person to a more fertile state. If the cause is anovulation from gonadotropic or sex steroidal deficiency, the patient can receive agents that stimulate ovulation. Of course, the ovary must be able to produce and release the mature ovum once stimulation occurs.

The two principle agents utilized to stimulate ovulation are clomiphene citrate and human menopausal gonadotropin. Clomiphene citrate (Clomid) is generally utilized when the estrogen levels are near normal but the gonadotropic follicle-stimulating hormone (FSH) and luteinizing hormone (LH) release is inadequate. Human menopausal gonadotropin (Menotropins, Pergonal) may be added to therapy when Clomid has failed to produce the desired effect. Pergonal, being a substitutive therapy rather than a stimulative one, would be used when there are low or absent gonadotropins and poor endogenous estrogen production.

Clomiphene Citrate (Clomid)

Clomid, a nonsteroid estrogen, appears to stimulate output of the pituitary gonadotropins (LH and FSH), which in turn stimulates the ripening of the graafian follicle. Chemically related to chlorotrianisene (TACE) and diethylstilbestrol, Clomid appears to displace estrogen from receptor sites in hypothalamus or pituitary, thus stimulating the LH peak (*AMA Drug Evaluations*). Clomid is used to induce ovulation in patients who are anovulatory as a result of hypothalamic dysfunction, in those who have polycystic ovaries or postpill amenorrhea, and in patients who ovulate rarely.

Adverse Effects   Abnormal cystic ovarian enlargement is the chief difficulty encountered. If cystic ovaries develop, additional therapy must wait until enlargment regresses naturally in 1 to 4 weeks. Other side effects are not usually serious, and the incidence is low with minimal doses. Between 5 and 10 percent of patients experience hot flashes as a result of the antiestrogenic effect. Dry vaginal mucosa, constipation or diarrhea, breast discomfort, nausea, vomiting, accentuated mittelschmerz, weight gain, loss of hair, and changes in menstrual bleeding have been reported. Women with polycystic ovaries are more sensitive to the drug and have a higher rate of multiple ovulation. There are no reports of congenital malformations or increase in abortion attributed to Clomid therapy (Huppert and Wallach, 1977). Clomid is contraindicated when ovarian cysts are already suspected, in malignant disease, or in ovarian failure (Haney and Hammond, 1977).

Dosage   50 mg qd for 5 days, beginning on day 5 of cycle (others recommend beginning on day 7). Before the second cycle is instituted the patient should be examined to be sure she has not conceived nor developed ovarian enlargement. If ovulation occurs without conception, six to nine courses are considered an adequate trial. If ovulation does not occur, the dose is raised to 100 mg for 5 days, and then to 150 and 200 mg. Some patients require up to 250 mg before ovulating (more than 250 mg is not given). [Manufacturers recommendations of a 100-mg limit for 5 days for 3 months is often exceeded without apparent difficulty (*AMA Drug Evaluations*).] In addition, "if therapy is begun with low doses and titrated increments are used, the multiple pregnancy rate will probably not be much greater than in the general population" (Huppert and Wallach, 1977).

Nursing Implications

1. Clients must be advised of the risks of multiple gestation.

2. Client should be taught how to keep an accurate basal body temperature chart so that sexual relations can occur at the time of expected ovulation.

3. Advise the client of the possible side effects, and instruct her to report any untoward reactions.

4. Teach the client early signs of pregnancy so that she can report a possible pregnancy.

Human Chorionic Gonadotropin

Human chorionic gonadotropin (HCG) is used to treat cryptorchidism in prepubertal boys because it appears to mimic LH in the male. To stimulate LH and ovulation in women, HCG is used in combination with Pergonal and Clomid. HCG may have some effect on maintaining the corpus luteum as well. Ovulation should occur within 24 h of HCG injection if urinary estrogen levels are adequate. The patient should be instructed carefully about timing of sexual intercourse on the day of the injection and during the following 2 days.

Basal body temperature will rise about 24 h after injection and persist for 2 weeks if conception does not take place. [This pattern is similar to a healthy secretory, postovulatory phase (Gemzell, 1977).]

Dosage   5000 U IM for 1 to 3 days, beginning 5 to 6 days after last dose of clomiphene; it is used with clomiphene-menotropins for unsuccessful cases.

Human Menopausal Gonadotropins (Menotropins, Pergonal)

Human menopausal gonadotropin (HMG) is extracted from the urine of postmenopausal women. Pergonal is a combination of FSH and LH in a 1/1 ratio. The hormones induce the growth and maturation of the graafian follicle. However, for ovulation to occur, HCG or a combination of clomiphene and HCG must also be given.

Adverse Effects   Symptons of ovarian hyperstimulation: *mild*—ovarian enlargement with lower abdominal discomfort (7 to 10 days); *severe*—hyperstimulation syndrome, which would include such signs and symptoms as weight gain, ovarian enlargement, and rarely, ascites, hypovolemia, hypercoagulability, oliguria, and pleural effusion (Haney and Hammond, 1977). Multiple gestation is more frequent than with Clomid.

Before any menotropins are given, the patient must be screened carefully to rule out uterine abnormalities, tubal problems, or pregnancy, and thyroid activity must be normal.

After therapy begins the patient must be seen every other day for up to 2 weeks after the HCG injection for signs of excessive ovarian stimulation. If hyperstimulation occurs, treatment must stop immediately.

Dosage   One ampul of Pergonal contains 75 IU of FSH and 75 IU of LH. One ampul is given daily for 9 to 12 days. Checks on the estrogenic activities of the patient (fern test, vaginal pH, and cervical smears) indicate the readiness of the graafian follicle. (Urinary estrogen levels should be in range of 50–150 μg/24 h. HCG is withheld if level is above 150 μg). HCG is then given. Therapy should not exceed 12 days during any cycle. If no ovulation occurs after three trials, dosage is increased to 150 IU each of LH and FSH.

Nursing Implications
1. The couple must be advised of the possibility of a 20 percent chance of multiple gestation.

2. The client must report untoward side effects.

3. The client must be able to attend the clinic or office daily for 14 days and then every other day for follow-up visits for evidence of success or failure.

HORMONES FOR CONTRACEPTION

Estrogens: General Considerations

The use of estrogens during the childbearing cycle is indicated for gonadal disorders such as amenorrhea and hypogonadism, for contraception (in conjunction with progesterone), and for preventing lactation by blocking the release of the lactogenic hormone.

Hormones should only be used during pregnancy under the close supervision and direction of a physician. Hormones have been shown to be teratogenic, as in cases of vaginal adenosis and adenocarcinoma in adolescent daughters whose mothers received diethylstilbestrol (DES) to thwart miscarriages. Recent studies of DES children are beginning to uncover genitourinary and psychosocial problems as well in male offspring (Yalom et al., 1973; Bibbo et al., 1977).

The natural estrogens—estradiol, estrone, and estriol—are steroids, whereas diethylstilbestrol, hexestrol, dienestrol, chlororianisene, and methallenestril are synthetic, nonsteroidal preparations. Overbach and Rodman note that natural estrogens can cause feminization and synthetic estrogens

Table 4-1   Results of an Excess of Estrogen and Progestogen

Estrogen	Progestogen
GASTROINTESTINAL	
Nausea, bloated feeling	Increased appetite, real weight gain
VASCULAR AND RENAL SYSTEMS	
Fluid retention, venous capillary engorgement	Depression, nervousness, fatigue
Occasional occurrence of spider nevi	
Headaches (migraine) and perhaps some elevation of blood pressure (?)	
A slight chance of thromboembolism in high-risk patients	
UTERUS	
Hypermenorrhea, myoma growth	Scanty menses
	Dysmenorrhea usually improved; sometimes breakthrough bleeding
VAGINA	
Mucorrhea, excess secretion	Reduction in lining thickness and secretions; more *Candida*, pruritus
BREASTS	
Mastalgia; possible enlargement of benign cysts	Regression of breast tissue
SKIN	
Chloasma (darkening of skin over nose and cheeks	Possible occurrence of acne

Table 4-1   Results of an Excess of Estrogen and Progestogen (Continued)

Estrogen	Progestogen
GLUCOSE METABOLISM	
Increased levels in fasting state	
Decreased glucose tolerance increased insulin response to glucose	

Source: Adapted from J. Nelson, "Clinical Evaluation of Side Effects of Current Contraceptives—Oral: Combined, Sequential," Journal of Reproductive Medicine, **6**:2, 1971.

(stilbestrols) can cause masculinization. Other studies indicate that androgens and oral progestins can cause virilization, and clitoral hypertrophy in the fetus.

Adverse Effects   The side effects of estrogens include change in libido, nausea, vomiting, dizziness, headaches, anorexia, malaise, diarrhea, skin rash, edema, weight gain (from increased salt retention), decreased glucose tolerance, hypercalcemia, and nitrogen retention. Estrogens may alter laboratory test results. Prolonged use may lead to amenorrhea (see Table 4–1).

Contraindications   Estrogens should not be administered where there is evidence or history of breast cancer, precancerous lesions, or genital tract cancer and should be used with caution in persons with a history of thrombophlebitis, cardiac, renal, and hepatic disease, asthma, migraines, epilepsy, and calcium–phosphorus imbalance. Estrogens should not be used in young girls whose long-bone growth is not completed.

Their use has also been contraindicated in breast-feeding mothers (even though small amounts tend to stimulate lactation) because of their possible future influence on the infant.

Main Drug Interactions

1. Anticoagulants—interferes with anticoagulant activity;

2. Antidiabetic agents—estrogen alters glucose tolerance; dosage adjustment required;

3. Barbiturates—increased liver metabolism induction of estrogen decreases estrogen effectiveness;

4. Corticosteroids—enhance anti-inflammatory activity;

5. Meperidine (Demerol)—increases effect of meperidine.

Progesterone and Progestins (Progestogens)

Progesterone is secreted during the luteal phase of the menstrual cycle and also during pregnancy by the placenta. However, naturally occurring progesterone is not suitable for use as a general contraceptive agent, since it is virtually ineffective when given orally because of its short duration of action. On the other hand, synthetic progestational agents (progestogens and progestins), including ethynodiol diacetate, chlormadinone acetate, medroxyprogesterone acetate, norethindrone, norethindrone acetate, norethynodrel, and norgestrel are effective oral agents and can be utilized for birth control. They are usually combined with estrogen to produce contraception, but two synthetic progestational agents—norethindrone and norgestrel—are being utilized alone to produce contraception. These are known as the mini-pills. Progestational agents are also used as intramuscular injections and subcutaneous implants for prolonged periods of contraception.

Action   Progesterone acts on the estrogen-primed endometrium to prepare it for nidation by a fertilized ovum. It also influences the cervix, vagina, and fallopian tubes in preparation for pregnancy. The cervical mucus changes in saline content and viscosity, and the vaginal cells change in cell composition much the way the endometrium changes under progestational influence. Whereas the estrogenic hormones increase fallopian tube contractility and probably cilia movement, progesterone has the opposite effect. Progesterone effects the reabsorption of sodium and water in the kidneys, exerts an influence on respiration, fat, carbohydrate, and protein metabolism, and changes the basal body temperature. Together with estrogen, it is also responsible for breast growth and development.

How progestogens act to prevent pregnancy is not fully understood. Several theories have been suggested, including (1) interference with endometrial buildup, causing it to be nonreceptive to the fertilized ovum; (2) reduction in the motility of the fallopian tube; (3) changing the character of the cervical mucus to resemble postovulatory mucus; and (4) suppression of FSH and LH at midcycle, rendering some women anovulatory (a variable effect).

Effectiveness   The overall failure rate for progestational contraceptives is 3 per 100 woman-years of use. The failure rate is higher (3.72/100) among new or "fresh" users who have not been on a steroidal contraceptive agent. The rate is 1.95/100 for those women who have been on other oral contraceptives and have changed to the mini-pill (Ortho, Syntex).

Adverse Effects   The adverse effects include changes in the menstrual flow and cycle length, spotting, breakthrough bleeding, amenorrhea, edema, weight changes, rash, mental depression, GI upsets, cholestatic jaundice, breast changes, changes in the cervical mucus and cervical erosion, chloasma or melasma, headaches, dizziness, increased body temperature, and perhaps, thrombotic disease.

The most common complaint which causes women to stop the mini-pill and change to another contraceptive seems to center on the changes in the menstrual cycle, such as spotting and irregular and unpredictable menses. When combined with estrogen in the birth-control pill, the side effects may increase (see Oral Contraceptives).

Progestational agents should not be utilized during pregnancy or lactation because of possible teratogenic effects to the fetus or possible unknown harm to the infant. Hence, progestational agents should be used with caution for pregnancy tests or for attempts to halt a threatened abortion. The evidence is not convincing that progesterone is even beneficial in attempting to stop a threatened abortion (Wentz, 1977).

Contraindications   The same contraindications for oral contraceptives apply to the progestogens (see p. 95).

Drug Interactions
   1. Phenobarbital—reduces effect of progesterone.

   2. Phenylbutazone—reduces effect of progesterone; on the other hand, progesterone prolongs or enhances the effect of phenylbutazone.

   3. Laboratory tests—progesterone may alter laboratory results in the following: GTT, 17-hydroxycorticosteroids, and 17-ketosteroids may have false-negative or lower results. Alkaline phosphate, cholesterol, hematocrit, serum iron, thyroxine values may have false-positive or higher readings.

Nursing Implications
   1. Clients should be given a complete physical examination and their history explored to be sure they qualify for progestational use. Pap smears should be done prior to therapy and periodically thereafter.

   2. Clients should be given the pamphlet insert and instructed to read and follow directions carefully.

   3. Side effects and untoward effects such as episodes of bleeding, spotting, yellowing of the sclera, or sudden weight gain should be reported.

   4. Clients should be told of the mental depression that can occur, particularly if there has been a history of mental depression.

   5. If laboratory tests must be done, the laboratory should be informed that the client is on progestational agents.

   6. If the client has missed two menstrual periods, the contraceptive agent should be stopped and another form of birth control utilized until pregnancy can be ruled out.

Contraceptive Combinations

The advent of the estrogen–progestogen oral contraceptive agent has brought freedom from unwanted pregnancies to millions of women. But "the pill" has also brought with it much controversy and confusion about its safe use. In the last few years, it has been implicated in thrombophlebitis, thrombosis, and strokes. Although some reports have tried to find a link, there is no conclusive evidence of any causal relationship with cancer (Berger and Fowler, 1977). However, the pill has been contraindicated in anyone with a history of breast or uterine cancer or tumors, genital bleeding, vascular damage, or problems such as hypertension, thrombophlebitis, or liver impairment. Planned Parenthood Federation of America and the U.S. Food and Drug Administration (FDA) caution women over 40 against taking the pill or any hormonal contraceptives because of the increased chances of heart attacks, blood clots, and strokes (Stern et al., 1976). Hormonal contraceptives are used with caution in very young teenagers, as they may interfere with normal steroidal patterns and perhaps alter growth and development. Pregnant women and lactating women should not take estrogenic or progestogenic hormones, as they could alter developmental patterns in the fetus and infant (Jost, 1975). The possible effects of hormones on breast-fed babies has not yet been determined.

Several other forms of hormonal contraceptives have been formulated in a search for fewer side effects and monthly doses, the morning-after pill for unprotected midcycle sexual engagement, and the once-a-month pill (synthetic estrogen often combined with progestogen). Injectable hormonal contraceptives include slow release of the estrogenic or progestational hormones after either intramuscular injection or implantation.

Action   The action is not completely understood. However, these agents are thought to act in one or more of the following ways: by suppressing the release of LH and FSH at midcycle, thus preventing ovulation; by altering the cervical mucus and endometrical receptiveness for the ovum; or by changing the motility of the tubal passageway.

Estrogen levels vary widely in different women and also vary during the menstrual cycle. Therefore, the key factor to consider is the average "estrogen profile," which is based on body build, history of menstrual cycles, energy and libido levels, hormone levels, and age and gives some indication of hyperestrogenic or hypoestrogenic states (see Table 4–2).

Estrogen-dominant tablets are prescribed for the hypoestrogenic woman, and progesterone-dominant are prescribed for the hyperestrogenic woman, the aim being to balance the hormonal levels. Progestogen is, in this case, considered to be an antiestrogen.

Beneficial side effects include a reduced menstrual flow, which can contribute to improvement of iron deficiency anemia. Many women feel free of the fear of an unwanted pregnancy and have an increase in libido, finding sexual activity more enjoyable. Often, other complaints such as dys-

Table 4-2 Estrogen Responses

Hyperestrogenic, 10–12%	Balanced, 76–80%	Hypoestrogenic, 10–12%
Heavy menstrual flow	Normal menses	Scanty menses at longer intervals
Large breasts	Normal contours	Small breasts
Tendency to gain weight	Normal weight	Boyish look
Premenstrual syndrome: Fluid retention Emotional lability Increased libido Increased vaginal secretion Mastalgia		Lower libido Thinner vaginal lining More vaginitis, pruritus
	Normal vaginal cytology and secretions	
Tendency toward fibroids		

Source: Adapted from J. Nelson, "Clinical Evaluation of Side Effects of Current Contraceptives—Oral: Combined, Sequential," *Journal of Reproductive Medicine*, 6:2, 1971.

menorrhea, acne, and premenstrual tension are decreased while the woman is on the pill.

Effectiveness The agents with the highest degree of reliability are the combined oral preparations and the injectable preparations. The rate of failure is low, with a rate of one to three pregnancies per 100 woman-years of use, and many failures are caused by user forgetfulness.

Adverse Effects Although infrequent with low-dose oral contraceptives, side effects include nausea (very common occurrence), vomiting, diarrhea, abdominal cramps, bloating, constipation, breakthrough bleeding, spotting, amenorrhea, breast changes, weight changes, edema, blood pressure alterations, chloasma or melasma, allergic skin rash, migraine, mental depression and changes in cervical erosion and secretions.

The oral contraceptives have also been associated with other side effects such as changes in libido, anorexia, headache, backache, fatigue, nervousness, dizziness, intolerance to contact lenses, hirsutism, loss of scalp hair, vaginitis, premenstrual-type syndrome, and hemorrhagic eruptions. Patients must be educated about symptoms to report. Their informed consent should be obtained after the enclosed drug information booklet has been read and questions answered.

If oral contraceptives are taken early in pregnancy, masculinization of the female fetus and congenital limb-reduction defects have been observed. The VACTERL (vertebral, anal, cardiac, tracheal, esophogeal, renal, limb) syndrome is the name given to the anomalies also noted in offspring exposed to oral contraceptives during organogenesis. (Wentz, 1977).

Dosage Whenever possible, women should be maintained on the lowest dosages of estrogen and progestogen. Since estrogen has been implicated in causing more of the serious side effects than its counterpart, progestogen, it is only logical that the lowest dosage of estrogen be utilized. When it was first manufactured, the birth-control pill contained up to 150 μg (0.15 mg) of estrogen, but today, several of the birth-control pills

Table 4-3   Oral Estrogen-Progestogen Contraceptives

Trade Name	Progestogen	Estrogen
Brevicon	Norethindrone, 0.5 mg	Ethinyl estradiol, 0.035 mg
Demulen	Ethynodiol diacetate, 1 mg	Ethinyl estradiol, 0.05 mg
Enovid	Norethynodrel, 2.5 mg	Mestranol, 0.1 mg
Enovid, 5 mg	Norethynodrel, 5 mg	Mestranol, 0.075 mg
Enovid, 10 mg	Norethynodrel, 10 mg	Mestranol, 0.15 mg
Loestrin 1/20	Norethindrone acetate, 1 mg	Ethinyl estradiol, 0.02 mg
Loestrin Fe 1/20	Same as Loestrin 1/20 with iron added	
Loestrin 1.5/30	Norethindrone acetate, 1.5 mg	Ethinyl estradiol, 0.03 mg
Lo/Ovral	Norgestrel, 0.3 mg	Ethinyl estradiol, 0.03 mg
Norinyl 1+50	Norethindrone, 1 mg	Mestranol, 0.05 mg
Norinyl 1+80	Norethindrone, 1 mg	Mestranol, 0.08 mg
Norinyl, 2 mg	Norethindrone, 2 mg	Mestranol, 0.1 mg
Norlestrin 1/50	Norethindrone acetate, 1 mg	Ethinyl estradiol, 0.05 mg
Norlestrin Fe 1/50	Same as Norlestrin 1/50 with iron added	
Norlestrin 2.5/50	Norethindrone acetate, 2.5 mg	Ethinyl estradiol, 0.05 mg
Norlestrin Fe 2.5/50	Same as Norlestrin 2.5/50 with iron added	
Ortho-Novum 1/50	Norethindrone, 1 mg	Mestranol, 0.05 mg
Ortho-Novum 1/80	Norethindrone, 1 mg	Mestranol, 0.08 mg
Ortho-Novum, 2 mg	Norethindrone, 2 mg	Mestranol, 0.1 mg
Ortho-Novum, 10 mg	Norethindrone, 10 mg	Mestranol, 0.06 mg
Ovcon- 35	Norethindrone, 0.4 mg	Ethinyl estradiol, 0.035 mg
Ovcon- 50	Norethindrone, 1 mg	Ethinyl estradiol, 0.05 mg
Ovral	Norgestrel, 0.5 mg	Ethinyl estradiol, 0.05 mg
Ovosiston	Chlormadinone acetate, 3 mg	Mestranol, 0.1 mg

Table 4-3   Oral Estrogen-Progestogen Contraceptives (*Continued*)

Trade Name	Progestogen	Estrogen
Ovulen	Ethynodiol diacetate, 1 mg	Mestranol, 0.1 mg
Zorane 1/20	Norethindrone acetate, 1 mg	Ethinyl estradiol, 0.02 mg
Zorane 1/50	Norethindrone acetate, 1 mg	Ethinyl estradiol, 0.05 mg
Zorane 1.5/30	Norethindrone acetate, 1.5 mg	Ethinyl estradiol, 0.03 mg

contain as little as 20 μg (0.02 mg) of estrogen (see Table 4–3).

Nursing Implications

1. Advise the client to read contraceptive package insert. Informed consent is important. Discuss questions.

2. If the client misses a pill, instruct her to take it immediately and continue on her regimen. If she misses 2 days or more, she should take 2 each day until she has caught up to her schedule and use an alternative method of birth control for the remainder of the cycle.

3. Instruct the client that breakthrough bleeding may occur and that she should report this to her physician or clinic.

4. The client should report any missed menstrual periods; if two menstrual periods are missed, the pill should be discontinued until pregnancy is ruled out.

5. Lactating and pregnant women should *not* take the pill.

6. Advise the client to report any untoward symptoms, including mood swings, blurred vision, headaches, etc. (see Table 4–1).

7. Teach the client the importance of obtaining periodic checkups and Pap smears.

8. If the client experiences nausea (morning sickness), advise her to take the pill in the morning rather than in the evening.

Mini-Pills

Norethindrone, 0.35 mg (Micronor, Nor-Q.D.)

> ACTION   It is thought that the action of norethindrone in preventing pregnancy is linked with changes in the cervical mucus, alteration of the tubal transport of the ovum through the tube, and changes in the endometrial lining (see discussion at beginning of the section).

> DOSAGE   One tablet daily beginning on day 1 of the menstrual cycle, every day of the year. If 1 tablet is missed, the user should take it as soon as she remembers, and then take her next dose at the regular time. If 2 tablets are missed, the user should take 1 tablet as soon as she remembers and then take her regularly scheduled tablet for that day. In addition, another form of birth control should be utilized. If more than 2 pills have been missed, the user should stop taking the mini-pill immediately and use another form of contraception (nonhormonal) until her menstrual period returns or pregnancy is ruled out. If her period has not appeared within 45 days after missing 1 or 2 pills, she should be checked to rule out pregnancy.

Norgestryl, 0.075 mg (Ovrette)   Same as norethindrone. (In addition, it is thought that Ovrette may inhibit gonadotropin production.)

Morning-after Pills

Conjugated Estrogens   (Amnestrogen, Conestrone, Estrifol, Genisis, Premarin)

> ACTION   Conjugated estrogenic hormones are prepared with water-soluble, conjugated estrogens (the principal estrogen being sodium estrone sulfate, 50 to 60 percent) extracted from the urine of pregnant mares. It is used after unprotected

intercourse, particularly after rape. Major side effects preclude its regular use. The effectiveness of the drug is thought to center on the alteration of the endometrium, suppression of the corpus luteum, and increased rate of transport of the ovum through the fallopian tube.

ADVERSE EFFECTS More than 50 percent of the clients utilizing conjugated estrogens experience side effects, including nausea and other GI tract disturbances, headache, menstrual disturbances and breast tenderness. Rash, anorexia, and leg cramps may also occur.

DOSAGE 5–10 mg qid for 5 days; should be given within 72 h of the unprotected intercourse.

NURSING IMPLICATIONS
1. Before any estrogenic agent is given, pregnancy should be ruled out. Because of the teratogenic activity in offspring, estrogens should not be given during pregnancy. If the client is already pregnant, the morning-after pill will probably not interrupt the pregnancy.

2. Caution the patient of the side effects that can be experienced.

3. If the client is pregnant and the estrogenic hormones are given, the option of abortion should be offered.

Diethylstilbestrol (DES, Stilbestrol) Diethylstilbestrol has the same action, adverse effects, and nursing implications as conjugated estrogens.

DOSAGE 25–50 mg bid for 5 days; should be given within 72 h of the unprotected intercourse.

Ethinyl estradiol (Estinyl, Feminone, Lynoral) Ethinyl estradiol has the same action, adverse effects, and nursing implications as conjugated estrogens.

DOSAGE 1–5 mg qid for 5 days; should be given within 72 h of unprotected intercourse.

Table 4-4 Drugs Used to Prevent Lactation

Drug	Action	Adverse Reaction	Dose	Nursing Implications
Chlorotrianisene (Tace, Tace 72)	Nonsteroid estrogen (synthetic); inhibits release of prolactin; prevents breast engorgement	Occasional: skin rash, nausea, vomiting, edema Rare: postpartum bleeding requiring treatment	Tace: 12 mg PO qid for 7 d; 25–50 mg PO q 6 h for 6 doses Tace 72: 72 mg PO bid for 2 d	1. Give first dose just after delivery. 2. Do not give if any question of breast-feeding. 3. Do not give with history of reproductive tract cancer or hepatic, renal, or cardiac disease.
Dienstrol (DV, Restrol, Synestrol)	Same	Same	0.5–1.5 mg PO qd for 3 d, then 0.5 mg for 7 d	1. Same as above. 2. Protect from light. 3. Instruct patient on home schedule.
Diethystilbestrol (DES, Stilbestrol)	Same	More severe and common—anorexia, nausea, vomiting, epigastric distress, diarrhea, dizziness headache, thirst, anxiety, insomnia. In puerperium, may be associated with thromboembolic disorder.	PO or IM, only postpartum, 5 mg qd or tid to total dose of 30 mg	1. Same as Tace 2. Do not give if patient has any history of thrombophlebitis
Ethinyl estradiol (Diogyn-E, Estinyl, Esteed, Eticylol, Feminone)	Same as Tace	Nausea, vomiting, headache, edema	0.5–1 mg PO qd for 3 d, then 0.1 mg for 7 d	1. Same as Tace 2. Remind patient of medication schedule at home

Drug	Action	Side effects	Dosage	Nursing considerations
Piperazine estrone sulfate (Ogen)	Steroid which inhibits prolactin and prevents breast engorgement	Same as other estrogens	3.75 mg PO q 4 h for first 20 h postpartum	Same as above
Methallenestril (Vallestril)	Same as Tace	Not as potent as other non-steroid estrogens; therefore, fewer side effects	20–40 mg PO qd for 5 d	Same as above

COMBINATION DRUGS

Drug	Action	Side effects	Dosage	Nursing considerations
Methyltestosterone/esterified estrogens (Estratest)	Inhibits lactogenic hormone, suppressing lactation	Minimal because of antagonism of hormones; breast tenderness or hirsutism may occur	Methyltestosterone: 1.25 mg; esterified estrogens; 2.5 mg. 1 tablet tid for 4 d, then 1 tablet qd for 10 d	1. Same as for other estrogens 2. Remind patient of dosage schedule at home
Testosterone enanthate/estradiol valerate (Deladumone OB, Ditate-DS)	Same as Estratest; premixed in sesame oil for gradual release	Virilization, incomplete suppression of engorgement, Rare: convulsions, jaundice, pain at injection site, and local dermatitis	Testosterone: 360 mg; estradiol: 16 mg; 2 ml IM at onset of 2nd stage or just after delivery	1. Same as other estrogens 2. Give via Z-track technique 3. Store at room temperature 4. Weight loss is slower after delivery

OTHER

Drug	Action	Side effects	Dosage	Nursing considerations
Pitocin nasal spray	Relieves breast engorgement in nonnursing mothers; stimulates "letdown" reflex, thus promoting milk ejection by contracting myoepithelium of mammary glands.	None	One spray delivers 1.7 U to nasal mucosa	1. Use 2 to 3 min prior to nursing infant 2. Intranasal spray most effective route 3. Useful especially when breasts are so engorged that infant cannot grasp nipple

Intramuscular Injections

Medroxyprogesterone Acetate (Depo-Provera)

> ACTION   The action of this synthetic progestational agent is thought to be the same as other progestational agents (see earlier discussion).
>
> ADVERSE EFFECTS   Same as with other progestational agents. Also, prolonged amenorrhea or infertility may occur with Depo-Provera.
>
> DOSAGE   150–300 mg IM every 3 to 6 months.
>
> NURSING IMPLICATIONS   Same as other progestogens. In addition, clients should be told of the possibility of permanent infertility. If the client is planning to conceive in the future, perhaps she should utilize another form of birth control.

HORMONES TO PREVENT LACTATION

> When the placenta separates from the wall of the uterus, there is an abrupt halt in the secretion of the placental hormones, particularly progesterone and estrogen. This seems to trigger the release of the lactogenic hormone, thus initiating the lactation process. The breasts have been prepared throughout pregnancy for the function of nourishing the newborn. However, many women choose to feed their infants by bottle and wish to reverse or halt the lactation process. In order to do this, a drug is usually prescribed, and if necessary, binders and ice packs or analgesics are used to relieve her discomfort.
>
> Estrogen and progestational agents, as well as androgens, are capable of preventing lactation, but estrogens are most frequently used. One of the most effective combinations for the suppression of lactation is testosterone coupled with estradiol valerate (*Deladumone-OB, Ditate-DS*). One of the most commonly employed oral estrogenic agents is chlorotrianisene (*Tace*). Table 4-4 lists drugs ued to prevent lactation.

Before any agent to suppress lactation is given, several points must be checked.

1. Be sure the patient is *not* going to breast-feed.

2. Before any estrogenic product is given, check the patient history for contraindications (see oral contraceptives).

3. Hormones should be given as close to delivery and placental separation as possible. Injections may be given just prior to the third stage of labor. Oral agents should be given as soon in the postpartum period as possible. Be sure the patient has reacted before giving her any oral medications.

BIBLIOGRAPHY

Berger, G.S., and W.C. Fowler, Jr.: "Exogenous Estrogens and Endometrial Carcinoma: Review and Comments for the Clinician," *Journal of Reproductive Medicine*, 18(4):177, 1977.

Bergersen, B.S., and A. Goth: *Pharmacology in Nursing*, C.B. Mosby, St. Louis, 1976.

Bibbo, M., et. al.: "Follow-up Study of Male and Female Offspring of DES Exposed Mothers," *Obstetrics and Gynecology*, 49:1, 1977.

Cohen, M.R.: "Endometriosis and Infertility," *Journal of Reproductive Medicine*, 18(3):120, 1977.

Garb, S.: "Guidelines to Avoiding Drug Interactions," *Contemporary Ob/Gyn*, 7(4):179–202, April 1976.

Garcia, C.R., and D.L. Rosenfeld: *Human Fertility: The Regulation of Reproduction*, F.A. Davis, Philadelphia, 1977.

*Gemzell, C.: "Induction of Ovulation with Human Gonadotropins," *Journal of Reproductive Medicine*, 18(4):155, 1977.

Haney, A.F., and C.B. Hammond: "Inducing Ovulation," *Contemporary Ob/Gyn*, 9(2):125–133, February 1977.

*Huppert, L.C., and E.F. Wallach: "Induction of Ovulation with Clomiphene Citrate," *Journal of Reproductive Medicine*, 18(5):201, 1977.

*Denotes particularly pertinent references.

*Jost, A.: "Hormonal Effects on Fetal Development: A Survey," *Clinical Pharmacology and Therapeutics*, **14**(4) part 2: 714–720, 1975.

Nora, J.J., and A.H. Nora: "Can The Pill Cause Defects?" *New England Journal of Medicine*, **291**:731, 1974.

Overbach, A.M., and M.J. Rodman: *Drugs Used with Neonates and During Pregnancy*, Medical Economics Company, Oradell, N.J., 1975.

Palmer, J.D., and R. Bressler: "Mechanism of Drug Interactions," *Contemporary Ob/Gyn*, **2**(3):86–90, 1974.

Speroff, L. (moderator): "Symposium: Workup on Menstrual Irregularities," *Contemporary Ob/Gyn*, **7**(2):132–182, February 1976.

Stortz, Laurie J.: "Unprescribed Drug Products and Pregnancy," *Journal of Obstetric, Gynecologic, and Neonatal Nursing*, **6**(4):9–13, July/August 1977.

Stern, M.P., et al.: "Cardiovascular Risk and Use of Estrogens or Estrogen-Progestogen Combinations," *Journal of American Medical Association*, **2350**(8):811–815, February 23, 1976.

Wentz, A.C.: "The Use of Estrogens and Progestins in Gynecologic Problems," *Clinical Obstetrics and Gynecology*, **20**(2):451–459, June 1977.

*Yalom, I.D., R. Green, and N. Fish: "Prenatal Exposure to Female Hormones: Effect on Psychosocial Development in Boys," *Archives of General Psychiatry*, **28**:554, 1973.

Drugs Used in Problem Pregnancies

Elizabeth J. Dickason
Paul A. Michelson

INFECTIOUS PROCESSES AND ANTIMICROBIALS

The incidence of infection as a cause of maternal morbidity and mortality has not diminished significantly over the last few years. Resistant strains of bacteria are more difficult to treat, and less common anaerobic bacteria are being implicated as causative agents. Increased awareness of modes of transfer and continued vigilance about aseptic practices in obstetrics are needed to help reduce problems.

Viral Infections

Viral infections may cause more severe illness when a woman is pregnant. Some evidence shows that during pandemics and epidemics, maternal and fetal deaths rose as a result of influenza infection. Polio carries a higher risk for a pregnant woman, with the incidence of paralysis and death increased compared with nonpregnant women of the same age. Most viruses have been shown to cross the placental membrane, and many have demonstrated teratogenic effects.

Bacterial Infections

Urinary Tract Infections   Changes in the genitourinary tract predispose toward an increased susceptibility to bacteriuria. Smooth muscle relaxation with dilated ureters and increased residual urine promote bacterial growth. *Escherichia coli* is most often implicated, but sometimes, bacteria more difficult to treat are the causative agents. Infection is common especially after delivery, when there has been trauma to the base of the bladder and overdistention of the bladder.

Vaginal Infections Increased blood supply to the vagina and cervix with changes in pH and glucose levels make the vaginal tract a more nourishing place for growth of organisms. *Candida vaginalis, Trichomonas vaginalis*, and *Hemophilus vaginalis* occur most often and are more resistant to treatment. *Candida* may increase, especially if the patient is treated with systemic antibiotics for infections elsewhere in the body.

Gonorrhea may involve mild infections of the lower genital tract with a vaginal discharge and dysuria. Pregnant women seem to be more resistant to gonococcal salpingo-oophoritis, perhaps as a result of the defensive character of the endocervical secretions. Syphilis acquired but treated before the sixteenth to eighteenth week may not infect the fetus, but after the eighteenth week, spirochetes can traverse the placenta to the infant.

Premature Rupture of Membranes Premature rupture of membranes of more than 12 to 24 hours' duration is associated with a high incidence of ascending infection. The longer the delay before delivery, the more likely will be the possibility of chorioamnionitis and subsequent endometritis. Most often, the bacteria are those which are normal residents of the vagina.

Frequent vaginal examinations and poor asepsis after membrane rupture can transfer exogenous bacteria and increase the likelihood of resident bacteria being inserted through the cervix. The risk of amnionitis is mainly to the infant, who may, under stress in utero, take a deep gasping breath, aspirating infected fluid deep within the respiratory tract. Swallowing also takes place in utero, and neonatal gastroenteritis has been reported as a result of bacteria in amniotic fluid. Prophylactic antibiotics may be ordered during labor to treat both mother and fetus.

Endometritis Endometritis may be a result of hemolytic streptococcal infections of group A or B. The onset is rapid, and the infectious process may become disseminated through lymphatic vessels to cause peritonitis and bacteremia. Mixed aerobic-anaerobic infections from normally resident bacteria in the vagina usually lead to less virulent, more localized infections of the episiotomy, lacerations, or endometrium. In severe cases, however, infection can progress to pelvic veins and cause thrombophlebitis with the rare complication of septic pulmonary emboli. In these cases, anticoagulant therapy accompanies antibiotic therapy. Antibiotic therapy is complicated by the presence of several organisms of different characteristics.

A very severe picture may be seen with infection caused by *Clostridium perfringens* or *Bacteroides fragilis*, both anaerobes. These bacteria may produce high fever, with renal failure, jaundice, and hemolysis.

Vaccination During Pregnancy

Information concerning the risk of immunization on the pregnant woman or her fetus can only serve as a guide, since many effects of both the disease and the vaccine are unknown. In general, live vaccines should not be given except when high susceptibility and exposure are greatly probable and the disease poses a greater threat than vaccination. No contraindication to the use of various toxoids exists, and they may be considered a practical step in antepartal care.

Vaccines are of three types:

1. Toxoids—preparations of chemically altered bacterial endotoxin;

2. Killed bacterial and viral vaccines—heat or chemically inactivated organisms;

Table 5-1   Vaccination During Pregnancy

	Risk from Disease to Pregnant Female	Risk from Disease to Fetus or Neonate
Tetanus-diphtheria	Tetanus mortality is 60%; diphtheria, 10%	Neonetal tetanus mortality is 60%
Poliomyelitis	No increased incidence in pregnancy	50% mortality in neonatal disease
Rubella	Low mortality not altered by pregnancy	High rate of abortion and congenital rubella syndrome in 1st trimester
Influenza	Possible increase in mortality to new strain	Possible increased abortion rate
Smallpox	Mortality, 90% during pregnancy	Possible increased abortion rate; congenital smallpox reported
Rabies	Near 100% fatal; not altered by pregnancy	Determined by maternal disease

Source: Adapted from *Vaccination During Pregnancy*, ACOG Technical Bulletin, Center for Disease Control, Atlanta, Georgia, March 1973.

Vaccine	Indication for Vaccination During Pregnancy	Dosage
Combined tetanus diphtheria toxoid preferred	Lack of primary series or no booster in 10 years	Primary: 3 doses at 1 to 2 month intervals, or booster dose 0.5 ml every 10 years
Live, attenuated virus vaccine	Not recommended routinely for adults in U.S. except in epidemics	Primary: 3 doses at 1 to 2 month intervals or booster dose
Live, attenuated virus vaccine	Contraindicated	—
Inactivated type A and B virus vaccines	Recommended only for patients with serious underlying disease	Primary: 2 doses 6 to 8 weeks apart ih early fall; booster: single dose
Live vaccinia virus vaccine	Not routinely recommended in U.S.; avoid in pregnancy	Live vaccinia immune globulin (0.3 ml/kg) with primary vaccination; revaccinate without vaccinia immune globulin
Killed virus vaccine	Pregnancy does not alter indications for prophylaxis	Consult public health agencies for indications and dosage

3. Live virus vaccines—viruses selected for their reduced virulence.

Various factors must be considered before immunization is performed. First, there should be confirmation of the pregnancy and a determination of gestational age, if possible. If a live virus vaccine is to be given, conception should be prevented for the subsequent 2 months because of the susceptibility of the embryo to teratogenic effect. Second, the patient should have an antibody determination to determine susceptibility. Third, it is preferable to reduce exposure when there is any question of fetal risk. Patients planning to travel to areas where plague, yellow fever, and smallpox are endemic should consider time of travel carefully. Fourth, evaluation of the risk of contracting a disease as compared with the risk of vaccination is the reponsibility of the physician. Table 5-1 lists the current recommendations from the Center for Disease Control.

The Aminoglycosides

The mechanism of action of the aminoglycoside antibiotics is not completely known, but action seems to be by interference in protein biosynthesis in the bacterial cell. Aminoglycosides are used in the treatment of serious systemic infections caused by susceptible organisms, mainly the gram-negative organisms, *E. coli*, *Pseudomonas*, *Proteus* (indole negative and positive), *Klebsiella*, *Serratia*, and enterobacteria resistant to less toxic antibiotics. Urinary tract infections respond especially well because of the high concentrations of antibiotic in the urine. Oral forms of kanamycin or neomycin are used mainly for GI tract antisepsis. In unusually severe staphlococcal infections in soft tissue or bone, some aminoglycosides may be employed (see Table 5-2).

Aminoglycosides are excreted unchanged, and an alkaline environment enhances activity. There is wide distribution in body fluids after parenteral administration or topical application to burns or open wounds but poor absorption from intact skin or the GI tract. Oral administration is therefore used primarily for GI tract antisepsis. Interactions are com-

Table 5-2   Aminoglycosides

Drug	Dosage	Comments
Amikacin (Amikin)	15 mg/kg IM, IV in 24 h in 2 to 4 divided doses; not to exceed 1.5 g per day	Same toxicities as kanamycin. It is the newest aminoglycoside. $T_{1/2}$ is 2 h; not protein-bound; excreted almost totally by the kidney. Active against several gentamycin-resistant strains.
Gentamycin (Garamycin)	3 to 5 mg IM, IV, in 24 h in 3 divided doses; IV dose is best given over a period of 1 to 2 h and no faster than in 30 min	IM administration may be painful; IV must be by intermittent infusion. Do not mix with any other drugs. Blood levels of 5–7 μg/ml considered best; over 12 μg/ml, toxicity occurs. $T_{1/2}$ is 2 h. Excreted unchanged in urine.
Kanamycin (Kantrex)	500 mg to 8 g PO qd for 2 d to reduce GI bacterial flora	Pre-GI surgery. In hepatic disease, reduces ammonia production in GI tract. Bacterial superinfection can occur with prolonged PO administration.
	15 mg/kg IM in 24 h in 2 to 4 divided doses; not to exceed 1.5 g qd	IM may be painful, give deeply, by Z track
	15–30 mg/kg IV in 24 h in 2 to 3 divided doses	Regulate IV flow rate carefully, run in slowly. Restrict treatment to 2 weeks or less.
Neomycin (Mycifradin Sulfate, Neobiotic)	50 mg/kg PO in 24 h in 4 divided doses	Use for severe diarrhea caused by enteropathogenic *E. coli*.
	100 mg/kg PO in 24 h	Higher doses for GI tract antisepsis, inhibition of nitrogen-forming bacteria in hepatic coma, cirrhosis.
	Topical application	Topical use for irrigation of wounds can lead to rapid absorption and distribution. Patients with renal disease can develop toxic levels.
Streptomycin	500 mg to 2 g IM qd in 2 to 4 divided doses, *or* 15–25 mg/kg in 2 divided doses for 7 to 10 d, then 1 g qd.	Used mainly for *Mycobacterium tuberculosis*, and with penicillin to treat *Streptococcus faecalis* or *S. viridans*. May enhance oral anticoagulants. Hypersensitive reactions, pain at injection site, paresthesias, and drug fever may occur. Give deep IM and rotate sites. Not used during pregnancy.

Table 5-2   Aminoglycosides (*Continued*)

Drug	Dosage	Comments
Tobramycin (Nebcin)	3–5 mg/kg IM, IV in 24 h in 3 divided doses for 7 to 10 d	Used in severe infections. Also affects providencia, citrobacter, and *P. aeruginosa*. May be combined with carbenicillin and cephalosporin; may produce enhanced effect with carbenicillin in *Pseudomonas* infection. Thrombophlebitis at injection site, increased bilirubin, and decreased hematocrit, platelets, and WBC may occur.

mon and can be serious with skeletal muscle relaxants, ethacrynic acid, and methoxyflurane. Cross-resistance may occur, as well as cross-sensitization within the family.

Adverse Effects   The most important toxicity involves the eighth cranial nerve. However, ototoxicity is more common at higher blood levels. High blood levels can produce vestibular damage, causing dizziness, tinnitus, and vertigo, while auditory effects occur less frequently, producing loss of high frequencies. Permanent deafness can occur with extended treatment. Renal toxicities include acute renal failure, oliguria, and increased BUN and serum creatinine levels. Early signs of kidney toxicity may include casts, albuminuria, and microscopic hematuria.

The possibility of ototoxicity and renal toxicity in the fetus has led to the use of aminoglycosides only when life-threatening infections occur during pregnancy.

Nursing Implications
1. Observe for signs of ototoxicity. Question patient daily about early signs of tinnitus, dizziness, or any degree of hearing loss.

2. Watch for signs of nephrotoxicity (decreasing urine output,

rising BUN and creatinine levels). Expect tests for serum levels of drug and creatinine to be ordered.

3. Never mix drug with any other in intravenous solutions.

Antifungal Agents

Amphotericin B (Fungizone)   Serious infections and meningitis caused by fungi such as *Aspergillus fumigatus*, *Coccidioides immitis*, *Cryptococcus neoformans*, *Histoplasma capsulatum*, *Blastomyces dermatitidis*, and *Candida albicans* respond to amphotericin B. The drug will cause potassium depletion (which may be enhanced by corticosteroids), facilitate the development of digitalis toxicity, and increase the effect of curarelike muscle relaxants.

ADVERSE EFFECTS   Intravenous administration may cause headache, fever, chills, cramps vomiting, or anaphylactoid reactions. Hypokalemia, nephrotoxicity, anemia, congestive heart failure, thrombophlebitis, and rashes may also occur. Safety in pregnancy has not been established, and the drug should not be used during the first trimester. Reactions may be reduced by lowering dosage, by slowing the infusion rate, and by giving antiemetics, antipyretics, and antihistamines.

DOSAGE   The drug must be reconstituted in sterile water without a bacteriostatic agent: 10 ml to 50 mg vial, then shake vial for 3 min. Then it is diluted in 250–500 ml 5% dextrose in water and given intravenously over a 6-h period, qd or qod. This regimen must continue over 1 or more months until effective. A test dose of 1 mg must be used for the first few days with dosage gradually increasing by 5–10 mg daily to maximum of 50 mg per day. Topical application of a 3% cream is used for dermatomycoses of *Candida* species.

NURSING IMPLICATIONS
1. Any patient given this agent must be observed for chills, fever, and other reactions.

2. Electrolytes and renal function must be closely monitored.

3. Check directions carefully, in-line intravenous filters may remove drug from suspension. Store in refrigerator.

Candicidin (Candeptin, Vanobid) Topically used for vaginal moniliasis, candicidin has very little toxicity. There may be slight local vulvar or perineal irritation in the presence of severe infection. Suppositories should be inserted manually during pregnancy; the use of an applicator is contraindicated. One suppository, inserted intravaginally in the morning and at night for 2 weeks, is usually effective.

Flucytosine (Ancobon) Flucytosine is used for infections produced by susceptible strains of *Candida* and *Cryptococcus*. Urinary tract fungal infections may respond because of the high concentrations in the urine. Systemic infections are treated with a combination of amphotericin B and 5-flucytosine. The mechanism of action is unknown.

Absorption is good through the GI tract, and the drug is widely distributed to body tissues and fluids. Impaired renal function produces higher blood levels.

ADVERSE EFFECTS Anemia with decreasing blood elements, nausea, vomiting, and diarrhea occur. Flucytosine has produced teratogenicity in rats because of metabolism to fluorouracil (anticancer pyrimidine antagonist); therefore, use during pregnancy is not wise.

DOSAGE 150 mg PO q 24 h in four divided doses.

NURSING IMPLICATIONS Hematocrit reading, white blood cells (WBC), and platelets should be monitored carefully as well as liver studies [increases in serum glutamic oxaloacetic transaminase (SGOT), serus glutamic pyruvic transaminase (SGPT), and alkaline phosphatase levels].

Griseofulvin (Fulvicin, Grisactin) Griseofulvin is used for cutaneous fungal infections of the skin, nails, and hair caused by strains of *Trichophyton*, *Microsporum*, and *Epidermophyton* (tinea, ringworm). Oral absorption is varied and occurs primarily in the duodenum, but high-fat meals increase absorption. The drug is concentrated in the skin, hair, nails, fat, liver, and skeletal muscle. Most is metabolized in the liver, with very little excreted unchanged.

Phenobarbital may decrease absorption of griseofulvin, producing lower serum levels. Griseofulvin may stimulate microsomal enzymes and alter oral anticoagulant effectiveness.

ADVERSE EFFECTS   Headache, nausea, vomiting ,excessive thirst, diarrhea, and oral candidiasis may occur. Rarely, rashes, serum sickness, leukopenia, and mental confusion have been reported. There have been reports of embryotoxic and teratogenic effects in mice and dogs; therefore, drug is not usually given during pregnancy.

DOSAGE   Micronized form desirable to reduce GI upset. 500 mg to 4 g PO, either qd or bid for 1 to 6 months.

NURSING IMPLICATIONS
1. Monitor renal, hepatic, and blood studies.

2. Observe for headache and GI disturbances.

Miconazole (Monistat)   Fungal infections, both topical and intravaginal, respond to miconazole. Local irritation and burning occasionally occur, with headache, hives, and skin rash reported. Safety in pregnancy has not been established, and use during the first trimester should be avoided.

DOSAGE   To treat vulvovaginal candidiasis: 5 g of 2% cream is inserted vaginally once at bedtime each night for 2 weeks.

NURSING IMPLICATIONS
1. Patients should be informed of the possibility of rash, hives, and irritation.

2. Careful insertion of applicator and abstinence from intercourse during treatment should be advised.

Nystatin (Mycostatin, Nilstat)   Nystatin is used orally in monilial infections of the GI tract. Cutaneous and vaginal infections respond to the cream, ointment, or vaginal suppositories. Gastrointestinal absorption is very poor, and no absorption occurs from intact skin and mucous membranes. Excretion is through the feces as unchanged drug (oral administration). Side effects are infrequent with nystatin, but mild nausea, vomiting, and diarrhea may occur. Hypersensitivity reactions can cause contact dermatitis.

DOSAGE   For oral and intestinal infections, instruct the patient to hold tablets in mouth before swallowing. One or two 500,000–1,000,000 U tablets tid. Cutaneous lesions are treated with powder, cream, or ointment. For vaginal candidiasis, vaginal suppositories (100,000 U) are inserted bid for 2 weeks. Sometimes, suppositories are ordered for 3 to 6 weeks prior to delivery to prevent thrush in the newborn.

NURSING IMPLICATIONS
1. Monitor for worsening of rash as a result of nystatin.

2. Proper instruction in administration of vaginal suppositories must be given.

Antitrichomonal Agents

Metronidazole (Flagyl)   Metronidazole is used as a systemic antitrichomonal agent in both men and women. Less common uses include treatment for amebic dysentery and amebic liver abscess. Gastrointestinal absorption is good, occurring in the small intestine. Most of the drug is excreted in the urine unchanged, and urine may be colored dark or red-brown. The drug crosses the placenta and is found in the breast milk; therefore it is not used unless other measures have proved inadequate, and use in the first trimester is not recommended.

ADVERSE EFFECTS   Some patients may experience Antibuse-type reactions (nausea, vomiting, flushing) from alcohol ingestion while on therapy. A patient taking Antibuse may develop confusion and psychotic problems. Otherwise, the incidence of side effects associated with oral therapy is low. Most often, nausea and sometimes abdominal cramps and diarrhea occur. Rarely, a metallic taste, color changes of the tongue, stomatitis, skin rashes, vaginal itching and burning, and ataxia are reported.

DOSAGE   250 mg PO tid for both men and women for 7 days. In acute amebic dysentery, 750 mg tid for 5 to 10 days.

The Cephalosporins

Cephalosporins are used for respiratory tract infections, skin and soft tissue infections, and urinary infections caused by gram-positive and gram-negative bacteria. They are highly protein-bound, and most of the drug is excreted unchanged in the urine. The drugs cross the placenta and are found in the cord blood and amniotic fluid. However, very low concentrations are found in the breast milk.

No specific drug interactions occur with cephalosporins, but a false-positive reaction for glucose may occur with Benedict's or Fehling's solution or with Clinitest tablets. Probenecid will reduce renal excretion.

Adverse Effects   There may be an increased incidence of adverse effects in patients allergic to penicillin. Drug fever, skin rashes, pruritis, and eosinophilia may occur. Gastrointestinal disturbances such as anorexia, nausea, vomiting, diarrhea, are common. A transient rise in SGOT, BUN, and alkaline phosphatase levels has been observed. Phlebitis is uncommon, but with some cephalosporins intramuscular injection causes severe pain.

There may be additive effects when these drugs are given with aminoglycosides or polymixins. A prolongation of prothrombin time and hypoprothrombinemia may occur; therefore, patients on anticoagulants should not be given cephalosporins.

Dosages and modes of administration are given in Table 5-3.

Table 5-3 Cephalosporins

Drug	Dosage	Comments
Cefazolin (Ancef, Kefzol)	250–500 mg IM q 8 h	Reconstitute with sterile water, shake well until dissolved. Solution stable only for 24 h.
	250–500 mg IV q 8 h	Dilute in 50–100 ml 5% dextrose in water.
Cephalexin (Keflex)	250–500 mg PO q 6 h for 10 d	Food delays absorption, but GI route preferred.
Cephaloridine (Loridine)	250–1000 mg IM q 6 to 8 h *or*	Given deep IM by Z track.
	500 mg dissolved in 5–10 ml water for IV injection, then added to 5% dextrose in water infusion	Administer either by continuous infusion or intermittently over a period of 3 to 4 min. Do not mix with other antibiotics.
Cephalothin (Keflin)	500 mg to 2 g IM q 4 to 6 h	Mix 1 g in 4 ml sterile water for IM use.
	4–6 g IV q 24 h in divided doses	Mix into at least 40 ml 5% dextrose in water solution for IV use.

Nursing Implications

1. Observe for GI disturbances or a change in Coombs' test.

2. Note false-positives with Clinitest and Benedict's solution.

3. Note when intramuscular administration causes pain; look for ways to alleviate discomfort.

The Erythromycins

The spectrum of the erythromycins is similar in many ways to that of penicillin and includes beta-hemolytic streptococci, pneumococci, *Corynobacterium diptheriae*, and some staphylococci. Absorption by the oral route is rapid and occurs mostly in the upper section of the small intestine. Absorption may be impaired or delayed if administered with food or acid drinks.

Erythromycin is excreted up to 15 percent unchanged in the urine but is also found in the bile, milk, and feces. Large concentrations occur in the liver and bile. Erythromycin and lincomycin may be antagonistic. As a bacteriostatic drug, it may inhibit the activity of bactericidal drugs such as the penicillins.

Adverse Effects   Primary adverse effects involve nausea, vomiting, and diarrhea. Intramuscular injection may be painful. Rash and anaphylactic reactions, as well as cholestatic hepatitis, occur very infrequently. Often, erythromycin is used in patients allergic to penicillin. The estolate salt has produced jaundice, and hepatic tests should be monitored.

Dosage requirements of the erythromycins are listed in Table 5-4.

Table 5-4   Erythromycins

Drug	Dosage	Comments
Erythromycin base (many brands)	250–500 mg PO q 6 h	Tablets have acid-resistant coating.
Erythromycin estolate or stearate	250–500 mg PO q 6 h	
Erythromycin ethylsuccinate	1 to 4 g PO, 100 mg IM q 4 to 12 h	May not be given SC or IV.
Erythromycin gluceptate	1–4 g IV in 4 divided doses	Reconstitute with sterile water and then add to IV solution of 5% dextrose in water for intermittent administration; must run over more than 20 min or vessel irritation occurs.
Erythromycin lactobionate	200–300 mg, IM, IV, q 6 to 8 h	Reconstitute with sterile water before adding to IV infusion.

The Penicillins

The penicillins act by inhibiting proper bacterial cell wall formation, which allows the production of defective cell wall structure. Penicillin is distributed to almost all body fluids and tissues. Smaller concentrations are found in cerebrospinal fluid (CSF), nerves, and muscles. Penicillins cross the placenta and are found in breast milk.

Probenecid will reduce the excretion of all penicillins, thus raising blood levels. Other drugs being given concomitantly will also increase penicillin's half-life, e.g., phenylbutazone, indomethacin, aspirin, and sulfinpyrazone.

When bactericidal drugs such as the penicillins are given together with bacteriostatic drugs, there may be an inhibition of the bactericidal drug action. Certain of the penicillins are acid-resistant and can be administered orally; others can be administered only parenterally. Some of the semisynthetic penicillins are not inhibited by penicillinase-producing bacteria. All the penicillins are most active against gram-positive organisms, but some gram-negative cocci and spirochetes can be effectively treated.

Adverse Effects   All the penicillins can produce hypersensitivity reactions that range from mild rashes to fatal anaphylactic shock. Other hypersensitivity reactions include hemolytic anemia, thrombocytopenia, leukopenia, interstitial nephritis, Jarisch-Herxheimer reaction in syphilitic patients, diarrhea, nausea, vomiting, and black hairy tongue. All patients must be monitored for allergy, and before the first dose, a history of reaction must be known. In addition, all patients must be screened for hepatic, renal, and hematologic changes during and after therapy. Serious superinfections may occur with resistant organisms, vaginitis may flare up, and gram-negative bacteria may flourish.

Table 5-5 lists the dosages of the penicillins.

Nursing Implications
1. Note carefully if drug is acid-resistant or if food interferes with absorption. Administer those types of penicillin 1 hour before meals or 2 hours after meals for best effect.

Table 5-5   Penicillins

Drug	Dosage	Comments
NATURAL PENICILLINS		
Penicillin G Potassium salt (Pentids)	600,000–3,000,000 U PO qd	Penicillin G is the first choice for severe infections by nonpenicillinase organisms. Partially inactivated by stomach acid, but can be given orally (one-third to one-fifth absorbed).
Sodium salt (Aqueous, Crystalline)	Up to 12,000,000 U IM qd, or in severe cases, up to 20,000,000 U by continuous IV infusion	IM administration is painful. Transient high levels are avoided by continuous IV infusion; excretion is rapid.
Procaine penicillin G (Crystacillin, Duracillin, Wycillin)	600,000–1,000,000 U IM qd in 1 or 2 doses for 10 to 14 d	IV administration may be fatal; watch carefully. Even though label says aqueous suspension, use IM route only.
Benzathine penicillin G	600,000–1,200,000 U IM qd, or for gonorrhea, 2,400,000 U divided, with ½ in each gluteus medius site	Long-lasting suspension in oil. For gonorrhea, precede IM administration by 1 g probenecid, ½ h before dose.
SEMISYNTHETIC PENICILLINS (PENICILLINASE-RESISTANT)		
Sodium cloxacillin (Tegopen)	500 mg to 1 g PO q 4 to 6 h, 1 h ac or 2 h pc	Maintains higher serum levels than other semisynthetic penicillins; protein-bound (90–94%). Identical to oxacillin in properties.
Sodium dicloxacillin (Dynapen, Veracillin)	250 mg to 1 g PO, q 4 to 6 h; for mild infections, 250 mg to 1 g, IM, q 6 h	Stable in gastric acid; slowly absorbed; excreted primarily from bile and recycled to some extent. More active against penicillinase-producing organisms than oxacillin.
Sodium methicillin (Staphcillin, Celbenin)	1 g in 1.5 ml water for IM injection q 4 to 6 h	Not acid-resistant; therefore, must be given IM or IV. Effective against all strains of *S. aureus*; 40% protein-bound; half excreted unchanged in urine, also in bile. Phlebitis after repeated IV doses. Painful IM, sterile abscesses have occurred.

Table 5-5   Penicillins (Continued)

Drug	Dosage	Comments
	1–2 g in 50 ml NaCl solution, IV, infused at a rate of 10 ml/min, given q 4 to 6 h	Solution unstable when mixed with water; store in refrigerator no longer than 4 days. IV solution must be used within 8 h. Do not mix with other drugs or into 5% dextrose in water infusion.
Sodium nafcillin (Unipen)	250 mg to 1 g PO q 4 to 6 h, given 1 h ac or 2 h pc	Highly resistant to penicillinase, and penicillin G-resistant strains respond. Absorption from GI tract irregular, but drug is given both PO and IM or IV. Major route of excretion is through bile.
	250 mg to 1 g IM, IV q 6 h	IM injection causes pain; thrombophlebitis may occur with IV route.
Sodium oxacillin (Prostaphlin)	500 mg PO, q 4 to 6 h ac	Effective against gram-positive organisms outside the staphlococci group and against penicillinase-producing staphlococci.
	500 mg to 1 g IM q 4 to 6 h	Food interferes with absorption; give before or well after meals.
	500 mg to 1 g IV q 3 to 4 h, well diluted, over a period of not less than 10 to 15 min	Dilute in NaCl solution for piggyback IV administration; do not mix with other drugs.
ACID-RESISTANT		
Potassium penicillin V (Pen-Vee, V-Cillin); potassium phenoxymethyl penicillin (Pen-Vee-K, V-Cillin K, Ledercillin VK)	125–500 mg PO q 4 to 6 h	Available only as oral tablets or capsules or powders or granules to put into oral solutions. Insoluble and stable in acid environments. Antibiotic spectrum identical to penicillin G. Food delays absorption.
Potassium phenethicillin (Darcel, Maxipen, Syncillin)	125–500 mg PO tid	Stable in gastric acid; absorption increased if given ac, but serum levels maintained longer if given with food. Follow physicians order as to timing of dosage.

Table 5-5   Penicillins (Continued)

Drug	Dosage	Comments
EXTENDED SPECTRUM		
Ampicillin (Omnipen, Polycillin)	250–500 mg PO q 6 h, 1 h ac or 2 h pc; 250–500 mg IM q 6 h	More effective against gram-negative strains than penicillin G. Urinary tract infections respond. Inactivated by penicillinase-producing bacteria. Absorbed readily from GI tract, 20% protein-bound, excreted rapidly into urine. Rashes occur frequently but are not signs of more severe reactions. Diarrhea is common.
Ampicillin sodium	250–500 mg IV q 6 h only when patient unable to take oral dose	
Amoxicillin (Amoxil, Polymox)	250–500 mg PO q 8 h	Resistant to gastric acid; not affected by presence of food. Spectrum is the same as ampicillin. Oral use only.
Carbenicillin (Geopen, Pyopen)	200–500 mg/kg IM, IV in 24 h; never more than 40 g in 24 h.	IM: reconstitute a 5 g vial with 9.5 ml sterile water. Never give more than 2 g in a single site. IV: dilute to at least 100 ml for piggyback intermittent infusion.
Carbenicillin indanyl sodium (Geocillin)	1 or 2 tablets (382 mg) PO qid	Active against Pseudomonas, anaerobic bacteria, and Proteus, especially. Given concomitantly with gentamycin for severe Pseudomonas infection, but do not mix drugs in solution together. PO preparation is acid stable and changed into carbenicillin. Useful for urinary tract infections.
Hetacillin (Versapen, Versapen-K)	225–450 mg PO q 6 h (capsules of 225, 450 mg available)	Converted into ampicillin in the body with same indications and adverse effects. Absorbed well from the GI tract. Suspension available as 112.5 mg/ml or 225 mg/5 ml.

2. Intramuscular administration must be deep using the Z track technique and is usually given in half doses, one in each gluteus medius site. Oil-based solvents will slow absorption time.

3. Intravenous administration must be monitored for slow rate of flow, since serum levels must be maintained. Excretion is rapid, primarily renal, and mostly unchanged.

4. Always check for a history of allergy before administration. Note such a history prominently on chart. All brands of natural or semisynthetic penicillin may cause allergic reactions.

5. Once administered, monitor for any signs of adverse effects, especially urticaria, edema, rash, diarrhea, and fever.

The Sulfonamides

The sulfonamides are used in the treatment of acute, non-obstructive urinary tract infections caused by *E. coli*, *Klebsiella*, *Aerobacter*, *S. aureus*, *P. mirabilis* and, less frequently, *P. vulgaris*. Sulfonamides increase the adverse effects of ethanol and further impair driving ability. Some local anesthetics, derivatives of PABA, may antagonize the bacteriostatic activity of sulfonamides. Antacids decrease the absorption by increasing the ionization of sulfonamides in the GI tract.

Adverse Effects   Gastrointestinal disturbances are common and include nausea, vomiting, stomatitis, and glossitis. Blood dyscrasias like leukopenia, eosinophilia, hemolytic anemia, thrombocytopenia, and aplastic anemia have been reported. Skin problems such as rash, pruritis, photosensitivity, and exfoliative dermatitis sometimes occur. Neurologic effects include ataxia, headache, dizziness, depression, confusion, and hallucinations. Jaundice and renal damage may also occur. Drug fever may develop from 7 to 10 days after administration, and crystalluria may form in an acid urine. Because of all these problems, sulfonamides are contraindicated during pregnancy. They pass the placenta, are excreted in milk, and may cause hyperbilirubinemia in the newborn. Cleft palate and bone abnormalities in offspring of pregnant rats and mice at high oral dosage have been reported.

Dosage requirements for the sulfonamides are given in Table 5-6.

Nursing Implications

1. Any patient on sulfonamides should be monitored for liver function and blood studies.

Table 5-6   Sulfonamides

Drug	Dosage	Comments
Sulfisoxazole (Gantrisin)	2–4 g PO initial dose, followed by 1–2 g q 4–6 h	Rapidly absorbed and eliminated. Effective urinary tract anti-infective. Gantrisin can be combined with phenazopyridine (a urinary tract analgesic) to form AZO Gantrisin. May be given IV or SC in the same dosage. Care must be taken to give infusion well diluted and slowly.
Sulfisoxazole diolamine	IV or SC, dose as above	
Sulfamethoxazole (Gantanol)	2 g PO initial dose, followed by 1 g bid or tid	Similar action and adverse effects as sulfisoxazole, but absorption and excretion are slower. More risk of crystalluria; therefore, forcing fluids is important. Also available as AZO Gantanol.
Sulfamethoxazole and trimethoprim (Bactrim, Septra)	Combined 400 mg/80 mg: 2 tablets q 12 h for 10–14 d; 8 tablets qd for 2 d for uncomplicated gonorrhea	Effective against a wide variety of gram-positive and gram-negative organisms. Used especially in acute and chronic urinary tract infections. Both cross placental membrane, and high concentrations are found in sputum, bile, milk. Same precautions as with other sulfonamides. Contraindicated during pregnancy, as trimethoprim is a folate antagonist.

2. Advise patients to drink extra fluids to prevent crystalluria and stone formation. Preparations containing phenazopyridine (AZO Gantrisin, AZO Ganatol) may produce an orange-red color in the urine.

3. Remind patient that exposure to sunlight or sunlamp may precipitate photosensitivity reactions.

The Tetracyclines

The tetracyclines are bacteriostatic, with a very broad antibacterial spectrum. Their greatest use is against gram-negative bacteria, gram-positive bacteria resistant to penicillin, and for patients allergic to other antibiotics. Rickettsia, mycoplasmas, and spirochetes are also susceptible.

Tetracyclines are absorbed orally, and peak serum levels occur in 2 to 4 hours. Heavy metal cations (Al, Ca, Mg, Fe) interfere significantly with absorption, and sodium bicarbonate will decrease absorption by increasing gastric pH. They are widely distributed in body tissues and fluids. Tetracyclines are found in breast milk, and cross the placenta with deposition in the fetal skeletal system, slowing bone growth. If given during pregnancy or if given to children in the first 6 to 8 years of life, permanent tooth discoloration and enamel defects occur. Partial excretion (unchanged) is through the urine, as well as through the bile and stool. Considerable recycling takes place, extending half-life.

Tetracyclines will produce false-positives when urine glucose levels are measured by Clinitest. False-negatives will occur with Clinistix and Tes-Tape.

Adverse Effects   Common side effects include nausea and vomiting, epigastric distress, bulky loose stools, diarrhea, vaginitis, glossitis, black hairy tongue, hoarseness, and fever. Hypersensitivity reactions may involve urticaria, rashes, anaphylaxis, pericarditis, and exacerbation of systemic lupus erythematosus. Sometimes, photosensitivity reactions occur, resulting in increased pigmentation. Enzyme elevations (SGOT, SGPT, alkaline phosphotase) and bilirubin increases may occur. Increased excretion of sodium and high BUN levels have been reported. Finally, cross-sensitization may occur between tetracyclines.

Dosage requirements for the tetracyclines are listed in Table 5-7.

Nursing Implications
1. Antacids, milk, and iron will interfere with absorption; give 1 hour before meals.

2. Remind the patient of possible photosensitivity reactions (exaggerated sunburn on exposure).

3. Remember possibility of false-positive or false-negative tests when testing for glycosuria.

4. Watch lab reports on renal function tests; observe for GI disturbances.

5. Caution patient against taking outdated capsules; the drug degrades quickly if stored improperly.

Table 5-7 Tetracyclines

Drug	Dosage	Comments
Demeclocycline (Declomycin)	600 mg q 24 h PO in 2 to 4 doses, 1 h ac or 2 h pc Gonorrhea: 600 mg, then 300 mg q 12 h for a total dose of 3 g	More likely to cause photosensitivity reactions than other tetracyclines. $T_{1/2}=12$ h.
Doxycycline (Vibramycin)	100 mg PO q 12 h first day, then 100 mg qd or 50 mg q 12 h Gonorrhea: 100 mg q 12 h for 2 to 4 d Syphilis: 100 mg q 12 h for 10 d	Enzyme inducers may speed liver metabolism of drug, decreasing half-life and efficacy. May delay blood coagulation and potentiate effect of coumarin like anticoagulants $T_{1/2}=15-17$ h.
Minocycline (Minocin, Vectrin)	200 mg initially, then 100 mg IV, PO q 12 h	Do not mix into IV solutions containing calcium because precipitation will occur. Reconstitute with sterile water, add to IV solution, and infuse over a 6-h period. Thrombophlebitis may occur. Vertigo may be observed. $T_{1/2}=17-19$ h.
Tetracycline hydrochloride (many brands: Achromycin, Tetracyn, Panmycin)	250–500 mg PO q 6 h	Least likely to cause photosensitivity.
	250 to 1000 mg IV q 12 h	IV rate not to exceed 2 mg per min. Dilute carefully according to directions.
	200 mg to 1 g IM daily in 2 to 3 divided doses	IM may be very painful; local anesthetic sometimes added. $T_{1/2}=8.5$ h.

Urinary Antiseptics

Methenamine Mandelate (Mandelamine)   Methenamine and its salts are used for urinary tract infections and infections caused by a neurogenic bladder. Bacteria are destroyed by the release of formaldehyde in an acidic urine. Absorption from the GI tract is good, and excretion into urine is rapid. Urine must be kept at a pH of 5.5 or lower, and drugs or foods which raise pH must be avoided. A diet with cranberry juice, plums, and prunes will assist in maintaining an acid urine. Vitamin C or methionine may be added to aid in keeping pH low.

ADVERSE EFFECTS   Adverse effects include nausea, vomiting, rashes, pruritis, bladder irritation, and hematuria. The SGOT and SGPT levels may become elevated. Formaldehyde in the urine interferes with estriol determination, and catecholamine readings may be artifically high. The hippurate salt (Hipprex) and the sulfosalicylate salt (Hexalet) in pregnancy have not been established as safe.

DOSAGE   1 g PO qid pc and hs. 500–1000 mg of ascorbic acid with each dose may be ordered.

NURSING IMPLICATIONS
1. Instruct patient to measure urinary acidity and to adjust acidity by food intake.

2. Observe patient for rashes and abnormal liver studies.

3. Encourage fluid intake.

Nalidixic Acid (Neg Gram)   Used for gram-negative organisms infecting the urinary tract, Neg Gram may become ineffective within a week, as bacterial resistance develops quickly. Eighty percent of the drug is excreted unchanged in the urine.

ADVERSE EFFECTS   Untoward effects are unusual but may include nausea, vomiting, dizziness, pruritis, rash, and urticaria. Patients with G6PD are most susceptible to the more severe effect of hemolytic anemia. Liver function tests may become elevated, and caution should be used in patients with liver or renal disease. Use is not recommended in the first trimester.

DOSAGE   500–1000 mg PO qid for 1 to 2 weeks. Reduce dosage after 2 weeks.

Nitrofurantoin (Furadantin, Macrodantin, and Others)   Used in the treatment of pyelonephritis, pyelitis, or cystitis, it inhibits *E. coli*, *S. aureus*, streptococci, enterococci, *Proteus*, and *Klebsiella*. Activity is increased in an acid urine. Gastrointestinal tract absorption is rapid and complete. Degradation products may color the urine brown. One-half the oral dose is excreted unchanged in urine, with excretion also occurring in the bile, feces, and milk.

ADVERSE EFFECTS   Gastrointestinal symptoms occur less often when macrocrystals are used or when drug is given with food. If nausea and vomiting occur with the parenteral form, a decrease in infusion rate alleviates the problem. Intramuscular administration may cause severe pain. Allergic reactions with chills, fever, pulmonary edema, and rashes have been reported. Other effects include headache and nystagmus, myalgias, arthralgias, increased SGOT and alkaline phosphatase levels, pulmonary fibrosis, leukopenia, cholestatic jaundice, and hemolytic anemia in G6PD patients. Safety in pregnancy has not been established, and use in pregnancy and during lactation is contraindicated.

DOSAGE   100 mg PO qid for 1 to 2 weeks; reduce dose to less than 400 mg q 24 h after this. 100–180 mg IM or IV q 12 h. Do not use IM route for more than 5 days, and dilute powder to give 60 mg/ml. For IV, dilute vial with at least 50 ml normal saline and give slowly by piggyback IV. Excessive heat or exposure to light will cause degradation. Solution must be used within 24 hours.

NURSING IMPLICATIONS
1. Inform patient that urine will appear brown.

2. Administer with food or milk, using macrocrystals where possible.

3. Observe for adverse effects of tingling in extremities, and monitor lab reports of renal and hematologic function.

Additional Antibiotics

Chloramphenicol (Chloromycetin) Many gram-positive and most gram-negative and anaerobic organisms are susceptible to the bacteriostatic effect of chloramphenicol. Because of its adverse effects, the drug is saved for severe infections such as typhoid fever, Rocky Mountain spotted fever, and psittacosis (parrot fever). It is well absorbed from the GI tract and is distributed to most body tissues and fluids, across the placenta, and into milk.

ADVERSE EFFECTS Interactions may occur which increase the effects of oral anticoagulants, phenytoin, and chlorpropamide. Serious adverse effects include aplastic anemia, hemorrhage, and jaundice. Gastrointestinal disturbances, stomatitis, cutaneous ulcerations, and peripheral neuritis have also occurred. Chloramphenicol given to the mother during the transitional period may adversely affect the infant during the early neonatal period.

DOSAGE 50–100 mg/kg PO in 24 h in four divided doses.

Clindamycin (Cleocin Hydrochloride and Cleocin Phosphate) Clindamycin is used in the treatment of anaerobic infections (especially *Bacteroides fragilis*) but is effective in diseases caused by streptococci, pneumococci, and staphlococci. Gastrointestinal absorption is good, with wide distribution to body tissues. It is excreted in urine, feces, and bile.

ADVERSE EFFECTS Gastrointestinal tract disturbances result in bloody diarrhea, pseudomembranous colitis, and abdominal pain. Sometimes, leukocytosis, eosinophilia, and transient leukopenia may be seen. Safety in pregnancy has not been established.

DOSAGE   150–450 mg PO q 6 h. Up to 600 mg IM per dose, and 600 mg IV q 6 h in severe illness (up to 4.8 g in 24 h). Always dilute IV medication to at least 6 mg/ml, and never administer as a bolus.

Colistimethate Sodium (Coly-Mycin M)   Coly-Mycin is active against almost all gram-negative organisms except *Proteus* and *Neisseria* and should be saved for severe infections. It must be given parenterally, and once in circulation, it passes the placental barrier and appears in bile and milk.

ADVERSE EFFECTS   Nephrotoxicity, manifested by azotemia, proteinuria, or oliguria with a rising serum creatinine level is a serious side effect. Transient paresthesias, pruritis, visual and speech disturbances, drug fever, dizziness, GI disturbances, and nystagmus may occur as well. Since this polymyxin drug is fairly toxic, other drugs should be used first.

DOSAGE   2.5–5 mg/kg IM or IV in 24 h in two to four divided doses. IM may cause pain at injection site. IV must be administered slowly over 3 to 5 min or given by diluted infusion.

Lincomycin (Lincocin)   Like the erythromycins, lincomycin is used to treat respiratory, soft tissue, urinary, and skin infections caused by group A, beta-hemolytic streptococci, pneumococci, and some strains of staphylococci. Food decreases absorption, but once in the circulation the drug enters most body tissues. Excretion occurs through urine, bile, milk, and feces.

ADVERSE EFFECTS   Lincomycin shares many of the same side effects as clindamycin. Severe diarrhea is an indication for stopping therapy. Monilial infections may flourish unless treated during the same period.

DOSAGE   500 mg PO q 6 to 8 h, given 1 h ac or 2 h pc. 600–1200 mg IM or 600 mg IV q 8 to 12 h diluted in 5% dextrose in water and given by intermittent infusion.

Polymyxin B Sulfate (Aerosporin)   Polymyxin B is used for most gram-negative bacteria and especially for *P. aeruginosa* infection of the urinary tract. It is bactericidal and can be administered by all routes except orally. Most of the drug is excreted unchanged through the kidney.

ADVERSE EFFECTS   Effects similar to colistimethate include nephrotoxicity and neurotoxicity. Signs of nephrotoxicity may manifest as albuminuria, azotemia, hematuria, and increased blood levels of the drug. Neurotoxicity may be manifested by dizziness, flushing mental confusion, irritability, nystagmus, muscle weakness, drowsiness, numbness, blurred vision, slurred speech, and ataxia. Safe use during pregnancy has not been established.

DOSAGE   15,000–25,000 U / kg IM or IV in 24 h or 1.5–2.5 mg/kg in divided doses. IM injection causes severe pain. IV must be given in intermittent controlled-volume infusion.

Spectinomycin (Trobicin)   Used only for acute gonorrheal infection in both men and women, this antibiotic is not effective in treating syphilis. There is rapid absorption after IM administration and active metabolites are excreted into the urine by glomerular filtration.

ADVERSE EFFECTS   The drug appears to be relatively nontoxic. Side effects reported include soreness at site of injection, urticaria, dizziness, nausea, chills, fever, and insomnia. Effects on the fetus and safe use in infants and children have not been established.

DOSAGE   2–4 g IM given Z track in divided doses, with half in each gluteus medius site.

ANTICOAGULANTS

The incidence of thromboembolic problems requiring anticoagulant therapy has been estimated to be 0.09 percent during pregnancy and 0.3 percent during recovery from birth

(Aaro and Jeurgens, 1971). The vascular changes of pregnancy contribute to this increased risk, in addition to the effect of pressure of the uterus on pelvic veins, which results in increased femoral venous pressure. Any infection or trauma as a result of delivery further increases risk.

Signs and symptoms of superficial vein thrombophlebitis are seen most often in the third trimester, when pregnancy pressure factors are highest. Some cases progress to or accompany more serious deep vein thrombus formation, which begins with a clump of platelets adhering to a roughened vein wall. The silent onset presents confusing signs until the thrombus is well enlarged. Formation may take from days to weeks to develop. Symptoms are aching pain in the thigh, calf, or foot, with unilateral edema. Pieces of this thrombus, with its long "tail" of fibrin and blood cells, can break off and travel to the lungs, causing pulmonary embolism. Treatment includes elevation of both legs at 30° to reduce edema and improve circulation. Heat is applied and absolute bed rest is maintained for 7–10 days after the acute phase. Anticoagulant therapy is begun at once and may be maintained for several months after delivery to ensure complete recovery.

Pulmonary embolus carries a risk of one death in every 7000 deliveries (Genton, 1974). Early signs may be vague: fatigue, fever, chills, coughing, vague chest pains, and a "fear of death." More overt signs are dyspnea, cyanosis, hemoptysis, and arrythmias progressing to respiratory failure. Large doses of anticoagulants are given intravenously to such patients.

Cardiac patients who have had valve prostheses or recurrent embolic problems may be on anticoagulant maintenance doses before and during pregnancy.

Heparin (Pan Heparin, Liquaemin, Lipohepin)

A fast-acting drug of large molecular weight, heparin retards the formation of fibrin by affecting the prothrombin–thrombin reaction, forming an antithrombin substance, and reducing the adhesiveness of platelets to increase clotting time. It is especially useful in pregnancy because of two factors: its large molecule does not cross the placenta, and it specifically counteracts the extra adhesiveness of platelets present in the late pregnancy and post-partum periods. Heparin has a very short half-life in the body, 1 to 3 hours depending on dose. About 25 percent of the drug is found unchanged in the urine, and the rest is handled by rapid protein binding and is metabolized in the liver. Heparin is best added to normal saline for intravenous infusion. It is not wise to add additional drugs to the same infusion.

Adverse Reactions   The main adverse reaction occurs from an overdose. The symptoms are bleeding from body orifices, or wounds, and petechiae and bruising under the skin. If the clotting time is followed carefully, overdose can be prevented. The specific antidote is protamine sulfate, administered 1.5 mg/1.0 mg (100 U) of heparin, by slow intravenous push.

Alopecia has been reported in some patients by 5 to 8 weeks after therapy was begun. The effect is reversible. Very few patients are hypersensitive, demonstrating urticaria, conjunctival itching and tearing, and fever.

There has been no adverse effect noted on the pregnancy. Heparin may be taken up to the time of labor and begun right after delivery. (Of course, nurses should check closely for extra vaginal bleeding and subinvolution.) No transfer across breast milk has been observed.

Preparation   Prepared from biological sources, heparin is measured in units with 1 U = approximately to 0.01 mg. Thus 100 U = 1 mg, and 10,000 U = 100 mg. Although usually ordered in units, dosage may be ordered by milligrams per kilogram as well.

Doses will vary daily, depending on patient condition and lab reports. A usual dose regimen is 10,000 U IV stat, then 8,000–10,000 units IV or SC q 8 h. In cases of pulmonary embolism, very high doses are given initially in the range of 20,000 U stat and 40,000–80,000 U by IV infusion qd.

Administration   When given subcutaneously, heparin should be injected at a 90° angle into the fat pad of the abdomen as in

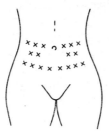

Figure 5-1   Sites for heparin injection.

Fig. 5-1. Rotate the sites systematically. Do not massage or inject into bruised areas, near a wound, or near umbilicus. Observe the area for formation of hematoma. Hematoma can be prevented by holding an ice cube over the site before and after injection.

Heparin is probably best administered intravenously. There are several acceptable methods: by slow intravenous push through a heparin lock; added to intravenous solutions in an episodic controlled-volume infusion; or mixed into intravenous fluids for continuous infusion, using an intravenous pump. In one study, patients on continuous infusion had less incidence of hemorrhage (Salzman et al., 1976). The heparin lock is used when the patient needs no other intravenous fluids.

Nursing Implications

1. Always check clotting time, being sure it has been drawn an hour prior to dosage time. The 5 to 10 minute control time will be increased when dosage is effective to two to three times the control, or 20 to 30 minutes. If clotting time is longer, it signals an overdose. Hold the medication, notifying physician. Other regimens use the partial thromboplastin time, 3 hours after a dose, once or twice a day. For this test, 29 to 35 seconds is the normal control, and time should be increased to 50 to 80 seconds for a desired level of therapy.

2. Observe patient for signs of bleeding, either internal or from mucous membranes and site of injection. Observe stool, urine, sputum, and gums. Look for petechiae and bruising.

3. Teach the patient home care and self-injection as necessary. Advise carrying an identification card with name, dose, physician's name, phone number, and hospital. Teach patient and family to recognize signs of overdose. Advise patient against taking nonprescription medications, such as those containing aspirin.

Coumarins

All the drugs in this family of anticoagulants act to inhibit production of prothrombin and factors, II, VII, IX, and X, thus lengthening prothrombin time from the normal 15 seconds. Coumarins are somewhat similar to vitamin K in structure and may also act to block vitamin K in the metabolic process.

Coumarins are easily absorbed from the GI tract, metabolized by the microsomal enzyme system in the liver, and excreted in the urine. Coumarins have a slower onset of effectiveness than heparin and a long half-life. The anticoagulant effect continues from 3 to 7 days after the drug has been discontinued.

Interactions   Drug interactions are common and are one of the drawbacks of coumarins. Other drugs affect coumarin action by competing for protein binding, by speeding liver enzyme processes, or by inhibiting vitamin K absorption in the intestine. The anticoagulant effect can be speeded or slowed, and when competing drugs are discontinued, a sudden overdose may occur. Table 5-8 lists some major drugs which may speed or slow the response to coumarins. Coumarins also affect other drugs; e.g., they increase the hypoglycemic effect of tolbutamide.

Adverse Effects   The major adverse effect is overdose, which results in bleeding from body cavities, wounds, or under the skin. The antidote is fresh whole blood transfusions plus large doses of vitamin K. The patient should be followed with frequent tests of prothrombin time.

Until recently, none of the coumarin family was used during pregnancy because of reported adverse effects on the fetus (Pettifor and Benson, 1975). Further study has demonstrated that a time element is critical. Coumarin derivatives are not used prior to the thirteenth week of pregnancy because of possible teratogenic effects nor after the thirty-sixth week because of their long-lasting effects. Some clinicians now use coumarins for extended therapy during the weeks 14 to 36 with no apparent adverse effects to date (Merrill and Verberg, 1976). Coumarins will transfer to breast milk and are not recommended during breast-feeding.

Nursing Implications

1. Always check prothrombin time prior to administration of drug, especially during initial period. A range of 22 to 35 seconds before plasma coagulation is the desired level of theraputic response. If the time is over 35 seconds, the patient may show signs of hemorrhage. Dosage should be omitted and the physician notified. Once well regulated, the prothrombin time is tested at regular intervals.

2. Observe patient for same signs of bleeding as with heparin overdose.

Table 5-8   Coumarin Interactions

Potentiate Response		Inhibit Response	
Drug	**Action**	**Drug**	**Action**
Sulfonamides Gram-negative antibiotics	Lower vitamin K production in intestine	Antacids Alcohol	Reduce oral absorption
Chloramphenicol Salicylates Phenylbutazone Phenytoin	Displace from protein-binding site	Barbiturates Glutethimide Meprobamate Thiazides	Speed up liver enzyme action, resulting in faster inactivation of oral anticoagulants

3. Instruct patient on home care, give identification card, and teach family to recognize signs of overdose. Be sure patient understands the importance of exact doses, keeping clinic appointments, and diet. (Deficiencies of vitamin C and protein and excess fats change drug effects.) Advise patient to keep alcohol consumption low and to avoid antacids, which hinder GI absorption, and home medications such as aspirin.

4. Patient should be given vitamin K tablets as a resource in case she shows signs of hemorrhage and cannot locate her physician or get to the hospital right away.

ANTICONVULSANTS

Epilepsy   The incidence of epilepsy in pregnant women has increased slowly as a result of better management of childhood epilepsy and is currently about 0.15 percent. Although epilepsy itself may not affect the fetus, there are serious questions about the effect of anticonvulsant therapy. Several studies have noted a higher incidence of birth defects, such as cleft lip and palate, and cardiac defects. Minor hand defects, wider fontanels, lower bridge of the nose, and epicanthal folds have been noted (Hansen and Smith, 1975). The effects are more likely to be present (2 to 4 percent in current studies) if the mother took anticonvulsants during the first trimester (Monson, 1973; Hill et al., 1974). Some studies have made a link between intrauterine growth retardation and anticonvulsants during the entire pregnancy. Fortunately, in most cases, there is no apparent effect. Since omitting anticonvulsants in women who need them might lead to fetal hypoxia with resultant brain damage, anticonvulsants continue to be given during pregnancy.

In pregnancy, the threshold for seizures is lowered, and the course of epilepsy may become somewhat erratic in formerly well-controlled patients. Since water retention normal to pregnancy may aggravate epilepsy, total weight gain should be monitored. Early signs of unusual edema must be reported to the physician. If convulsions first occur toward the end of pregnancy, diagnosis may be difficult at first, since a variety of factors can precipitate convulsions. A major concern will be to distinguish between epilepsy that first occurs during later pregnancy and preeclampsia-eclampsia.

Once diagnosis is made, the patient is placed on antiepileptic medication alone or with an accompanying sedative. In a state of continuous seizures (status epilepticus) intravenous diazepam is administered.

Phenytoin (Dilantin)   Useful for grand mal, focal, and psychomotor seizures, phenytoin appears to retard the electrical stimulation in the brain which triggers seizures. It is also a folic acid antagonist, an action which may have some effect in inhibiting seizures. Folic acid antagonism is being studied for its effect on the growing fetus, and folic acid levels (8 ng/ml is normal) are measured in pregnant women taking this drug.

Phenytoin has a long half-life in the body; therefore normally oral doses twice a day will maintain an adequate level of medication. Phenytoin is absorbed easily from the GI tract, metabolized by the microsomal enzymes in the liver, and excreted in the urine.

Phenytoin has an enzyme-inducing effect, speeding metabolism of certain drugs in the liver. As a result, usual doses of those drugs may have to be altered. Other drugs inhibit or slow the metabolism of phenytoin, thus causing higher doses to remain in the body. The dose of anticonvulsant should be decreased when given concurrently with such potentiating drugs.

ADVERSE EFFECTS   Adverse effects include ataxia, drowsiness, or irritability. Effects on the eye may be nystagmus and diplopia. Swelling of gum tissue (gingival hyperplasia) is particularly troublesome. Fortunately, gum tissue regresses when the drug is withdrawn. Hirsutism and skin rashes are seen in some patients. Nausea and vomiting may be helped by taking pills with meals and increasing fluid intake. Phenytoin, when given parenterally, may cause vertigo, nausea, and cardiac arrythmias in addition to the above effects.

DOSAGE   Oral medication is administered on a slowly increasing dosage scale until optimal effect is achieved at blood serum levels of 10–20 μg/ml. Higher blood levels precipitate adverse effects. Since patients react differently to phenytoin, depending on age and other concurrent medication, adult dosage may range from 100–600 mg qd. Phenytoin sodium injectable dosage of 150–250 mg may be injected by IV push at a slow rate of 50 mg/min. IM dosage is not commonly used but may be ordered, especially before neurosurgery.

NURSING IMPLICATIONS
1. Observe drug effects closely: drowsiness, ataxia, seizure incidence when drug first being regulated.

2. Promote safety of patient from injury due to seizures, obtain history, and elicit patient's understanding of situation.

3. Administer drug with meals; observe for nausea; encourage fluid intake.

4. Encourage good oral hygiene because of gingival hyperplasia.

5. Be sure patient understands medication regime and realizes need to continue medication without abrupt withdrawal.

6. Interpret epilepsy as a controllable problem. Help patient face fears of social disapproval. Provide patient with an identification card with name, doctor, and medication listed.

7. Be alert to patient's fears about effect of drug on infant, especially if she is a newly diagnosed epileptic. Be aware of physician's interpretation of drug effect. Patient should be fully informed as to risks (FDA, 1974).

Mephenytoin (Mesantoin)   Mephenytoin causes more sedation than phenytoin but is less effective. It may be chosen, however, because it does not cause gum hyperplasia. It may depress bone marrow; therefore, regular blood tests are mandatory.

DOSAGE   Oral tablets of 100 mg are given bid or tid for an average dose of 400–600 mg qd.

NURSING IMPLICATIONS   Precautions are similar to those of phenytoin, and nurses should be aware of the current complete blood cell count.

Trimethadion (Tridione)   Trimethadion is in the oxazolidine family and is given specifically for petit mal seizures.

ADVERSE EFFECTS   Nausea, vomiting, blurred vision, light sensitivity, and depression of bone marrow are the major adverse effects. Given early in pregnancy, trimethadione has been associated with facial and cardiac defects (German, 1970).

DOSAGE   Trimethadion is given orally in 900–1200 mg divided doses tid or qid.

Antiepileptic drugs that are not usually given during pregnancy because of their adverse side effects include acetazolamide (Diamox), phensuximide (Miltonin), methsuximide (Celontin), and ethosuximide (Zarotin). When a patient already maintained on one of these drugs becomes pregnant, the physician must weigh the benefit-to-risk ratio in making a decision about prescription.

Sedatives Useful in Raising Seizure Threshold

Phenobarbital   Phenobarbital is the most common barbiturate used as an anticonvulsive drug. The mechanism of action is unknown, but effects are those caused from a uniform distribution within the central nervous system and will, depending on dosage, cause effects from mild sedation to coma. Phenobarbital raises the threshold for seizures and reduces the tonic phase of a convulsion. Thus, it is primarily useful in grand mal, focal, or psychomotor seizures and in preeclampsia-eclampsia.

The drug is distributed to all body tissues, including the brain and across the placenta to the fetus. Protein binding is low in comparison to other barbiturates. It is metabolized by the liver and excreted by the kidney.

It has the effect of stimulating enzyme production in microsomal liver tissue, which results in speeded metabolism of coumarin anticoagulants, bilirubin, phenytoin, digitoxin, chlorpromazine, cortisol, and several other drugs not used during pregnancy. This drug interaction can be useful or detrimental but must be accounted for in dosage and observation of effects. Bilirubin metabolism in the newborn may be speeded by the use of phenobarbital for the mother prior to birth (see Chapter 7). If urine is highly alkaline, phenobarbital excretion is delayed.

ADVERSE REACTIONS   When phenobarbital is used over a long period, the nurse must expect that a certain tolerance will develop. Side effects may develop, especially after the drug is metabolized, and withdrawal symptoms may occur. Rashes may also occur. Ataxia and sedation may result from larger doses.

DOSAGE   Oral: 30–100 mg bid or tid as an anticonvulsant in preeclampsia; 15–30 mg bid or tid in epilepsy; 100–200 mg hs for hypnotic effect.
    IM or IV: Larger doses are administered in crisis situations of status epilepticus and eclampsia.

NURSING IMPLICATIONS
1. Patient must be educated about drug effects and side effects. The patient must be taught about maintaining daily dosage and avoiding sudden withdrawal.

2. Protect the patient from injury with side rails, and assist with feeding, toilet, etc.

3. Report observations of drug interactions and side effects.

4. Be alert to report to nursery if mother has been receiving drug.

Magnesium Sulfate Injection   The Mg^{2+} ion has the properties of depressing central nervous system function, especially at the neuromuscular junction it acts to reduce muscle excitability. The result is depression of deep tendon reflexes and reduction of the possibility of convulsions. The Mg^{2+} ion also depresses smooth

Table 5-9   Additional Sedatives Utilized in Epilepsy

Drug	Daily Dosage	Comments
Mephobarbital (Mebaral)	0.2–0.8 g PO	Metabolized to phenobarbital in body. Fewer side effects.
Metharbital (Gemonil)	300 mg PO qd in divided doses	
Primidone (Mysoline)	0.25–1.5 g PO	Often given with phenobarbital. Synergistic effect with anticonvulsants; therefore, watch side effects. Adverse effects include ataxia, headaches, sedation, decrease in vitamin K formation. Hemorrhage in infant. Drowsiness if mother breast-feeds.

and cardiac muscle, and toxic doses may lead to cardiorespiratory arrest. Uterine function may also be diminished with large doses. Magnesium sulfate increases cerebral blood flow and peripheral vasodilation (the patient may appear flushed), an effect which may assist slightly in lowering the elevation of arterial blood pressure. In large doses, magnesium sulfate has been used for an osmotic diuretic, thus indirectly assisting in reducing generalized edema, but currently, other agents such as mannitol are used. In low or moderate dosage, however, magnesium sulfate has an antidiuretic, sodium-retaining effect.

The drug is absorbed fairly rapidly from muscle tissue, and plasma concentrations in the fetus will rapidly become the same as in the mother. It is excreted by the kidneys unchanged. In severe preeclampsia with oliguria, if urinary output is less than 30 ml per hour, a cumulative dose may further depress muscle response.

ADVERSE REACTION   Intramuscular administration must be deep, since subcutaneous tissue will be highly irritated, with swelling and pain as a result. The effective dose level is very close to the toxic level and is only achieved by careful observation and monitoring of the condition. Blood levels of

Mg^{2+} at 4 meq/L or more are signs of effective dose, but above 10 meq/L, toxic effects will occur (Greenhill, 1974).

DOSAGE 1 g of magnesium sulfate contains approximately 8 meq of Mg^{2+}. Available in ampuls of 10, 20, and 50% solution, each dose must be calculated according to grams per 100 ml. (Percent solution always means grams per 100 ml unless otherwise specified.) Thus, for example, if a 20% solution is the best concentration to choose, the dose is 20 g contained in 100 ml of solution.

To complicate things further, IV orders are often written with a time factor added. For example: add 4 g of magnesium sulfate to 500 ml 5% dextrose in water and run IV to give 1 g per hour. (Check administration set for drops (gtt) per milliliter and regulate IV accordingly after calculating milliliters per minute.)

IM dosage is always ordered in grams, but because of the volume, a 50% solution is chosen. Because it is very concentrated, it is painful to the patient. Often 1 ml of 1% procaine is added (if the patient has no allergy). IM injection is always by Z track, with a long enough needle to penetrate deep muscle tissue.

NURSING IMPLICATIONS

1. Frequently monitor vital signs, remembering effect on cardiac muscle and vascular system.

2. Always check three parameters *before* administration. Omit dose, and report to physician if patient's condition shows cumulative toxic effects of respirations under 12 breaths per minute, absent knee jerk reflexes, urine output below 30 ml per hour.

3. Rotate sites; mark site on Kardex and bedside chart.

4. If intravenous route is used, observe site carefully for early signs of infiltration, and use infusion pump to monitor rate of flow.

5. Be sure patient has a Foley catheter inserted with hourly urometer attached. Maintain intake and output recording on an hourly basis.

6. Always have calcium gluconate 20% ready as an antagonist. Ampul and syringe should be kept at patient's bedside.

DRUGS USED FOR ASTHMA AND HYPERSENSITIVITY STATES

Pregnancy does not change allergic states unless the stress of pregnancy aggravates emotional factors involved in the disease. In that case, the first trimester, with the usual ambivalence toward pregnancy, could be a period of aggravated symptoms. During the last few weeks of pregnancy, when the enlarged uterus presses on the diaphragm, patients with compromised breathing may be further affected. Nasal stuffiness caused by normal hyperemia of nasal tissues may aggravate symptoms of hay fever.

The incidence of asthma in pregnant women is estimated to be about 1 percent (Weinberger and Hendeles, 1976, p. 1172). Management is the same in pregnancy as in the nonpregnant state. Use of bronchodilators, antihistamines, and mild sedatives can continue, but a desensitization program should not usually be begun during pregnancy (Rovinsky, 1976, p. 799). Prevention of respiratory illness and prompt treatment with antibiotics of any infection is important.

On admission for labor, it is important to note a history of asthma and avoid any respiratory depressants, anticholinergics or respiratory irritants. Local or regional anesthesia is recommended.

Care of the infant during transition will be modified by the effect of maternal drugs such as phenobarbital and corticosteroids. Iodides should be avoided during pregnancy as much as possible.

Adrenergic Agents

Adrenergic agents are alpha- and/or beta-receptor stimulants (Sympathomimetics) and therefore have, as a group, a wide array of effects. The primary purpose for their use in allergic states is their powerful vasoconstrictor and smooth muscle dilator effects. Many of the adrenergic agents have positive effects on cardiac function and are useful in raising blood

Table 5-10 Adrenergic Agents

Drug	Daily Dosage	Comments
Ephedrine sulfate	20–50 mg PO q 4 h; 20–50 mg IM	Prophylaxis against asthmatic attack. Long-lasting effect. Useful in hay fever, mild bronchospasm. Positive inotropic, chronotropic effect on heart. Anxiety, insomnia, tremors, headache, nausea and vomiting, anorexia, and palpitations with high doses. Common ingredient in many nonprescription drugs.
Epinephrine (Adrenalin)	1/1000 solution 0.2–0.5 ml SC, IM q 5 to 20 min until relief; 1% solution/inhalation or in oil, 0.2–1 ml hs	Alpha- and beta-receptor stimulant. Drug of choice for acute allergic response. Cardiac stimulant, vasoconstrictor, bronchodilator. Reduces bronchial secretions but causes CNS effects of wakefulness, tremor, irritability. With chronic use, often combined with phenobarbital. Added to local anesthetic to prolong action. Do not use with isoproterenol or propranolol. Promotes hyperglycemia in diabetics. Use tuberculin syringe to measure accurately. Monitor vital signs. Found in nonprescription nasal sprays.
Isoproterenol (Isuprel, Norisodrine, Aludrine)	Hand-held nebulizer: 1/100, 1/200 solution for inhalation 5 to 6 times day; cardiovascular stimulant: 1/5,000 solution 0.2 mg IM, SC, intracardiac, or 0.5–5 μg/min infusion diluted in 5% dextrose in water	Potent bronchodilator and lowers peripheral vascular resistance. Increases myocardial efficiency. Inotropic, chronotropic action on heart—used with cardiac arrest, atrioventricular block. Nausea and vomiting may occur. Inhalation may result in pink color of saliva. Palpitation, arrythmias, tremor, and headache occur with overuse. Caution patient. Tolerance develops.
Metaproterenol (Alupent, Metaprel)	20 mg PO tid; inhalant powder: 0.65 mg q 2 min, 3 times (hold breath a few seconds after inhaling)	Beta$_2$ stimulant, similar to isoproterenol, except less likely to cause cardiac stimulation. Fewer adverse effects. Protect from light. Safety during pregnancy has not yet been fully established.
Phenylephrine hydrochloride (Neo-Synephrine)	10–25 mg PO; 1–10 mg IM; 0.25% solution topical	An alpha-receptor stimulant and therefore a powerful vasoconstrictor. Used parenterally in treatment of hypotension and topically to relieve nasal congestion. Same

Table 5-10 Adrenergic Agents (Continued)

Drug	Daily Dose	Comments
		adverse effects as other adrenergics, except little effect on CNS. Commonly found in nonprescription nasal sprays.
Pseudoephedrine hydrochloride (Sudafed, Novafed)	30–60 mg PO tid or qid	No effect on blood pressure, only mild stimulation of CNS. Symptomatic relief of nasal and sinus congestion, colds, hay fever, and mild asthma. Reduce dose if nervousness, insomnia, restlessness occurs. Common in nonprescription preparations. Not used for asthma.
Salbutamol (Albuterol, Vetolin)	Metered aerosol of 0.1 mg per dose	Selective beta$_2$-receptor stimulant, relaxes smooth muscle of bronchi, uterus, and vascular supply to muscle. Equal to Isuprel in bronchodilation, but much less cardiac stimulation. Used to delay labor (see Chap. 6).
Terbutaline (Brethine, Brincanyl)	2.5–5 mg PO q 6 h 3 times; 0.25 mg SC, may repeat once in 4 h (solution 1/1000)	Beta$_2$-adrenergic agent; bronchial, vascular, and uterine smooth muscle dilation. Duration of action longer than ephedrine (4 to 8 h). Used in chronic obstructive pulmonary disease and asthma. Side effects same as other adrenergic agents.

ADJUNCTIVE AGENT

Drug	Daily Dose	Comments
Cromolyn sodium (Aarane, Intal)	Inhalation only. 20 mg capsule opened into spinhaler qid	Blocks histamine release and slow-reacting substance of anaphylaxis (SRS-A). Not an antihistamine or adrenergic drug, but is useful in prophylaxis of asthma and chronic allergy. Excreted mostly unchanged in urine and feces. Patient must be taught inhaling procedure carefully. Adverse effects are local irritation of throat and bronchi from powder. Safety in pregnancy has not been established. May take up to 1 month for beneficial effects to appear. Very few side effects. No effect in acute attacks.

Table 5-11 Drug Mixtures

Ingredients	Isuprel	Marax	Tedral	Verequad
ADRENERGIC AGENT				
Isoproterenol	2.5 mg			
Ephedrine	12.0 mg	25 mg	24 mg	24 mg
BARBITURATE				
Phenobarbital	6.0 mg		8 mg	8 mg
THEOPHYLLINE	45.0 mg	130 mg	130 mg	130 mg
ANTIHISTAMINE				
Hydroxyzine hydrochloride		10 mg		
EXPECTORANT				
Potassium iodide	150 mg			
Glycerolguaiacolate				100 mg

pressure and strengthening myocardial function in cases of hypotension and cardiac failure.

Side effects commonly include central nervous system stimulation, with restlessness, tremors, anxiety, insomnia, headache, and irritability. In chronic administration, these drugs are often given with phenobarbital or another sedative. Table 5-10 lists drug dosage and effects.

Mixtures of drugs may provide good control for asthmatics. Of the more than 30 mixtures available, some sample drugs and their ingredients are listed in Table 5-11. Those containing iodides should be used with extreme caution during pregnancy; usually, other drugs are substituted. Nursing implications are included in the comments of Table 5-10.

Antihistamines

Antihistamines antagonize histamine by competing for receptor sites. A large number of drugs have antihistaminic action, acting to inhibit histaminic effects of (1) smooth muscle constriction, (2) arteriolar and capillary dilation, (3) increased capillary permeability (edema), and (4) increased secretion from exocrine glands. There may also be central nervous system depression with some agents. Thus, these drugs are useful in allergic conditions in which symptoms are precipitated by excess release of histamine, especially allergic rhinitis (hay fever), perennial rhinitis, allergic dermatitis, and motion sickness. They are common ingredients of nonprescription cold and hay fever remedies and sedative preparations (see Table 3-5).

Adverse Effects   Drowsiness and additive effects with alcohol, barbiturates, tranquilizers, and other central nervous system depressants occur. Central nervous system stimulation may occur with excess doses, resulting in insomnia, restlessness, nervousness, and tremors. Drying of mucus secretions may not be advisable when purulent material should be coughed out; therefore, asthmatics may be hindered in recovery by antihistamines. Because of smooth muscle effects, voiding may be difficult, and gastrointestinal disturbances may occur.

Daily dosage requirements for some selected antihistamines are listed in Table 5-12.

Nursing Implications

1. Warn patient about drowsiness affecting mental alertness when driving or working with machinery.

2. Additive effects with alcohol and sedatives should be explained to patient.

3. Work with patient to identify allergies and ways of preventing episodes.

4. Teach patient to recognize signs and to decrease dose if drying effect thickens bronchial secretion, which then cannot be coughed up.

Table 5-12 Selected Antihistamines

Drug	Daily Dosage	Comments
Diphenhydramine hydrochloride (Benadryl)	25–50 mg PO,IM,IV tid, qid	Anticholinergic antitussive, antiemetic, and sedative effects. Used for local mild allergic rash and transfusion reactions. Sometimes used for intractable insomnia in elderly or chronically ill; not used for asthma. No contraindication during pregnancy, but may hinder lactation.
Dimenhydrinate (Dramamine)	50 mg PO, rectally, IM IV: dilute and inject over 2 min	Prevents nausea, vomiting, and vertigo of motion sickness. Duration of effect, 4 h. Available without a prescription.
Tripelennamine hydrochloride (Pyribenzamine)	25–50 mg PO; topical ointment, 2%	Seasonal and perennial rhinitis and transfusion reaction accompanying epinephrine. Side effects increased by alcohol, barbiturates, other CNS depressants. Not used for asthma because of atropinelike effects. Causes some drowsiness. *Avoid* during lactation. Less likely to cause sedation than diphenhydramine.
Citrate form	37.5 mg/5 ml liquid, 10 ml PO	
Chlorpheniramine maleate (Chlor-Trimeton, Teldrin)	2–4 mg PO tid, qid; 10–20 mg IM	Seasonal and perennial rhinitis, allergic conjunctivitis and dermatitis, blood transfusion reactions, and anaphylactic reactions with epinephrine, after acute phase. Adverse reactions of drowsiness and anticholinergic effects. Some hypotension with IM administration.
Hydroxyzine hydrochloride (Vistaril); hydroxyzine pamoate (Atarax)		An antihistamine with strong antianxiety action. Hydroxyzine is used primarily during labor and delivery (see Chap. 6).
PHENOTHIAZINE		
Promethazine hydrochloride (Phenergan)		Prominent sedative and antiemetic action. Phenergan is used primarily during labor and delivery (see Chap. 6).

Corticosteroids and Corticotropin (ACTH)

ACTH regulates the production of adrenocorticosteroids, which have glucocorticoid activity (cortisol, hydrocortisone, prednisone) and/or mineralocorticoid activity (desoxycorticosterone, aldosterone). These substances influence every tissue of the body and are secreted rhythmically during a 24-hour period. Higher peaks are found during stress periods, up to 10 times the usual output.

Their major actions are (1) anti-inflammatory; (2) potentiation of norepinephrine and vasoconstriction to maintain normal blood pressure; (3) participation in metabolism of fats, carbohydrates, and proteins and regulation of electrolyte balance (can contribute to hyperglycemia and glycosuria or loss of minerals); (4) an immunosuppressant, antiallergenic effect; (5) production of increased energy; they act synergistically with epinephrine and norepinephrine during stress.

Corticosteroids are used in bronchial asthma and other chronic allergic disorders as well as in a wide variety of other deficiency states and collagen diseases. Since they participate in the stress response, they are not usually used for stress-induced illness (peptic ulcer) or for diabetes.

Women in premature labor may be given cortisol (betamethsone, dexamethasone) therapy for 24 to 48 hours prior to delivery (Mead, 1977), since some improvement has been noted in lecithin/sphingomyelin (L/S) ratio, with cortisol acting as a stimulant to surfactant production (at least 48 hours are needed to induce surfactant release).

Adverse Effects   Endocrine imbalance, electrolyte and mineral imbalance, and loss of protein from body tissues may occur. Gastrointestinal tract disturbances may be aggravated, and because of anti-inflammatory action, infections may become severe, although masked. Diabetes may be aggravated. Numerous other adverse effects are possible with excessive doses, and the least possible dosage should be utilized for the shortest possible period.

Corticosteroids administered during pregnancy have not had definitely adverse effects, with the exception of some indication of increased cleft palate, but cleft lip and palate are seen commonly in certain strains of mice receiving such drugs. Infants of mothers who have received corticosteroids over a long period should be observed for signs of hypoadrenalism in the neonatal period.

Dosage   Varies widely and must be adjusted to each patient's response. Alternate day therapy (ADT) appears to provide the safest timing, allowing for the adrenals to function more normally every other day (see Table 5-13).

Nursing Implications
1. Be alert for multiple adverse reactions

2. Corticosteroids may increase incidence of infections. Maintain aseptic techniques. Observe for signs and symptoms.

3. When used with patients who have chronic diseases, note dosage carefully, as it may be decreased. Increased sensitivity may be present to hyperglycemia, hypertension, edema, sodium retention, potassium depletion, metabolic alkalosis, mental confusion and psychosis.

4. Be alert for and check drug interactions.

5. Avoid abrupt withdrawal of medication, which must be tapered.

Table 5-13   Approximate Corticosteroid Activity Equivalents

Corticosteroid	Dosage	Glucocorticoid/Mineralocorticoid Activity (M / m = + + / +)
Cortisone	25 mg	G / M
Hydrocortisone	20 mg	G / M
Betamethasone	0.6 mg	G / -
Dexamethasone	0.75 mg	G / -
Methylprednisolone	4 mg	G / -
Prednisolone	5 mg	G / m
Prednisone	5 mg	G / m

CARDIOVASCULAR DRUGS

One fourth of all nonobstetric causes of maternal mortality are due to cardiac disease (Romney, 1976, p. 778). A woman with rheumatic heart disease, congential cardiac defects, hypertensive heart disease, or coronary artery disease may have her symptoms aggravated by the cardiovascular changes normal to pregnancy. Preexisting functional deficits may become worse, and embolic complications or arrythmias may occur.

Cardiac Glycosides

All cardiac glycosides work to increase the force of the myocardial contractions and are selected for two basic reasons: (1) to control ventricular rate in atrial fibrillation or flutter, and (2) to treat congestive heart failure by strengthening myocardial contraction. Effects result from two different mechanisms: changes in calcium stores in myocardial muscle cells and changes in sodium and potassium transport in and out of the muscle cell. Calcium, sodium, and potassium serum concentrations are therefore important to digitalis effectiveness. Calcium and digitalis are synergistic; therefore increases in Ca^{2+} levels may result in arrhythmias in a digitalized patient. On the other hand, potassium and digitalis are antagonistic, and hypokalemia may result in increased digitalis sensitivity. Administration of K^+ often counteracts toxic effects (DiPalma, 1976, p. 226).

Digitalislike drugs also produce some smooth muscle contraction of peripheral arteries and veins and may have an effect on labor contractions, for digitalis appears to cause an earlier onset and a shorter duration of labor. As Miller and Greenblatt (1976) note, "the evidence suggests that digitalis improved myometrial contractibility in the cardiac patient as it improved myocardial function."

Differences between drugs in this family lie in their absorption rates, half lives, routes of metabolism and excretion, and their degree of protein binding. Dosage is individualized, and therapeutic levels are very near toxic levels. Therefore, close observation of patients is important, and the range of adverse effects must be taught to patients. To achieve a steady-state therapeutic level of a cardiac glycoside, five half-lives must have elapsed, unless a loading dose is used to begin therapy. Thus, a patient must be observed especially carefully during the initial period of therapy (6 to 10 days for digoxin and 30 to 45 days for digitoxin; Miller and Greenblatt, 1976, p. 180) when maintenance doses only are used.

Metabolism differs between digoxin and digitoxin. Digoxin is easily filtered at the glomerulus and poorly reabsorbed. Eighty percent is excreted through the kidney, and the half-life is about 34 hours. Digitoxin, in contrast, is highly protein-bound and metabolized more extensively before being excreted into the bile. From 20 to 35 percent of digitoxin undergoes enterohepatic recycling, resulting in an extended duration of drug effect in the body ($T_{1/2} = 7$ days). Physiologic changes of pregnancy would affect this recycling and would also increase the digoxin excretion rate. As a result of increased sensitivity, the dosage of digitalis like drugs may be slightly reduced during pregnancy.

Adverse Effects   Adverse effects may occur when potassium is depleted after diruetic therapy, nausea or vomiting, or prolonged administration of corticosteroids. Any condition reducing urine output, causing variable absorption from the GI tract, or reducing metabolic rate would also precipitate toxic symptoms. Toxic signs begin to occur when serum levels rise above the following therapeutic levels: digoxin, 0.9–2.2 ng/ml; digitoxin, 12–28 ng/ml (Miller and Greenblatt, 1976, p. 181).

Adverse effects are demonstrated as electrocardiographic (ECG) changes in rate and rhythm: premature ventricular beats, atrial tachycardia with block, ventricular tachycardia, atrioventricular block, etc. In fact, almost any arrhythmia can be caused by digitalis glycoside toxicity; therefore, differential diagnosis may be difficult. Symptoms of toxicity may be confused with preeclampsia or other illness during pregnancy, and usually ECG evaluation is necessary to diagnose toxic responses to these drugs. Anorexia is usually the earliest sign of toxicity, and nausea, vomiting, diarrhea, headache, and malaise are other common warnings of toxicity. Visual symptoms may include white halos on dark objects and disturbances in yellow and green colors. The measurement of a pulse rate of 60 beats per minute as the lower limit of normal for the cardiac patient is not usually a valid criteria for omitting a dose during pregnancy because of normal increase over the baseline of approximately 15 beats per minute during pregnancy. The pulse level for omission of a dose should be ordered specifically for each pregnant patient.

Digitalislike drugs traverse the placenta in varying amounts as demonstrated in lab experiments. When the human mother is on a maintenance dose, equilibrium with the fetus is reached. Usually, no adverse effects are noted in the human infant; however, careful observation for signs of possible toxicity is necessary during the period after birth.

Drugs used to diminish toxic effects are potassium (PO or IV), phenytoin, lidocaine, propranolol, quinidine, and procainamide, all drugs in the antirrhythmic category.

Cardiac glycosides are compared in Table 5-14. Pay particular attention to the wide variation in dosage: digitoxin is one thousand times as strong as digitalis, so that 1 mg of digitoxin equals 1 g of digitalis.

Nursing Implications

1. Observe for signs of toxicity or ineffective dosage levels when patient is hospitalized to monitor cardiac strain, digitalis and electrolyte levels, and thyroid and kidney function.

2. Expect dosage to be adjusted if any superimposed illness occurs.

3. Pay special attention to vital signs, and use nursing interventions to reduce stress, prevent infection, and monitor for signs of thrombophlebitis.

4. Prevent supine and postural hypotension by careful positioning.

5. Monitor intake and output. Especially note that infusion of large amounts of glucose and water may cause hypokalemia. Observe carefully during induction or during any infusion. Use carefully controlled rate of flow.

Table 5-14 Cardiac Glycosides

Drug	Daily Dosage	Comments
DIGITALIS PURPUREA (PURPLE FOXGLOVE)		
Digitalis leaf (Digifortis)	50–100 mg PO qd	PO use only
Digitoxin (Crystodigin, Unidigin, Purodigin)	0.1–0.2 mg PO	1 mg equals strength of 1 g of digitalis. Slow onset of action; average $T_{1/2}$ of 7 d. Well absorbed PO.
Gitalin (Gitaligin)	0.25–0.75 mg PO, IM, IV	Action same as digitalis. Protect IV solution from light. Well absorbed PO.
DIGITALIS LANATA (WHITE FOXGLOVE)		
Digilanid (lanatoside A, C)	0.67–1.33 mg PO, IM, IV (0.33-mg tablets)	Actions similar to digitalis.
Acetyldigitoxin (lanatoside A, Acylanid)	0.1–0.2 mg	Actions similar to digitoxin but more rapid onset.
Digoxin (lanatoside C, Lanoxin)	0.5–1.5 mg PO, IM, IV	Rapid onset of action; $T_{1/2}$ is 36 h. Protect from light.
Lanatoside C (Cedilanid)	0.5–1.5 mg PO	Poorly absorbed from GI tract although only given PO.
Deslanoside injection (Cedilanid-D, deacetyllanatoside C)	0.4 mg IM, IV	More soluble, only for IM, IV use. Used in emergencies since onset of action is rapid.
STROPHANTHUS GRATUS		
Oubain (G-strophanthin)	—	Action similar to digitalis. IV use only. Very rapid onset of action, so used in emergency when patient has not used digitalis therapy during the past 3 wk. Not used for maintenance therapy. Oral dose of one of above drugs begun as soon as possible.

DRUGS USED FOR HYPERTENSIVE STATES

Hypertension in pregnancy may result from chronic disease present before conception, or it may be an effect of physiologic changes for a particular patient. Classification has not been uniform, and statistics vary, depending on methods of identifying each type of hypertension.

Universally, hypertension has been the cause of an increased incidence of fetal and neonatal mortality and has resulted in increased morbidity due to abruptio placenta, premature labor, and chronic fetal distress, with intrauterine growth retardation among many other complications. Therapy is aimed at reducing blood pressure, promoting renal and uterine circulation, and preventing premature labor, eclampsia, and cerebrovascular and cardiovascular accidents.

Preeclampsia

Recently, it has been determined that sodium is lost rather than excessively retained during pregnancy, and thus the preeclamptic state may partially reflect the body's desperate attempt to retain sodium. Therefore, both sodium restriction and diurectics are no longer routine parts of treatment. Bed rest in a lateral recumbent position, a high-protein diet, and fluid intake are used for the patient until evidence occurs that a more acute situation is developing (Lindheimer and Katz, 1973).

Medication will be necessary in a number of cases when there has been no preventive care or when there is little warning of severe preeclamptic signs. Sedatives (phenobarbital), anticonvulsants (magnesium sulfate), and antihypertensive drugs are usually effective in reducing pressure levels. In preeclampsia, diuretics may be used only on a trial basis to reduce excessive edema, but electrolyte imbalance in mother and newborn must be closely monitored.

Most antihypertensive drugs affect peripheral vascular resistance in order to reduce the force of the heartbeat in maintainance of circulation. "Patients may require multiple drugs to attack the major sites of peripheral vascular resistance; the central vasomotor sympathetic center, the peripheral sympathetic nervous system, and the arteriolar smooth muscle directly" (Kelly, 1976).

Chronic Hypertension

Although they reduce maternal complications, hypotensive drugs have not significantly increased circulation to the placenta in cases of chronic hypertension. Thus, any medication used for chronic hypertension can be expected only to alleviate maternal symptoms but not to significantly improve fetal condition.

Maternal estriols are monitored frequently after the week 32 and may remain low in spite of bed rest and treatment. In severe cases, the infant may have to be delivered as soon as L/S ratios indicate lung maturity, for the infant already suffering from chronic distress must receive specialized care in a neonatal intensive care unit.

Women with chronic hypertension may enter pregnancy or be diagnosed in early weeks with a diastolic pressure of 90 mm Hg or above. In such cases, after a trial bed rest period, a mild antihypertensive is usually prescribed, and diuretics may be made part of the control regimen. When hypertension is diagnosed late in the third trimester, more rapid results are needed, and intravenous medication may be used initially to control pressures before adding oral medication.

The most seriously ill patient is the chronic hypertensive with superimposed preeclampsia. Such a case may be an emergency and certainly always is a very high risk situation.

Propranolol Hydrochloride (Inderal) By competing with beta-adrenergic agonists at their receptor sites, beta blocking agents such as propranolol cause a variety of effects on the heart, the vascular system, and the central nervous system. The decrease in force and frequency of cardiac contraction reduces cardiac output, and a response of peripheral vasoconstriction occurs, followed by a decrease in total peripheral resistance. These mechanisms, along with some influence on renin secretion, appear partially to explain the decrease in blood pressure, but the entire mechanism is still unknown. Arrythmias are reduced by the effect of the drug on myocardial cell electrical activity. Propranolol has been used in a variety of conditions including thyrotoxicosis, hypertension, severe angina, and cardiac arrythmias. It is synergistic with diuretics and vasodilators and interacts with a number of drugs (DiPalma, 1976, p. 225).

ADVERSE EFFECTS   Because propranolol has a direct effect on autonomic responses, it has been shown to have several adverse effects during pregnancy.

1. Increases muscle tone of the uterus, reducing circulation. Thus, chronic use may lead to a small placenta and a growth-retarded infant.

2. Impairs responses of the infant to anoxia just after birth and causes postnatal bradycardia and hypoglycemia from which the infant usually recovers by 4 to 5 days of life, with supportive care.

3. Complicates anesthetic management during delivery because of myocardial responses to the drug

4. Reduces contractility of the uterus, prolonging labor (Gladstone et al., 1975).

In any patient, propranolol causes a variety of effects on the heart, GI tract, and central nervous system, illustrated most commonly by cold extremities, nausea, indigestion, diarrhea, fatigue, insomnia, vivid dreams, and rarely, by urinary retention and skin rashes. Bradycardia and postural hypotension may occur as well as bronchoconstriction and bronchospasm. In addition, it may mask or intensify hypoglycemia. Because of all these side effects, propranolol is not usually ordered for asthmatics and diabetics and only very cautiously during pregnancy.

DOSAGE   10–30 mg PO ac tid and hs.

NURSING IMPLICATIONS
1. If a pregnant woman has been receiving propranolol therapy, as may be necessary in a few cases, be alert to adverse effects on labor progress and neonatal adjustment.

2. Administer drug on time and note the occurrence of any side effects. Always check for drug interactions on enclosed manufacturers instructions before administering additional drugs.

Sympathetic Blocking Agents

Other sympathetic blocking agents are used for hypertensive patients (the sympathetic system works to cause vasoconstriction). Reserpine, methyldopa, and guanethidine are the most commonly prescribed. Although not without problems, they may be prescribed for pregnant women with chronic hypertension. These drugs act by interfering with sympathetic impulses to the adrenergic nerves in blood vessels. Systolic and diastolic pressures are lowered by reduction of peripheral vascular resistance, and plasma renin levels are reduced. The blood flow to the kidney and uterus appears to remain normal, a fact especially important in pregnancy.

Adverse Effects The general adverse effects of these drugs are depression, sedation, bradycardia, and sodium retention. Use during pregnancy has been as necessary, with special precautions taken during labor and for the neonate. Lactation is not advisable, as the drugs transfer into milk and may cause sedation and nasal congestion (reserpine) in the infant.

Nursing Implications for All Antihypertensive Drugs
1. Observe for signs of depression, insomnia, or excessive drowsiness. Explain drug effects to patient and family.

2. Place patient in side-lying position for rest in last trimester to promote diuresis. Encourage fluid intake, and observe for edema.

3. Monitor vital signs, and note bradycardia or hypotension, especially.

4. Observe for GI tract distress or constipation.

5. Weigh patients carefully; especially note effect if diuretic is added to regimen.

6. Observe patient for edema, since many antihypertensives promote sodium retention. Diuretics may be necessary.

Reserpine (Many Trade Names)   Reserpine, a rauwolfia alkaloid is useful in mild to moderate hypertension. There is a slow onset of effect, with desired levels reached after 2 weeks of therapy. Because of a long half-life, the drug continues its effect 2 to 3 days after the last dose, and the depletion of norepinephrine persists for about 2 weeks. These points must be noted when changing medication or preparing a patient for surgery. Because general or local anesthetics greatly potentiate the antihypertensive effect, the drug is usually discontinued 2 weeks prior to surgery. The stress of labor may also contribute to potentiation of hypotensive effect.

ADVERSE EFFECTS   Reserpine may cause postural hypotension, bradycardia, fatigue, sedation, depression, lethargy, headache, and dizziness. Less common are nasal congestion, weight gain, nausea, GI tract disturbances, nightmares, and muscular pain.

DOSAGE   0.25–0.5 mg PO initially, then reduced to 0.1–0.25 mg daily. 1–5 mg IM, IV only in emergencies. Onset of action still is slow, and peak is at 2 to 3 hours.

NURSING IMPLICATIONS
1. In addition to general observations listed above, nasal congestion is an especial side effect of reserpine. The nursery personnel should be notified of maternal drug use and observe infant carefully for respiratory difficulty (newborns are nose-breathers).

2. Monitoring for drug response in emergency situations should be carefully carried out; 2 to 3 hours after administration is a critical observation period at peak of effect.

Methyldopa (Aldomet)   Methyldopa reduces the blood pressure by relaxing arterioles but does so apparently because of central action. It is used in moderate to severe hypertension. Since there are minimal side effects and an absence of adverse effects on blood flow to the uterus and kidneys, methyldopa is being selected more frequently for use during pregnancy. Slow onset of action, even with intravenous administration

(2 to 3 hours), indicates that its usefulness in hypertensive emergencies is modified by the time interval. A single oral dose will peak at 4 to 6 hours and persist for 24 hours.

ADVERSE EFFECTS The major effect is sedation, although methylodopa appears to lighten sleep and increase the amount of REM (rapid eye movement) sleep. It may mask fever from infections and may cause mild hypothermia. (Persistent drowsiness may be difficult for a patient returning to normal activities after first introduction to the drug.) Depression, sodium retention, and constipation are other common adverse effects. Postural hypotension, dizziness, and weakness may occur during the early weeks of therapy. Finally, some patients have had a direct Coombs' reaction change to positive during therapy, a change which persisted for many months (Woods and Brinkman, 1973).

DOSAGE 0.5–2.0 g per day PO in three divided doses. 250–500 mg diluted in 100 ml 5% dextrose in water; IV infusion to run over 30 to 60 min.

NURSING IMPLICATIONS
1. Prevent postural hypotension by careful change of position and by rising slowly. Teach patient to maintain side-lying position in late pregnancy when resting.

2. Observe urine for specific gravity and color change (may develop blue color) while always observing patient for edema.

3. Monitor blood pressure closely with intravenous infusion. Wait 3 hours for maximal effect to occur.

4. Note Coombs' test report, especially if infant demonstrates jaundice. Confusion may occur as to cause of Coombs' positive reaction.

Guanethidine Sulfate (Ismelin Sulfate) Guanethidine sulfate is used in moderate to severe hypertension, usually accompanied by a diuretic for control of fluid retention. The effect is mostly an orthostatic one; therefore, it is not usually used during pregnancy unless the patient is already regulated on the drug.

It acts to inhibit responses to sympathetic adrenergic nerve endings. Chronic administration depletes the tissue concentration of norepinephrine. It is necessary to allow 2 to 7 days for full therapeutic effect.

ADVERSE EFFECT   Sedation, dry mouth, and orthostatic hypotension are major effects. There is rebound hypertension when the medication is discontinued which is severe enough to cause hypertensive crises.

DOSAGE   400 mg–2.0 mg daily in four divided doses (2.4 mg is maximum dose).

Vasodilators

In hypertensive crises, intravenous vasodilators may be employed for short-term therapy until adjunct antihypertensives can take effect.

Hydralazine (Apresoline)   The major action of hydralazine is direct relaxation of vascular smooth muscles, especially arterioles; thus, postural hypotension is less common than in drugs which cause generalized vasodilation. When given in preeclamptic states, it may be helpful in overcoming vasoconstriction of renal arterioles. The drug is potentiated by anesthetics, ethacrynic acid, and MAO inhibitors. When combined with thiazides, diastolic pressures are further reduced and toxic effects minimized. Use is usually for short periods.

ADVERSE EFFECTS   There are numerous side effects, some of which can be reduced by concurrent medication with thiazides or beta-adrenergic blockers. Major effects are chills, fever, depression, and in patients with coronary insufficiency, exacerbation of anginal pain. Headache, palpitations, dizziness, nausea and vomiting, anxiety, tachycardia, and dry mouth and sweating are common effects. Propranolol may be utilized to block the reflex tachycardia of hydralazine. Other rare effects are flushing, tearing, conjuctivitis, parasthesias, tremors, and muscle cramping. High doses (greater than 200 mg) have resulted in symptoms of rheumatoid arthritis.

DOSAGE   Initial: 10 mg PO qid, up to 50 mg qid. 20–40 mg IV or IM, with effect 10 to 80 min after dose.

NURSING IMPLICATIONS
1. Monitor vital signs closely, noting onset of effect and maximal peak effect with parenteral use. If there is precipitous fall in blood pressure, hypoxic stress may occur in the fetus.
2. Check list of interacting medications carefully before introducing a new drug.

Diazoxide (Hyperstat IV)   Related to the thiazide family but without diuretic action, diazoxide relaxes smooth muscle in peripheral arterioles. Cardiac output rises, and renal and uterine blood flow remains constant after an initial decrease. Diazoxide relaxes smooth muscle and is a powerful relaxant of myometrial tissue; thus, labor may be interrupted or inhibited, and oxytocics may be needed to maintain normal contractions (Romanklewicz, 1977).

ADVERSE EFFECTS   Acts strongly to retain sodium and water; therefore it must usually be given with a diuretic. Strong protein-binding action may displace other drugs and may affect infant in the immediate recovery period by increasing bilirubin level. It also may cause thrombocytopenia and hyperglycemia in infant. Postural hypotension occurs when it is given concurrently with diuretics or other antihypertensives. Severe hypotension may occur; in such cases, elevation of legs and/or administration of norepinephrine will diminish hypotension. The drug causes unexplained hyperglycemia, and insulin levels in a diabetic must be adjusted carefully, following blood sugar levels.

Other side effects are nausea, flushing, tachycardia, abdominal discomfort, and sedation. Warmth and burning along the vein may occur and persist for 1 to 2 hours, since the solution is highly alkaline. Extravasation should be prevented.

ADMINISTRATION   Given only as a bolus, 300 mg (5 mg/kg) within 10 s, or effectiveness is lost. The drug is 90 percent protein-bound; therefore, if administered slowly, little free drug will be in the circulation to achieve vasodilating effect. Duration of effect is 12 h or less. The blood pressure must be taken every 1 to 2 min during immediate period, every 5 min until stabilized, then every hour until the 12-h period is over. Additional doses will be given according to patient responses.

NURSING IMPLICATIONS
1. Any patient receiving diazoxide must be monitored intensively for vital signs, FHT, and character of labor.

2. Check urine for glucose and volume.

3. Be sure intravenous has not infiltrated. Apply warm/cold compresses to alleviate burning sensation along vein.

4. Inform nursery of drug use and time if mother was in transitional period.

Sodium Nitroprusside (Nipride)   Used only intravenously in hypertensive emergencies, nitroprusside relaxes both arterial and venous smooth muscle. It has an immediate effect, reducing blood pressure within 1 to 2 minutes, but the effect only persists as long as the infusion is flowing. A patient must be weaned off nitroprusside while beginning another antihypertensive. If the infusion is stopped suddenly, the blood pressure will rise to prior levels within 10 minutes. Undesirable levels of hypotension can be corrected by slowing the infusion.

ADVERSE EFFECTS   All adverse effects are caused by vasodilation: tachycardia (30 percent increase in beats per minute), nasal congestion, flushing, nausea, and weakness, and all can be alleviated by slowing the rate of flow. The metabolite, thiocyanate, can rise to toxic levels with continued infusion; therefore, cyanide serum levels should be monitored in mother and later in infant.

ADMINISTRATION   Only use fresh solution, mix powder in 2–3 ml of 5% dextrose in water and then add to 500 ml of 5% dextrose in water. Since the mixture decomposes in light, the intravenous bottle must be wrapped in foil or heavy paper. Brown or blue color indicates a light effect. The solution should be discarded when this occurs and always after 4 h have elapsed since mixing. Always use a constant infusion pump and a tandem intravenous line.

DOSAGE   0.5–8.0 µg/kg per minute titrated to blood pressure response.

NURSING IMPLICATIONS
1. Do not allow patient to sit or stand during infusion.

2. Check fluid frequently for signs of light effect.

3. Monitor maternal and fetal vital signs frequently. Look for signs of reduced uterine blood flow with hypoxic effect on infant. Monitor flow rate of pump. Do not allow intravenous to infiltrate.

Trimethaphan (Arfonad)   A drug only for hypertensive emergencies, trimethaphen causes ganglionic blockade and peripheral vasodilation, resulting in pooling of blood in the extremities. It liberates histamine and thus should be used with caution in allergic patients.

An extremely potent drug, it is always used after careful dilution and is administered by the physician. There may be additive effects with other antihypertensive drugs, and it should not be used with regional anesthesia. Too radical a drop in blood pressure may jeopardize the fetus.

ADMINISTRATION   Dilute ampul with 5% dextrose in water to make 1 mg/ml. Begin administration by constant infusion pump at 3–4 ml per minute; titrate to patient response with constant blood pressure monitoring.

NURSING IMPLICATIONS
1. Keep patient in side-lying position. Do not allow to sit or stand.

2. Monitor fetal and maternal vital signs frequently.

3. Do not allow intravenous to infiltrate.

DIURETICS

The changes of pregnancy affect sodium balance markedly, and intervention with diuretics can upset a delicate balance. A state of hypervolemia exists naturally, one which in a nonpregnant state would trigger diuresis. In adjusting to this total increase of 6–8 L of body water, there are a number of mechanisms which promote increased sodium excretion and a number of others which prevent sodium excretion. Among other changes, the glomerular filtration rate rises to reflect the 50 percent increase in renal blood flow; thus the sodium load to be filtered is increased from 5000 to 10,000 meq per day (Lindheimer and Katz, 1973, p. 892). To tamper with these mechanisms by salt restriction or diuretics may introduce iatrogenic problems. A number of authorities now recommend only fluids and bed rest in a lateral recumbent position to treat any mild edema during pregnancy. The lateral position promotes the best renal blood flow by removing the pressure of the enlarged uterus, and water is a natural physiologic diuretic.

Most pregnant women experience dependent edema in the last trimester, reflecting physical factors of increased femoral venous pressure and uterine pressure on blood flow in upright and supine positions. Diuretics for this type of edema are no longer recommended. However, diuretics are the first line of treatment for the hypertension not associated with pregnancy. A conflict of benefit-to-risk may arise, therefore, when a woman who has been stabilized on a thiazide becomes pregnant.

Diuretics mainly increase urine flow by increasing excretion or preventing the reabsorption of sodium ions. Some also cause potassium, chloride, and bicarbonate loss. Only thiazides and furosemide are the drugs of choice for high-risk situations during pregnancy.

Agents that Inhibit Reabsorption of Sodium

Mercurials (Mercaptomerin, Thiomerin)   Mercurials are no longer used during pregnancy or lactation because of the potentially toxic character of mercurial metabolites.

Benzothiadiazines (Thiazides)   Thiazides are sulfonamide derivatives which, as a group, are utilized frequently in the control of hypertension. Indirectly, they reduce peripheral vascular resistance, while directly they promote excretion of Na^+, K^+, Cl^-, and sometimes HCO_3^-. Thiazides inhibit the reabsorption of Na^+, Cl^-, and water. Changes in pH do not affect drug action.

Absorption is good from the GI tract, and oral doses are more commonly used than parenteral ones. Duration of action ranges from 6 to 36 hours. Excretion is into the glomerular filtrate and by tubular secretion, with a small portion of the drug excreted into the bile.

ADVERSE EFFECTS   Most adverse effects result from electrolyte imbalance, particularly hyponatremia, and hypokalemia. Magnesium excretion is also enhanced. Fatigue, weakness, anorexia, heartburn, nausea and vomiting, cramps, diarrhea, or constipation may accompany poorly controlled electrolyte balance. A maculopapular skin rash may occur in allergic patients. Drugs may augment the effect of digitalis by promoting potassium loss, and potassium replacement is necessary in those cases. Thiazides also may cause a rise in blood glucose levels and aggravate preexisting diabetes through an unknown mechanism.

USE IN PREGNANCY   Thiazides are now only used in cases of cardiac or chronic hypertensive disease, with trial doses sometimes given for severe preeclamptic patients. Transfer across the placenta is easy, and adverse effects on fluid balance in the neonate, in addition to thrombocytopenia and elevated bilirubin levels, can be observed. Dosage requirements for thiazides are listed in Table 5-15.

Table 5-15 Thiazide and Related Drugs Used as Diuretics and for Hypertension

Drug	Daily Dosage	Comments
Chloro- thiazide* (Diuril)	0.5–2.0 g PO qd or bid	Duration short, 6 to 12 h; omit drug 1 or 2 times per week to avoid hypokalemia, hyponatremia. Take with potassium-bearing foods.
Hydrochloro- thiazide* (Esidrix, Hydrodiuril, Oretic)	25–100 mg qd or bid	Duration 6 to 12 h; administer in A.M. Interrupt medication 1 or 2 times per week.
Benzthiazide (Exna, Aquapres)	50–100 mg PO	18 to 24 h duration.
Hydroflu- methiazide (Saluron)	50–100 mg PO	18 to 24 h duration.
Bendroflu- methiazide (Naturetin)	2.5–10 mg PO	Administer every other day to prevent electrolyte imbalance; duration 24+ h.
Methyclothiazide (Enduron)	2.5–10 mg PO	
Trichlorme- thiazide (Naqua, Methahydrin)	2–4 mg PO	Duration longer than 24 h; Usually give every other day, duration 36 h.
Polythiazide (Reverse)	2–4 mg PO	
Chlorthalidone* (Hygroton)	50–100 mg PO	Give with food; 72 h duration; potentiates hypotensive agents.
SULFONAMIDES		
Quinethazone (Hydromox)	50–100 mg PO	Sulfonamides with similar action and side effects as thiazides. Look for gout in some patients. Duration 12–24 h.
Methlazone (Zaroxolyn)	2.5–5 mg PO	

*Most commonly used.

Furosemide and Ethacrynic Acid

Furosemide and ethacrynic acid are the most potent diuretics currently available and are almost identical in their actions, although dosage regimens vary. However, ethacrynic acid has not been used in pregnant patients because of its potent nature and the likelihood of causing severe electrolyte imbalance. Furosemide is used only in hypertensive crises or in pulmonary edema emergencies, and then only for very brief periods.

Furosemide (Lasix)   Furosemide inhibits the reabsorption of sodium in proximal, distal tubules and in the loop of Henle. Onset of action with oral medication is within 1 hour, peak is in the second hour and duration is 6 to 8 hours. Intravenous onset is within 5 minutes, peak is at 30 minutes, and duration is 2 hours.

ADVERSE EFFECTS   Lasix has caused fetal abnormalities in animals when administered during the period of organogenesis; therefore, use in pregnancy should only be in situations where the benefit to the mother outweighs the risk to the fetus. Since the structure is related to sulfonamides, any patient with such an allergy should not receive Lasix. Electrolyte depletion is the major cause of side effects: weakness, dizziness, lethargy, leg cramps, anorexia, nausea/vomiting, and mental confusion. It potentiates antihypertensives; therefore, those doses should be reduced. Elevation of BUN and uric acid levels may be seen, especially when dehydration occurs. Transient deafness and tinnitus have occurred when doses exceeded 20–40 mg daily. Do not give with cephaloridine or aminoglycosides. Discontinue drug 1 week prior to surgery, since curare derivatives are greatly enhanced by Lasix.

In many instances, Lasix-induced diuresis may be accompanied by weakness, fatigue, lightheadedness, thirst, increased perspiration, bladder spasm, and muscle cramps. Transient pain after intramuscular injection has been reported.

DOSAGE   Severe pulmonary edema: 20–80 mg PO repeated

only after 8 h; intermittent dosage, 2 to 4 days, then 3 days rest.

Hypertension: 20–40 mg for one dose IM or IV over a period of 1 to 2 min. A second dose can be given 2 h later. Replace with oral administration as soon as possible. 40 mg PO bid. Reduce dosage of antihypertensives by 50 percent. Reduce dosage of Lasix as soon as possible.

NURSING IMPLICATIONS

1. In acute situations, the patient will be on indwelling Foley catheter. Measure hourly output of urine, especially if on nephrotoxic drugs.

2. Monitor vital signs closely, especially if on digitalis or antihypertensive therapy. Look for potentiation of those medications.

3. Watch fluid intake carefully; prevent dehydration. Weigh daily.

4. Expect fetus to be affected by drug and acutely compromised by poor placental function due to chronic stress.

5. Serum electrolytes, BUN, uric acid, CO_2, calcium, and blood glucose levels should be checked frequently.

6. Observe for liver damage, blood dyscrasias, or other idiosyncratic responses.

7. Observe for transient deafness or tinnitus, especially when given with aminoglycosides.

Potassium-Sparing Diuretics

Spirolactone (Aldactone); Triamterene (Dyrenium) These diuretics are used in adjunct therapy with thiazides because they act differently on the distal tubule to promote potassium reabsorption while inhibiting sodium reabsorption. Although there are relatively few side effects, neither drug is used commonly during pregnancy. These drugs are not given with potassium supplements.

Agents That Inhibit Carbonic Anhydrase

Acetozolamide (Diamox)   Acetazolamide is a drug of the aromatic sulfonamide group which increases renal sodium and bicarbonate excretion. It produces alkaline urine with loss of Na^+, K^+, and HCO_3^- ions. The Cl^- ion is reabsorbed, and as a result, plasma bicarbonate decreases, and the patient may develop metabolic acidosis. Rarely used in pregnancy, this weak diuretic has been used for patients with petit mal epilepsy and for premenstrual tension. Patients who might have had the drug prescribed for those conditions should be cautioned against using it on their own during pregnancy.

Osmotic Diuretics

Mannitol (Osmitrol)   Mannitol is a pharmocologically inert substance which is excreted without being metabolized and is not reabsorbed by the tubules. It increases water loss by demanding dilution of a hypertonic fluid as it passes through the tubules. Intravenous infusions increase blood volume by pulling fluid into the vascular compartment. The resultant state of hyponatremia and hyperosmolality then promotes diuresis. Water is lost, and Na^+ ions may also be excreted in larger amounts. Mannitol is used to increase urine formation in states of preeclampsia where oliguria is present.

DOSAGE   25–200 g per day for IV use only; administration by slow infusion to keep the urine output above 30–50 ml per hour. If 100 g in 24 h does not produce a 100 ml per hour diuresis, a more potent diuretic should be used.

Agents That Increase Glomerular Filtration Rates

Xanthines   Xanthine diuretics include theophylline, caffeine, and theobromine. However, theophylline (and aminophylline) are used primarily for their bronchodilating effect rather than for their diuretic effect. These drugs increase cardiac output and thus improve renal blood flow. They are thought to inhibit sodium reabsorption in tubules.

Aminophylline   Aminophylline is utilized in situations of congestive heart failure and in bronchial asthma attacks since its action is to relax smooth muscle while stimulating cardiac muscle. (Therapeutic level about 15 μg/ml.)

ADVERSE EFFECTS   Central nervous system stimulation, severe persistent vomiting, fever, and hematemesis occur. Cardiovascular effects of palpitation, flushing, arrythmias, and circulatory collapse if intravenous infusion too rapid have been reported.

DOSAGE   100–200 mg PO tid (absorption may be erratic). 125–500 mg rectally (repeated doses may be irritating). 250–500 mg IV (slowly, over 3 to 5 min, repeat up to tid). If administered as infusion, load with 5.6 mg/kg over 30 min, then 1 mg/kg per hour.

NURSING IMPLICATIONS
1. Monitor vital signs carefully.

2. Rate of intravenous flow is critical.

3. Rectal suppositories will be unevenly absorbed if feces is present. Oral absorption is erratic.

4. Observe for adverse effects.

Dyphylline (Airet, Dilor, NeoThylline)   Dyphylline is a theophylline derivative with same condition as aminophylline and theophylline. It is less irritating to the GI tract and can be given intramuscularly.

DOSAGE   300 mg PO q 6 to 8 h. 250–500 mg IM tid.

Theophylline (Agualin, SloPhyllin, and Others)   Theophylline is not well absorbed from the GI tract and is used more frequently for rectal administration.

DOSAGE   160 mg PO q 6 h. 250–500 mg rectally q 8 to 12 h.

ANTIDIABETIC DRUGS

The incidence of diabetes is increasing as quality obstetric care allows high-risk diabetics to complete pregnancy and their infants to recover safely from birth. When careful control of hyperglycemia and ketonuria has been achieved throughout pregnancy, the perinatal mortality has been as low as 5 to 12 percent, as compared to the rate with poor control of 5 to 40 percent (White, 1975, p. 5).

Ketonuria may be more damaging than maternal hypoglycemia or hyperglycemia. Studies have shown that ketonuria, occurring at any phase of pregnancy, was associated with significantly lower infant IQ than in controls (Greene, 1975).

The infant of a diabetic does not provide insulin for its mother (since insulin does not cross the placenta). Instead, in response to maternal hyperglycemia, the fetus experiences pancreatic hypertrophy and, although it may tolerate episodes of fetal hypoglycemia (20–40 mg/100 ml) better than an adult, excessive maternal hyperglycemia will increase the fetal fat/glycogen stores.

The large baby is most often a product of uncontrolled class A diabetic or insulin-dependent diabetic who is consistently hyperglycemic. In contrast, the very severe diabetic may have a growth-retarded infant, compromised by severe maternal disease and placental dysfunction.

Diabetics of class A (gestational, latent, or stress-induced) usually do not require insulin or oral antidiabetic agents for control. However, careful control of diet and exercise is important to prevent the consistent hyperglycemia. Some groups are using small doses of insulin for these mothers in an attempt to improve fetal condition. The class A diabetic is usually diagnosed by an abnormal glucose tolerance test. The most accurate readings are thought to be achieved with IVGTT plus 2-hour postprandial blood glucose readings, since GI absorption of glucose may be delayed (see Chap. 2). There can be false-positive results with either method, however. Glycosuria may occur during pregnancy even for a nondiabetic (Baker et al., 1968); therefore, reliance strictly on urine levels is inadequate. Treatment is usually aimed at maintaining a normal 2-hour, postprandial blood glucose reading of 120 mg/100 ml (Greene, 1975), even with some glycosuria.

Insulin   Insulin is normally released constantly by the pancreatic beta cells, with the rate changing in response to blood glucose levels. It is protein-bound to some extent but is not stored for long periods in body tissue. Insulin is metabolized by an insulinase–anti-insulinase system in liver, kidney, and muscle, whose functions do not appear to be altered by diabetes (DiPalma, 1976, p. 305).

Insulin controls the cellular uptake of glucose for energy or storage as glycogen. In the presence of hypoglycemia, epinephrine plus *glucagon*, another pancreatic hormone, promotes the change of glycogen to glucose. Glucagon and occasionally epinephrine may therefore be administered to counteract insulin-induced hypoglycemia.

Adverse Effects   Insulin itself is too large a protein to cross the placenta to affect the fetus. Therefore, adverse effects during pregnancy result from insulin–glucose imbalance with hypo-hyperglycemic changes affecting ketonemia and transfer of nutrients to the fetus. A few patients experience allergic reactions to protein-containing mixtures, and others appear resistant to the drug. Main interactions are listed in Table 5-16.

Dosage   Different concentrations of insulin, 40 U, 80 U, and 100 U, have been available, but insulin is now being widely marketed as 100 U/ml in an attempt to standardize dosage and syringes as well as to minimize the amount the patient must inject. A 1 ml tuberculin syringe may be used or a specifically marked 100 U insulin syringe (Fig. 5-2). Dosage must be individualized for each patient and will vary through each period of pregnancy and during recovery. Subcutaneous injection must be deep, with sites carefully rotated to reduce tissue reaction (see Fig. B-3). Table 5-17 lists insulin preparations.

Table 5-16   Insulin–Drug Interactions

Increase Activity (Potentiate Hypoglycemia)	Decrease Activity (Potentiate Hyperglycemia)
Alcohol	Epinephrine
Anabolic steroids	Furosemide
Anticoagulants (except heparin)	Corticosteroids
Antineoplastics (displaces from protein binding)	Isoniazid (large doses)
Beta-adrenergic blockers	Oral contraceptives (increase blood glucose levels)
Isoniazid (small doses)	Thiazide diuretics
MAO inhibitors	Thyroid preparations
Methamphetamine	
Oral diabetic agents	
Phenylbutazone	
Propranolol	
Salicylates	
Sulfonamides	
Sulfonylureas	

Source: Adapted from E.W. Martin, *Hazards of Medication*, J.B. Lippincott, Philadelphia, 1971, p. 638.

Nursing Implications

1. Every patient on insulin therapy must be educated about every aspect of diabetes control, diet management, and insulin therapy.

2. Pregnant patients must learn how pregnancy changes the metabolic pattern of insulin and be on guard for hypo-hyperglycemia and ketonuria.

3. Ketonuria must be avoided, but some glycosuria is acceptable. When severe diabetics spill too much glucose, it must be replaced in the diet (Greene, 1975).

4. Always use "double-voided" specimen for any cover insulin or regulation of insulin. (Empty bladder, drink fluids, and void again in one-half hour; test second specimen.)

5. Screening urine testing should be done with agents specific for glucose, since lactosuria is common in later pregnancy (Nelson, 1974).

   a. Glucose oxidase method (Clinistix, Diastix, Tes-Tape) tests for glucose only. It does not discriminate well between mild and heavy sugar; therefore, for quantitative testing, an insulin-dependent diabetic should use the method below as well.

   b. Copper reduction method (Clinitest) picks up lactose, and all reducing sugars. Use for insulin-dependent diabetic when amount of insulin needed for coverage is important to detect (quantitatively more accurate). Tes-Tape is qualitative.

6. Be alert to changes in insulin needs during labor and after delivery. Be sure patient is re-regulated on standard home-care dose before discharge.

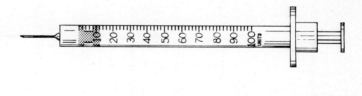

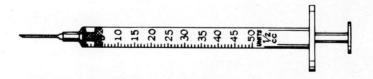

Figure 5-2   Syringes, 0.5 and 1.0 ml, calibrated for 100U insulin.

Table 5-17 Insulin Preparations

Insulin	Effect Begins	Peak	Duration	Indications	Comments
CRYSTALLINE ZINC					
Regular insulin	Fast ½ to 1 h	2 to 3 h	6 to 8 h	Emergencies, during surgery, delivery, and to supplement other insulins	IV as ordered. SC, 15 to 20 min ac. Can mix with all other preparations.
ZINC AND PROTEIN SUSPENSIONS					
Isophane insulin suspension (NPH insulin)	Intermediate 1 to 1½ h	8 to 12 h	24 h	Maintenance	Cloudy solution. Mix only with regular insulin. SC only, 1 h ac. Lilly insulin can be mixed with all.
Protamine zinc insulin suspension (PZI)	Long-acting 4 to 8 h	14 to 20 h	36 h+	Maintenance	Mix only with regular insulin. Give deep SC, 1 h ac. Hypoglycemia may show first as extreme fatigue.
Globin zinc insulin	Intermediate 2 h	8 to 16 h	24 h	Maintenance	Rarely used. Clear yellowish solution. SC only, 1 h ac.
ZINC SUSPENSIONS WITHOUT PROTEIN (LENTE INSULINS)					
Semilente					
Prompt insulin zinc suspension	Fast ½ to 1 h	5 to 7 h	12 to 16 h	No protein; may be ordered for patients with protein sensitivity	Give deep SC, 30 to 45 min ac. Mix only with lente preparations or with regular insulin.
Insulin zinc suspension	Intermediate 1 to 1½ h	8 to 12 h	24 h	Maintenance	Mixture of 30% semilente 70% ultralente. Give deep SC, 1 h ac. Variations can be custom mixed.
Ultralente					
Extended insulin zinc suspension	Long-acting 4 to 8 h	16 to 18 h	36 h+	Maintenance	Usually give deep SC, 1 h ac.

Oral Antidiabetic Agents

Sulfonylureas appear to stimulate synthesis and release of endogenous insulin. Thus, if the patient has no pancreatic beta cells, these drugs are ineffective. Biguanide derivatives, in contrast, act by increasing peripheral utilization of glucose and have been given in combination with sulfonylureas or insulin (see Table 5-18).

Table 5-18 Oral Antidiabetic Agents

Drug	Daily Dose	Comments
SULFONYLUREAS		
Aceto-hexamide (Dymelor)	0.25–1.5 g divided into 1 or 2 doses. Twice as potent as tolbutamide. Safety in pregnancy has not been established.	Peak 3 h, duration 12 to 24 h. Reduces glucose output from liver. May combine with insulin.
Chlorpro-pamide (Diabi-nese)	100–500 mg qd. Six times as potent as tolbutamide. Safety in pregnancy has not been established.	Peak 4 to 10 h, duration 60 h. Long $T_{1/2}$; therefore effect persists after drug d/c. Prolongs action of sedatives, hypnotics. More frequent side effects. Test urine for sugar/acetone three times a day during initial 6 weeks of therapy.
Tolazamide (Tolinase)	0.1–0.75 g qd. Not recommended during pregnancy. Five to six times as potent as tolbutamide.	Peak 4 to 6 h, duration 12–14 h. Test urine for sugar/acetone tid.
Tolbutamide (Orinase)	0.5–2 g divided in 2 to 3 doses daily pc. Animal toxicity shown. Not recommended during pregnancy, especially 1st trimester.	Peak 4 to 6 h, duration 12 h. Sometimes gives false-positive albumin in urine. May be given with insulin.
BIGUANIDE DERIVATIVES		
Phenformin hydrochloride (DBI)	Being removed from market as of October 1977.	Acts by increasing peripheral utilization of glucose. Adverse effects outweigh benefits.

Adverse Effects   None of the four sulfonylureas in use as antidiabetic agents has been completely cleared for use during pregnancy. Teratogenic effects have been noted in large doses in lab animals but have not been proven in humans. There is concern about the effect of such drugs on hyperinsulinemia and hyperglycemia in the fetus and newborn. One study of chlorpropamide use during pregnancy found improved control of chemical diabetes in the mother but no change in fetal outcome. As a result of the long duration of effect, serious hypoglycemia developed in many infants (Sutherland, 1973).

Biguanide derivatives are being removed from the market because of drug-related deaths. In addition, studies have implicated such drugs in fetal anomalies. When a patient has been regulated on these antidiabetic agents prior to pregnancy, it is wiser to discontinue treatment before the woman wishes to conceive.

Sulfonylureas, especially chlorpropamide, cause disulframlike reactions when taken with alcohol and may precipitate photosensitivity. They may cause gastric upsets, headache, tinnitus, and some allergic reactions. Control of insulin levels is uneven, and some patients cannot utilize these agents. In some instances, they have been combined with insulin to reduce insulin dosage.

THYROID AND ANTITHYROID AGENTS

Thyroid Dysfunction

Pregnancy induces a 15 to 20 percent elevation of basal metabolism with some symptoms of slightly increased thyroid hormone production: increased pulse and cardiac output, less ability to tolerate heat, more flushing of the skin. However, true hyperthyroidism (20 to 60 percent above normal) is fairly uncommon, occurring, according to Niswander and Gordon (1972), in about 0.19 percent of all pregnant women. There is a slight increase in low birth weight and in neonatal mortality in infants of those women (Buiron, 1975).

A number of different approaches are currently being

used, all of which must consider the fact the fetal thyroid is beginning to function by the fourteenth week of life and drugs given to inhibit maternal thyroid function will cross to the fetus and may depress thyroid growth. Excessive maternal antithyroid medication may result in the development of neonatal goiter and hypothyroidism or may inhibit mental development. Long-acting thyroid-stimulating hormone (LATS) has been found in cord blood of infants with thyrotoxicosis, a transient disease thought to be the result of transplacental passage of LATS when high levels are present in the mother (Fisher, 1975).

The fetal thyroid functions independently of maternal function, since very little (0.01 percent) of total thyroxine used by the fetus is from maternal origin (Majtaba and Burrow, 1975). Unless fetal thyroid function has been affected by antithyroid medication, by iodine deficiency, or by excessive maternal iodide intake, the newborn should be in an euthyroid state at birth.

Iodides are not recommended during pregnancy because as little as 12 mg daily may cause fetal goiter, (Fisher, 1975). Radioactive iodides are prohibited during pregnancy and should not be given to women who wish to become pregnant, since the radioactive iodide will be taken up selectively, will be excreted slowly, and may damage the fetal thyroid development. Surgery, which may be necessary in severe cases, can be done best during the second trimester without harm to the fetus.

In response to estrogen levels, there is an increase in thyroxine-binding globulin (TBG) during pregnancy. As a result the protein-bound iodine (PBI) changes from the normal rate of 4–8 μg/100 ml to 6–12 μg/100 ml, but the free metabolically active hormone level remains the same. In only a few cases, additional thyroid replacement may be necessary for women who have been slightly hypothyroid prior to pregnancy.

The hypothyroid condition frequently underlies infertility, so that a woman would rarely be discovered to be hypothyroid after pregnancy has begun. However, women on controlled

Table 5-19 Thyroid Agents

Drug	Daily Dose	Comments
Thyroid hormone (Thyrar, Throcrine); dessicated animal thyroid	60–180 mg qd	Slow onset of action. Increase initial dose every 1 to 3 wk until daily minimum dose is reached.
Thyroglobulin (Proloid)	30–180 mg qd	Slow onset of action. As potent as thyroid, but contains two of the three fractions of the thyroid hormone: (T_3) triiodothyronine and (T_4) thyroxine
Levothyroxine sodium (Lithyroxine Sodium, Synthroid, Letter, Titroid)	100–400 μg qd	PO or IV. Slower onset but longer lasting effect than liothyronine.
Liothyronine sodium (Cytomel)	25–100 μg qd	Rapid onset of action, short duration. Crosses placenta more easily, more potent than thyroxine.
Liotrix (Euthyroid, Thyrolar), combination in 4/1 ratio of T_3 and T_4	Levothyroxine 60–180 μg qd; liothyronine 15–45 μg qd	Patient must not switch medication brand, as there are different dosage forms.

maintenance thyroid doses may become pregnant. Thyroid doses should be carefully regulated and may have to be increased during the first trimester and decreased in later pregnancy.

There are varying opinions about the best method of therapy. Three current alternatives are found: minimal doses of antithyroid hormone, full doses of antithyroid hormone plus supplemental thyroid hormone, and surgery. Dosage levels for thyroid agents are given in Table 5–19.

Antithyroid Agents

Antithyroid agents temporarily depress synthesis of the thyroid hormone but do not affect hormone already formed in the thyroid gland. Adverse effects are dose-related and include prothrombin deficiency, leukopenia, rash, fever, lymph node enlargement in the neck, loss of taste, hepatitis, and lower extremity edema. Antithyroid medication is contraindicated with cardiovascular disease. Antithyroids pass easily into milk; therefore, lactation is not advisable. Antithyroid medication may affect insulin response, may potentiate anticoagulants, and may cause digitalis preparations to be metabolized more quickly. Table 5-20 lists dosage requirements for thyroid agents.

Table 5-20 Antithyroid Agents

Drug	Daily Dose	Comments
Propylthiouracil (PTU)	200 mg qd or less in first trimester. 100 mg qd or less in second and third trimesters.	Most commonly prescribed, dose must be regulated by response in trimesters, never more than 300 mg qd given during pregnancy.
Methothiouracil (Methiacil, Muracil, Thimecil)	30–200 mg qd	Crosses placenta easily. More potent than PTU; not used so commonly during pregnancy.
Methimazole (Tapazole)	10–30 mg qd	Ten times stronger than PTU. Crosses placenta easily. Some incidence of scalp defects in infants at birth.
Carbimazole (Neomercazole)	2.5–20 mg qd	Used more commonly in Great Britain.
Potassium perchlorate	250 mg tid initially; 300 mg qd maintenance.	Interferes with iodine-retaining process in the gland. Administer with food to reduce gastric irritation.

Nursing Implications

1. Observe for normal progression through trimesters, as mother is at some risk for abortion, premature labor, and preeclampsia.

2. Observe for signs of thyrotoxicosis: increase in pulse, temperature, restlessness, anxiety, and muscle weakness.

3. Teach patient importance of regular intervals in doses. Teach patient to recognize signs of ineffective dosage and to report signs of infection or adverse effects.

4. Be alert to observe infant for thyrotoxicosis or hypothyroidism in first few weeks after birth. Notify nursery of mother's medication level during transition period.

BIBLIOGRAPHY

Aara, Leonard A., and John L. Jeurgens: "Thrombophlebitis Associated with Pregnancy," *American Journal of Obstetrics and Gynecology*, 109(8):1128, 1971.

Amstey, M.D.: "Immunization in Pregnancy," *Clinical Obstetrics and Gynecology*, 19:47, 1976.

Armstrong, D., M.H. Grillo, D.B. Louria, and L. Smith: *Infectious Disease: Diagnosis and Treatment*, Medlow Press, New York, 1975.

Baker, D.P., J.R. Hutchinson, and D.L. Vaughn: "Comparison of Standard Oral and Rapid Intravenous Glucose Tolerance Tests in Pregnancy," *Obstetrics and Gynecology*, 31:475, 1968.

Burrow, G.N.: "The Thyroid in Pregnancy," *Medical Clinics of North America*, 59(5): 1089, September 1975.

Cluff, L.E., G.J. Caranasos, and R.B. Stewart: *Clinical Problems with Drugs, Major Problems in Internal Medicine*, W.B. Saunders, Philadelphia, 1975, vol. 5.

Coid, C.R.: "Infection in Pregnancy and Impaired Fetal Growth," *Proceedings of the Royal Society of Medicine*, 69:1, 1976.

"Criteria and Techniques for the Diagnosis of Gonorrhea," Center for Disease Control, U.S. Public Health Service, Atlanta, Georgia, 1974.

Davies, P.S.: "Maternal and Fetal Infection," *Clinics in Obstetrics and Gynecology*. 1:17, 1974.

DiPalma, J.R.: *Basic Pharmacology in Medicine*, McGraw-Hill, New York, 1976.

Fisher, D.A.: "Thyroid Function in the Fetus and Newborn," *Medical Clinics of North America*, 59(5):1102, September 1975.

Fletcher, H.P.: "The Oral Hypoglycemic Drugs: Pro and Con," *American Journal of Nursing*, 76(4):596, 1976.

Genton, E.: "Guidelines for Heparin Therapy," *Annals of Internal Medicine*, 80:77–82, 1974.

Gladstone, G.R., A. Horsdof, and W.M. Gusony: "Propranolol Administration During Pregnancy: Effects on the Fetus," *Journal of Pediatrics*, 86:962–964, June 1975.

Greene, J.W.: "Diabetes Mellitus in Pregnancy," *Mt. Sinai Journal of Medicine of NY*, 42(5):401, September 10, 1975.

Greenhill, J.P., and E.A. Friedman: *Obstetrics*, W.B. Saunders, Philadelphia, 1974.

Hansen, James W., and David W. Smith: "The Fetal Hydantoin Syndrome," *Journal of Pediatrics*, 87(2):285, August 1975.

Hansten, Philip: *Drug Interactions*, 3d ed., Lea & Febiger, Philadelphia, 1975.

Hill, Reba, M. et al.: "Infants Exposed in Utero to Antiepileptic Drugs," *American Journal of Diseases of Children*, 127(5):645, May 1974.

Immunization During Pregnancy, ACOG Technical Bulletin, Center for Disease Control, U.S. Public Health Service, Atlanta, Georgia, March 1973.

Kelly, K.L.: "Beta Blockers in Hypertension: A Review," *American Journal of Hospital Pharmacy* 33:1284–1290, December, 1976.

Ledger, William: "Infectious Disease," in S.L. Romney (ed.), *Obstetrics and Gynecology: The Health Care of Women*, McGraw-Hill, New York, 1975, chap 28, pp. 440–473.

Levison, M.E., and D. Kaye: "Anaerobic Infections II. Clinical Syndromes and Their Management," *Drug Therapy*, pp. 65–78, April 1976.

Lindheimer, M.D., and A.I. Katz: "Sodium and Diuretics in Pregnancy," *New England Journal of Medicine*, **288**:891, 1973.

Majtaba, Q., and G. N. Burrow: "Treatment of Hypothyroidism in Pregnancy with Propylthimacil and Methemazole," *Obstetrics and Gynecology*, **46**(3):282, September 1975.

Martin, E.W.: *Hazards of Medication*, J.B. Lippincott, Philadelphia, 1971.

*Mead, P. and J.F. Clapp III: "The Use of Betamethasone and Timed Delivery in the Management of Premature Rupture of the Membranes," *Journal of Reproductive Medicine*, **19**(1): 3–7, July 1977.

Merrill, Kent L., and Daniel J. Verberg: "The Choice of Long-Term Anticoagulants for the Pregnant Patient," *Obstetrics and Gynecology*, **47**(6):711, June 1976.

Metronidazole (Flagyl) Warning, FDA Drug Bulletin, April-May 1976.

Miller, R.R., and D.J. Greenblatt: "Clinical Use of Digitalis Glycosides," *American Journal of Hospital Pharmacy* **33**:179–185, February 1976.

Monit, C.R.G.: "Viral Vaccination in Pregnancy," *Infectious Diseases in Obstetrics and Gynecology*, pp. 345–356, 1974.

Monson, Richard R.: "Diphenylhydantoin and Selected Congenital Malformations," *New England Journal of Medicine*, **289**:1049, 1973.

Nelson, J.: "Glucose Urine Testing Systems," *Drug Intelligence and Clinical Pharmacology*, **8**:422, July 1974.

*Newton, D.W., A.O. Nichols, and M. Newton: "You Can Minimize the Hazards of Corticosteroids," *Nursing '77*, **7**(6):26–33, 1977.

Niswander, Kenneth R., and Myron Gordon: *The Women and Their Pregnancies*, The Collaborative Perinatal Study of the National Institute of Neurobiological Diseases and Stroke, W. B. Saunders, Philadelphia, 1972.

Pettifor, J.M., and R. Benson: "Congenital Malformations Associated with the Administration of Oral Anticoagulants during Pregnancy," *Pediatric Pharmacology and Theraputics*, **86**(3):459, 1975.

*Denotes particularly pertinent references.

Pridemore, B.R. et al.: "Management of Anticoagulant Therapy During and After Pregnancy," *British Journal of Obstetrics and Gynecology*, **82**:740, 1975.

Romanklewicz, J.A.: "Pharmacology and Clinical Use of Drugs in Hypertensive Emergencies," *American Journal of Hospital Pharmacy*, **34**:185–193, February 1977.

Romney, S.L.: *Obstetrics and Gynecology: The Health Care of Women*, McGraw-Hill, New York 1976.

Rovinsky, J.J.: "Diseases Complicating Pregnancy," in S. Romney (ed.), *Obstetrics and Gynecology: The Health Care of Women*, McGraw-Hill, New York, 1976.

Salzman, Edwin W. et al.: "Management of Heparin Therapy," *New England Journal of Medicine*, **292**(20):1046, May 15, 1976.

Schatz, M. et al.: "Corticosteroid Therapy for the Pregnant Asthmatic Patient," *Journal of the American Medical Association*, **233**:804, 1975.

Sutherland, H.W., J.M. Stowers, and J.D. Comack: *British Medical Journal*, 3:9, 1973.

Weaver, J.B., and J.F. Pearson: "Influence of Digitalis on Time of Onset and Duration of Labor," *British Medical Journal* 3:519, 1973.

*Weinberger, M., and L. Hendeles: "Pharmacotherapy of Asthma," *American Journal of Hospital Pharmacy*, **33**:1071–1080, October 1976.

White, P. "What It Means To Be Female and Diabetic," *Diabetes Forecast*, November-December 1975.

Woods, J.R., and C.R. Brinkman III: "The Treatment of Gestational Hypertension," *Journal of Reproductive Medicine*, **15**(5):195, 1973.

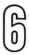

Drugs Used During Labor and Delivery

Elizabeth J. Dickason

Both the timing and the dosage of drugs given during labor govern the degree of drug effect observed in the infant after birth. Some indication of fetal effect can be observed with internal or external monitoring, but persisting effects of sedatives, analgesics, and anesthetics may not be seen then nor in the immediate response of the newborn infant. These persisting effects on the newborn during the recovery period are discussed in Chapter 8.

It is evident that psychologic preparation has helped women to go less fearfully through the childbirth process. Anticipatory education and the presence of a significant support person may decrease both fear of the unknown and anxiety, factors which can compound pain perception. Thus, every effort of the staff should be directed toward providing an environment which will allow the couple to approach labor with confidence. Support should be provided as necessary so that intervention with drug therapy may be kept at a minimum.

BARBITURATES

Barbiturates are not used commonly today because the adverse effects on the newborn are more widely recognized. Long-term depression of newborn responses and delayed maternal bonding and infant adaptation to feeding have been recognized after women received barbiturates (100–200 mg) routinely during active labor. Occasionally, if a woman enters the hospital in very early labor, a sedative may be prescribed to allow sleep. In such cases, there is enough time for drug metabolism before active labor and delivery ensues.

Barbiturates often act as antianalgesics, causing restlessness in the presence of pain. They reduce REM sleep and are quickly habituating. In fact, their use as sedatives is diminishing in general hospitals because of multiple drug interactions and adverse effects of chronic use. Tranquilizing agents are thought to be equally effective in assisting patients to rest (Greenblatt and Shader, 1972).

In large doses, barbiturates depress respirations in the mother and the newborn infant. Since they rapidly traverse the placenta, fetal levels may be high at birth, and prolonged metabolism times may extend effects well into the recovery period (see Fig. 7-2). Barbiturates induce enzyme activity in both mother and fetus (see Chapter 7). Phenobarbital is used commonly for long periods prior to labor in both epileptic and preeclamptic patients. In such cases, doses of potentiating drugs such as analgesics, antianxiety agents, and anesthetics must be reduced.

POTENT ANALGESICS

Morphine Sulfate

Morphine is the parent analgesic whose effectiveness in alleviating pain is the standard against which synthetic narcotics are measured. It is a powerful respiratory depressant, an effect which limits its use in labor. However, each of the drugs in Table 6-1, in equianalgesic doses, may have almost equally depressant action on respirations. Duration of action for intramuscular morphine is 4 to 5 hours. In obstetrics, use of morphine has been limited mainly to crises such as severe preeclampsia or acute pulmonary edema. Postoperatively, it is rarely utilized except for severe pain, as it is too powerful an analgesic for pain resulting from normal childbirth.

Adverse Effects Among numerous adverse effects are central nervous system depression and sedation in varying degrees. Eu-

Table 6-1   Approximately Equianalgesic Dosages

Morphine	10 mg
Oxymorphone	1.0–1.5 mg
Oxycodone	10–15 mg
Meperidine	100 mg
Alphaprodine	40–60 mg
Anileridine	25–30 mg
Pentazocine	20 mg

phoria, dizziness, warmth, itching and urticaria and nausea and vomiting are other common side effects. Postural hypotension can occur, so patients should be cautioned about changing positions rapidly. Spasms of smooth muscle of the intestine, biliary tract, and urinary tract occur, and oliguria may be present. It has addicting potential, and doses should be diminished as soon as possible and a less powerful analgesic substituted.

Dosage   5–15 mg SC q 3 to 4 h. 2.5–15 mg IV diluted in 5 ml normal saline, injected slowly over 4 to 5 min.

Nursing Implications

1. Observe for side effects, especially respiratory depression.

2. Monitor vital signs frequently, since patient is usually critically ill.

3. Observe for maximal analgesic effect 20 minutes after intravenous administration and 30 to 60 minutes after subcutaneous administration.

Oxymorphone Hydrochloride (Numorphan Hydrochloride)   A semisynthetic derivative of morphine, oxymorphone has similar action and side effects. However, there may be more nausea and vomiting and less antitussive effect.

DOSAGE   Labor: 0.5–1 mg IM. 0.5 mg IV diluted in saline, injected slowly.
Postoperative: 1–1.5 mg SC, q 4 to 6 h.

Oxycodone with APC (Percodan)   Oxycodone is a codeine analogue with greater analgesic effect and addicting potential. It is available only as a mixture with aspirin, phenacetin, and caffeine (Percodan). Use in obstetrics is mainly for postoperative pain as an intermediate analgesic.

ADVERSE EFFECTS   Nausea and vomiting and drowsiness are infrequent in usual doses. Dizziness and constipation may occur. Respiratory depression is rare. Dependence on Percodan may occur, and doses should be tapered as soon as possible.

DOSAGE   One tablet q 6 h pc or with milk. (Each tablet contains: oxycodone hydrochloride, 4.5 mg; oxycodone terephthalate, 0.38 mg; aspirin, 224 mg; phenacetin, 160 mg; caffeine, 32 mg.)

NURSING IMPLICATIONS
1. Check for aspirin or codeine sensitivity before giving.

2. Give with food or milk.

3. Space doses correctly and taper as soon as is feasible.

Phenylpiperidine Derivatives

Meperidine (Demerol, Pethoid, Pethidine)   Meperidine acts in many ways similar to morphine and although less effective to relieve severe pain, it has equally depressant effects on respiration at equianalgesic doses. The best effect is obtained 30 to 50 minutes after intramuscular injection and duration is 2 to 4 hours.

Uterine activity may be increased, while maternal restlessness and oxygen consumption are decreased. Observation of uterine contractions (especially when oxytocin is being utilized) and fetal responses are therefore important, for labor proceeds, but symptoms may belie the advancing cervical dilatation.

ADVERSE EFFECTS   Because of a positive effect on smooth

muscle, meperidine may cause biliary tract spasm and initiate vomiting. Because of central nervous system depression, doses are reduced when the patient is hypotensive or concurrently receiving potentiating drugs. Postural hypotension and tachycardia (when intravenous route is used) may occur.

Meperidine has long been used for analgesia during labor. Until the time–dose relationship was clarified, doses were large and given whenever the patient appeared to need medication. Now it has been determined that doses of 75–100 mg given intramuscularly, cause the greatest neonatal depression in infants born 1 to 3 hours after injection, with the peak coming at 2 hours. Meperidine given intravenously has a "safe period" of only a few minutes, as levels in the fetus rise to 70 percent of maternal levels within 6 minutes (Schinder and Moya, 1974). The delay in full development of signs of depression is probably caused by slow fetal metabolism of meperidine to the active metabolites, normeperidine, normeperidic acid, and meperidic acid. Although respiratory depression diminishes with time, persistant effects of these active metabolites has been noted by Brackbill et al. (1974), with demonstrated adverse effects on infant neurobehavioral adjustment in the first month of life.

With dosage over 50 mg, enough time must be allowed for maternal disposition of meperidine (>4 h) prior to birth so that equilibrated levels in the fetal circulation can drop into an ineffective range. If given closer to birth time, dosage should remain under 50 mg. Intramuscular injection has a slower uptake in the fetus and less placental transfer and may be the preferred route. Some observers have noted, however, that a small dose (25 mg) of intravenous meperidine, when titrated with patient's needs and repeated in 5 to 10 minutes if necessary, has been effective (McDonald, 1977).

In some settings heavy doses are still utilized during labor (average 350 mg, range 150–1000 mg). In these cases it has been shown that newborn oxygen saturation was lowered, and spontaneous correction of acidosis was slower, probably as a result of drug-induced hypoventilation (Dancis 1974, p. 141). One minute Apgar scores were 7 or below in 36 percent of these heavily medicated infants.

DOSAGE   IV: 25 mg diluted in 5 ml saline, injected slowly over 1 to 1.5 min. Repeat in 10 min if necessary.

IM: 25–50 mg (within 1 h of delivery or 3 to 4 h before delivery).

Postoperative: 50–100 mg IM q 3 to 4 h.

Precaution: SC injection may result in abscess formation.

NURSING IMPLICATIONS

1. Utilize all possible nonpharmacologic means of support for the patient during labor.

2. Be alert for effect of drug on progress of labor and on oxygen levels. Observe vital signs.

3. When giving intravenously, be sure drug is diluted and given slowly.

4. Work together with physician to educate the frightened or demanding patient about adverse effects of large doses.

5. Observe infant carefully at birth. Remember dose-time relationships and that initial Apgar score does not correlate with long range meperidine effects.

Alphaprodine (Nisentil)   Nisentil is related to meperidine but has a more rapid onset of action and a duration of only 2 hours (intramuscular route). Duration of effect when given intravenously is only one-half hour to 1 hour. Adverse effects are similar to meperidine. It has a greater potential for respiratory depression, however, and the last dose should be administered more than 2 hours before birth. The newborn must be observed carefully during the first period after birth. A narcotic antagonist (naloxone) should be available if the mother experiences respiratory depression and, of course, for the infant. As a precaution, some units combine dosage of 50 mg of Nisentil with 1 mg of levallorphan tartrate (Lorfan) for the mother.

DOSAGE   20–30 mg IV, slowly over 3 to 4 min. 20–60 mg SC; may be repeated in 2 h if not near time of birth.

Anileridine (Leritine)   Anileridine is formed by a slight modification of meperidine structure and has similar adverse effects and precautions. Respiratory depression in the mother equals that of meperidine, but effects on the infant may be more severe. Duration of effect is 2 to 4 hours. For these reasons, Leritine is not often used in labor. Respiratory depression resulting from anileridine is antagonized by naloxone.

Benzomorphan Derivative

Pentazocine (Talwin)   Pentazocine, an nonnarcotic analgesic, has been utilized in obstetrics, for it crosses the placenta less readily than meperidine, and respiratory depression is about one-half that of morphine. Talwin is both an analgesic and a narcotic antagonist (with about 1/50 the effect of naloxone). It may reverse the effect of concurrently administered narcotics. Interestingly, naloxone acts as its specific antagonist if depression does occur, whereas other antagonists are ineffective.

Talwin is not under the Drug Abuse Prevention and Control Act (1970) but has been noted to have potential for psychic and physical dependence. Therefore, caution as to drug access is necessary.

Central nervous system effects include analgesia and depression of respirations. Large doses cause cardiovascular effects of slight hypertension and tachycardia. Duration of effect is 1 to 3 hours (intramuscular route) and 2 to 6 hours (oral route).

ADVERSE EFFECTS   Sweating, sedation, dizziness, nausea, euphoria, and rarely, hallucinations and nightmares occur. Sclerosis of skin and subcutaneous tissue has occurred with chronic use of the subcutaneous route; therefore, this route is not recommended.

DOSAGE   30 mg IM as a single dose during labor. 20 mg IV, may be repeated in 2 to 3 h. Do not mix other drugs in syringe.

ANTIANXIETY AGENTS

Antihistamines

Hydroxyzine   A useful antianxiety agent with antihistaminic qualities, hydroxyzine calms the patient without impairing mental alertness. It is used in obstetrics mainly before and after delivery to allay anxiety, prevent nausea and vomiting, and potentiate narcotic analgesic or barbiturate doses. Narcotic or barbiturate dosage can be reduced 50 percent when hydroxyzine (Vistaril) accompanies the dose.

ADVERSE EFFECTS   Drowsiness and dryness of the mouth at high doses may occur. It is relatively free of toxic effects. Precautions with parenteral medication include injection only into deep muscle of gluteus or into vastus lateralis by Z-track technique. In correct doses, there appear to be no adverse effects in the infant during recovery.

Benzodiazepines

Benzodiazepines are prescribed more often than any other drugs in our society. Effective antianxiety drugs with few side effects, they can also be used to reduce muscle tension and spasm and to induce sleep, and they are moderately effective as anticonvulsants. Although effects are not fully understood, certain effects are thought to occur in the central nervous system, which results in a reduction in inhibition and thus anxiety. Interestingly, in some psychiatric patients, treatment has resulted in increased hostility and violence rather than calming, perhaps because of release of "anxiety-bound" hostility (Greenblatt and Shader, 1972). Chlordiazepoxide is not recommended during pregnancy, labor, or lactation (Milkovich and Van Den Berg, 1974).

Adverse Effects   Physical dependence occurs only when very large daily doses are ingested. Abrupt withdrawal then leads to agitation, insomnia, anorexia, increased psychosis, and grand mal seizures. In obstetric doses, adverse effects are not usually noted in the mother, and attention centers on the fetal and neonatal effects (see diazepam). Maternal ataxia, drowsiness, and lethargy are main side effects. Some skin rashes, nausea, and increased sensitivity to alcohol have been noted.

The chronic use of benzodiazepines should be noted if a woman wishes to become pregnant, and withdrawal should be attempted prior to conception. If taken consistently during pregnancy, the infant will show adverse signs and need careful care while withdrawing from the drug effect (see Chapter 8).

Diazepam   Although it is not recommended for use during organogenesis or for chronic administration, diazepam can be used as a premedication before general anesthesia, either orally or intravenously, and as an intravenous induction agent before general anesthesia. Diazepam's use in labor and delivery as an adjunct to analgesia has been quite common and has apparently been effective in reducing analgesic doses. However, recent studies have demonstrated (1) clearly adverse effects in the infant if the mother receives more than 30 mg within 15 hours of delivery and (2) a loss of normal beat-to-beat variability and an increase in tachycardia as noted on the fetal monitor (Mandelli et al., 1975). For these reasons, diazepam is being widely discontinued as a drug for labor. However, it is still used effectively if given just prior to delivery or just after delivery, when it acts as an effective calming agent for the mother. Studies have been shown that within 12 minutes after intravenous administration, diazepam was found to have higher cord blood levels than maternal plasma levels (Mandelli et al., 1975). The drug accumulates in fetal brain, lungs, heart, and liver and, being highly lipid-soluble, is highly protein-bound. Diazepam has been thought to displace bilirubin, although recently it has been demonstrated that the parenteral solvent propylene glycol may cause this effect. It is metabolized slowly, having a maternal $T_{1/2}$ between 20 and 40 hours and an infant $T_{1/2}$ of 21 to 45.9 hours. It is not completely eliminated for up to a week in the mother and for 8 to 10 days in the infant.

The younger the infant's gestational age, the more hazardous the effects of diazepam. Prolonged lethargy, hypotonia, hypoactivity, respiratory depression, failure to suck, and depressed reflexes have continued up to 72 hours after birth. When the affected infants were subjected to cold stress, the expected metabolic adjustment did not readily take place. In addition, even with a thermoneutral environment, a number of the infants observed had rectal temperatures of 35°C or below in the first 12 hours (Cree et al., 1973).

Benzodiazepines are not recommended during lactation, as enough drug crosses into milk to affect the infant, causing lethargy and poor sucking reflexes.

Carbamates

Meprobamate (Equanil, Miltown) is not recommended during pregnancy and lactation. Properties are very similar to barbiturates, as it suppresses REM sleep and causes some muscle relaxation. It may aggravate grand mal epilepsy, and abrupt withdrawal after chronic use results in convulsions. Meprobamate induces microsomal activity and has many drug interactions. Tolerance and physical dependence occur.

Phenothiazines

Phenothiazine derivatives have a wide variety of effects on central and peripheral nervous systems and on endocrine and metabolic functions. Effects vary because of differing chemical configurations, and drugs are chosen for the strength of these varying effects. The classic example of the family, chlorpromazine (Thorazine) is utilized in psychiatric disorders in high doses to reduce severe disturbance. Other drugs in this family have low antipsychotic effects but higher antiemetic, antihistaminic, and adrenergic or cholinergic blocking effects. Selection is made on the basis of effectiveness, degree of adverse reactions, and/or lack of production of the major effects listed in Table 6-2.

Use During Pregnancy   Studies of animals have shown some untoward effects in offspring when the parent was treated with tranquilizers. Learning and motor ability was impaired, and higher than usual numbers of offspring were born dead or died in the weaning period (Thornburg and Moore, 1976). In

Table 6-2   Common Phenothiazine Effects

Effects	Nursing Implications
1. Depresses CNS and blocks dopamine receptors in the brain with larger doses, thus reducing psychotic behavior such as delusions, hallucinations, and agitation (chlorpromarone, thioridazine).	Effective agents to reduce severe anxiety states and psychotic behavior manifestations.
2. Depresses vomiting center and chemoreceptor zone (prochlorperazine).	Control of some kinds of vomiting. Caution should be taken not to mask symptoms of serious illness.
3. Alters temperature-regulating mechanisms, causing hyperthermia or hypothermia (all).	Patients must be taught to protect themselves from extremes of heat and cold. Infants of these mothers should be observed closely for hypothermia.
4. Causes antipruretic effects due to antihistaminic effects (trimeprazine).	Other drugs are more effective to achieve this effect.
5. Depression of hypothalmus, thus releasing lactogenic hormone (all).	Long-term therapy may cause lactation (galactorrhea).
6. Alters endocrine balance and delays ovulation (all).	Large doses may delay both ovulation and cause amenorrhea.
7. Releases melanocyte-stimulating hormone from pituitary (all).	Skin pigmentation may darken; gray pigmentation may appear on areas of body.
8. Potentiates barbiturates, narcotics and alcohol, hypotensive agents, tranquilizers, atropine, sedatives (all).	Warn patient not to mix alcohol and phenothiazines. Controlled use during labor lowers need for narcotic.
9. Alters muscle tone, either causing extrapyramidal symptoms or reducing tone (primarily fluorine-substituted phenothiazines like trifluoperazine).	Not seen in small doses, but fairly common in children and adults receiving daily doses.
10. Causes orthostatic hypotension (all).	May contribute toward hypotension during labor. Watch patient position.

Table 6-2   Common Phenothiazine Effects (Continued)

Effects	Nursing Implications
11. Causes allergic reactions of dermatitis, jaundice, agranulocytosis, and photosensitivity (all).	Not usual in small doses in labor. Contact dermatitis may occur in nurse handling drug. Patients on drug should protect skin from sun.

human infants no studies have indicated clear-cut teratogenic effects of phenothiazines. Women receiving chronic antipsychotic doses may have infants who must be supported through the withdrawal period. During this period, inhibition of bonding and early adaptation might be hindered. More importantly, the time it takes to finally excrete some of the phenothiazines (up to 18 months) may be inordinately long, even in adults. Because of basically unknown long-term effects on the infant, unless the patient is in need of antipsychotic therapy, the following phenothiazines are not usually prescribed during pregnancy or labor: chlorpromazine (Thorazine), thioridazine hydrochloride (Mellaril), fluphenazine (Permitil, Prolixin), trifluoperazine hydrochloride (Stelazine), prochlorperazine (Compazine), and trimeprazine (Temaril).

The usual use for the remaining phenothiazines is in adjunct therapy with narcotic analgesics during labor. These assist in reduction of tension and provide some antiemetic effect as well. All drugs used may contribute to a transient hypotension, with a few instances of hypertension. Some stimulate respirations, thus counteracting meperidine inhibition, while others have a slight depressive effect on respirations. In the small doses used, no adverse effects should occur, but precautions should always be taken to observe hypersensitivity reactions and to observe infant responses after birth.

Dosage requirements for the phenothiazines and other antianxiety agents, including antihistamines and benzodiazepines, are listed in Table 6-3.

Table 6-3   Antianxiety Agents

Agent	Dosage	Comments
ANTIHISTAMINES		
Hydroxyzine hydrochloride (Atarax)	25–150 mg PO	Not usually used during pregnancy, but no well-recognized adverse effects have as yet been discovered.
Hydroxyzine pamoate (Vistaril)	25–150 mg PO	
Hydroxyzine hydrochloride (Vistaril IM)	25–150 mg IM *only*	Has been used as adjunct with analgesia during labor; reduces nausea, potentiates narcotic. After high doses, observe infant for sedation.
BENZODIAZEPINES		
Diazepam (Valium)	2–10 mg PO 2 to 4 times daily	Extensive tissue distribution lengthens $T_{1/2}$ to 20 to 40 h.
Diazepam injectable (solvent is propylene glycol)	2–20 mg IM or IV preoperatively, preinduction and for control of seizures.	IM: inject deeply into muscle, use Z track. IV: inject *slowly*, never faster than 5 mg per min. Avoid extravasation, for phlebitis, sloughing can occur. Do not dilute in IV fluid. Be alert for apnea and cardiac arrest. Reduce narcotic dosage by one-third when accompanying Valium.
Oxazepam (Serax) (Metabolite of Diazepam)	10–15 mg 3 to 4 times daily. PO only.	Especially useful in mild depression; has greater safety factors than those above. Conjugated with glucuronide, if in mother's system, may affect infant bilirubin levels after birth. $T_{1/2}$ 3 to 21 h.
Flurazepam (Dalmane)	15–30 mg PO hs	Hypnotic use only. Metabolized rapidly to metabolite, which has long half-life. Side effects: dizziness, drowsiness, ataxia in elderly; headache, heartburn, nausea and vomiting, constipation, apprehension, irritability. Dependency possible. May be used infrequently to induce sleep in postpartal period. Small reduction in REM time during sleep.
PHENOTHIAZINES		
Promazine (Sparine)	25–50 mg IM, IV	Excellent analgesia and sedation when combined with a narcotic during labor.

Table 6-3   Antianxiety Agents (*Continued*)

Agent	Dosage	Comments
		However, may cause labile hypotension or hypertension. Into fetal circulation by 2 min, with higher concentration at 4 to 8 min than in mother.
Prometh-azine (Phen-ergan)	25–50 mg IM, IV	Causes extra sedation with narcotic analgesic combination. Stimulates respirations. Prevents nausea and vomiting and relieves anxiety. However, also may have some transient hypotension but milder than promazine. Enters fetal blood and equilibrates by 15 min. Rare impairment of platelet aggregation in newborn.
Propio-mazine (Largon)	20 mg IM, IV	May cause some respiratory depression in adult. No adverse effects noted in infant. May cause hypotension. Avoid combination with other drugs.
Triflupro-mazine hydro-chloride (Vesprin)	During pregnancy for severe nausea and vomiting: 20–30 mg PO; 5–15 mg IM deep; 1–3 mg IV. Labor: 15 mg q 4 h IM or only at delivery, 8 mg IV once.	Many drug interactions. Check literature. Useful for severe nausea, vomiting, anxiety during pregnancy. However, benefits should outweigh risks. Do not use if solution is pink-tinged or discolored. Urine may become darker.

CHOLINERGIC BLOCKING DRUGS (ANTICHOLINERGICS)

Atropine and scopolamine in usual doses inhibit transmissions at parasympathetic nerve endings and thus inhibit secretions of saliva, tears, and sweat, and mucus secretions of respiratory and GI tracts and of the pancreas. Smooth muscle tone is somewhat relaxed, and cardiac rate is first slowed and then shows an increase. Both atropine and scopolamine are used as preoperative medications in combination with a narcotic or an ataractic.

Atropine   During anesthesia, additional doses of atropine have been used for a vagal blocking effect to counteract untoward cardiovascular effects of hypotension and bradycardia. [Although commonly supposed, atropine, either intravenous or intramuscular administration in preanesthetic doses (0.4 mg), does not increase intraocular pressure and can be safely administered to patients with wide angle glaucoma (Goodman and Gilman, 1975). However, eye drops or ointments applied locally are absolutely contraindicated for patients with any type of glaucoma.]

Scopolamine

Scopolamine has a hypnotic effect and, combined with a narcotic in correct doses, can obliterate memory for labor and delivery. Problems arise in maintaining correct effective levels, since the duration of action differs from the analgesic. During the period of diminishing narcotic effect, the persistent effect of scopolamine causes varying degrees of restlessness, excitability, and delirium. Such restlessness indicates that analgesia is incomplete and contributes to maternal exhaustion. The patient must either receive more analgesic (depending on the imminence of delivery) or have constant attendance with restraints applied to prevent injury. Patients in this phase have pulled out intravenous catheters, monitors, and climbed over side rails in an attempt to "get out of here." The mother further demonstrates flushing of skin, dry lips and tongue, and rambling, incoherent speech. Although generally forgetful of the entire experience, she will remember any threatening negative statements. On recovery, she often expresses guilt feelings about being "so difficult, talking too much."

Although for years nurses have regarded the effects of scopolamine as untoward during labor, what has finally reduced its use is the evidence on the fetal monitor record that the heartbeat moves into tachycardia and loses its beat-to-beat variability, thus masking signs of possible fetal hypoxia. Based on these findings, a number of units are no longer using scopolamine. Where it is still in use, the nurse has a special role in protecting the patient from injury by providing continuous monitoring.

Table 6-4   **Anticholinergics**

Drug	Daily Dosage	Comments
Atropine	0.2–0.6 mg IM, IV	Inhibits secretions, reduces smooth muscle tone, increases heart rate, dilates pupils, stimulates CNS, and then causes depression. Some peripheral vasodilation (flushing). Some inhibition of micturition postoperatively.
	0.2–0.6 mg PO	Used in peptic ulcer, and Parkinson's disease. Small doses occur in cold remedies.
Scopolamine	0.1–0.6 mg PO	Oral doses used for motion sickness and nonprescription sleeping medications.
	0.2–0.6 mg IM, IV	Powerful sedative or hypnotic action IM, IV. Causes amnesia when combined with narcotic. Raises FHT and erases beat-to-beat variability.

Nursing Implications

1. Inform patient of drying effect of both drugs. Provide mouth care as needed.

2. Anticipate the amnesic effects of scopolamine and provide for patient safety.

3. Note fetal heart rate before and after atropine and scopolamine administration. Note time of administration on monitor record.

4. Do not discuss patient in her hearing. Explain each procedure even if patient appears asleep.

5. Notify nursery of drugs given during labor.

6. Voiding may be inhibited by larger doses (urinary retention).

ANESTHETICS

Local and Regional Anesthesia

During labor, pain of uterine contractions and cervical dilation is transmitted to the posterior roots of the eleventh and twelfth thoracic nerves. Pain of descent and expulsion of the fetus travels by way of the posterior roots of the second, third, and fourth sacral nerves. Local anesthetics have been used effectively after active labor has begun to reduce or eliminate labor discomfort without affecting quality of uterine contractions and can also be used to achieve higher levels of anesthesia for cesarean section either by lumbar epidural, or spinal anesthesia.

Although quite effective for the mother, local anesthetics may cause some problems in the fetus and neonate, since all local anesthetics are absorbed quickly into maternal plasma. Metabolic rates vary, with *amides* (lidocaine, mepivacaine, dibucaine, bupivicaine, prilocaine) being more slowly metabolized than *esters* (procaine, cloroprocaine, tetracaine, cocaine). The rate of transfer across the placental membrane is governed by this metabolic rate in addition to the drug's molecular weight, the pH at which it remains a free nonionized base, and the degree of protein binding and lipid solubility. A number of the esters are metabolized so rapidly that there is negligible placental transfer. Most of the amides transfer freely to the fetus, each rate governed mainly by the degree of protein binding. The search has been for a substance that will transfer less quickly as a result of being highly protein-bound, ionized, and of larger molecular weight or as a result of being rapidly metabolized. Currently the amide, bupivacaine, which is 90 percent bound in maternal plasma and the ester, Nesacaine, which is rapidly metabolized in maternal plasma, are most frequently used in obstetrics.

Table 6-5 contains more information about specific regional anesthetics.

Adverse Effects   In adults, local anesthetics may cause varying degrees of vasodilation with sustained hypotension. A depressive effect on the myocardium reduces myocardial excitability and contractility, an effect that can be used therapeutically in cardiac arrythmias, e.g., lidocaine and procainamide.

Since local anesthetics easily cross the blood-brain barrier if absorbed in very large amounts, the result can be central nervous system stimulation with excitement, apprehension, disorientation, tremors, and convulsions. Hypersensitivity is unusual and involves allergic dermatitis, asthmatic attacks, or anaphylactoid reactions. Since hypersensitive reactions, although rare, can be extremely hazardous, test doses are always given prior to full injection. Ester-type anesthetics are most likely to precipitate problems. Patients should therefore be queried about prior experience with or reactions to local anesthesia, and amides can be substituted when any questions arise. Repeated contact with local anesthetic solution can be sensitizing, causing skin reactions in medical personnel.

Studies have shown that in the fetus, there is an additive effect when hypoxia and acidosis are present. Since there are normally higher concentrations of drug in fetal brain, liver, and heart, adverse effects are more severe in compromised infants. The chief adverse effect has been myocardial depression, resulting in marked bradycardia. Varying degrees of bradycardia are observed in as many as 70 percent of all cases of local anesthetic administration during labor, with the most marked instances after paracervical block (Barton, 1974).

In spite of high Apgar scores, studies have shown that during recovery, there were significant differences in the newborn neurobehavioral responses after the mother received a normal dose of local anesthetic (Scanlon et al., 1974). In that study, birth weight, gestational age, Apgar scores, pH of umbilical artery blood, routine physical examinations, and hospital courses were identical and normal in both control and lumbar epidural groups. Significant differences were found in muscle control and tone, but little difference was found in more complex habituation responses.

In another report, administration of local–regional anesthesia correlated significantly with decreased motor maturity and greater irritability during the first 24 hours of life (Standley et al., 1974). These studies have not delineated long-term effects, but point out the problems in the first 24 hours of life. The goal in obstetric medication with local anesthetics continues to be the use of the smallest effective dose of a substance which is least able to cross the placental barrier to affect the infant.

Table 6-5 Regional Anesthesia

Type of Anesthesia	Period of Labor	Location of Injection	Comments	Precautions
Paracervical block (uterosacral block)	First stage: active dilation, phase of maximum slope.	Hypogastric nerve plexus and ganglia beside cervix in each lateral fornix. Anesthesia to 2nd, 3rd, 4th sacral nerves and 11th, 12th thoracic nerves	Relieves pain of dilation but not perineal pain. Effective for 1 to 2 h. Does not inhibit uterine contractions. Because of direct absorption of local anesthetic into maternal system and transfer across placenta, has a negative inotropic, chromotropic, and dromotropic effect on fetal heart. Not used in any case of chronic fetal distress or prematurity.	Check FHT prior to and frequently after administration. Monitor closely for 30 min. Check fetal scalp vein pH whenever bradycardia persists. Bradycardia and late decelerations occur in 30 to 70% of cases. Recovery usually without any lasting effect, but cesarean section necessary if longer than 15 to 18 min or pH falling. Uterine hypertonicity may result if myometrium is infiltrated.
Pudendal block	Second stage: expulsive phase	Pudendal nerves above and behind ischial spines. Anesthesia to 2nd, 3rd, 4th sacral nerves	Blocks sensation to entire perineum but not to uterus. Must allow 5 to 10 min for anesthetic to take full effect. Additional local to site of episiotomy. Does not cover pain of manual extraction of placenta or mid-forceps delivery. Recovery takes place within 1 h.	May have one-sided effect if placement is incorrect. Aspiration for blood important as area is very vascular. Usually quite safe for mother and infant.

Table 6-5 Regional Anesthesia (Continued)

Type of Anesthesia	Period of Labor	Location of Injection	Comments	Precautions
Peridural block: Caudal (continuous)	First stage: active labor, phase of maximum slope through second stage	Insertion into sacral cornua, low block to 2nd, 3rd, 4th sacral nerves, higher block to 10th thoracic to 5th sacral. Blocks cervical and perineal pain, depending on dose and location of catheter.	Patient in knee-chest position or lateral decubitus. Test dose always administered with 5 min wait for response. Plastic cannula taped in place for future additional doses. When each dose is administered, check for bilateral anesthesia, vasodilation in legs, and toe temperature. Patient will not have sensation to bear down. Must be coached. Recovery complete by 2 to 3 h, depending on dose and type of medication.	After dose is given, patient turned supine to distribute medication to both sides. Then may assume semi-Fowler's position. Check that catheter taping is secure. Watch for hypotension in first adjustment period; elevate legs to correct. Watch for vena cava compression. During recovery, no urge to void. Delayed recovery of sphincter control may persist after full recovery or leg movement. Watch for bladder distention.
Lumbar epidural (continuous) for vaginal delivery or cesarean section	First stage: active labor through second stage	Insertion at interspace between 2nd, 3rd, or 4th lumbar, depending on desired location of catheter Anesthesia for cesarean section to 6th and 7th thoracic by insertion of catheter up toward 1st lumbar.	Lateral decubitus position with neck flexed. Contractions are not impaired, but sensation to bear down is obliterated. Check effectiveness of anesthesia and signs for hypotension q 5 min for first 20 min.	After catheter inserted and taped, semisitting position while 2 ml test dose inserted. Observe for vena cava compression and hypotension (see above for caudal). Administer IV fluids and oxygen to prevent further hypotension and hypoxia in infant. Postural hypotension possible during recovery as well as voiding problems (see above).

Subarachnoid block	Second stage or just prior to delivery	Insertion of needle at 4th lumbar through dura into spinal fluid.	Does not block contractions, but no urge to push. Must be coached.	Hypotension most common complication due to vena cava compression. Must position uterus with a lateral tilt.
Saddle block (low spinal)		Hyperbaric solution used to allow anesthetic to gravitate down toward sacral area. Anesthesia 10th thoracic to 5th sacral at level of umbilicus.	Administered in a sitting position—remain upright 90 to 120 s for solution to descend, then place supine with neck flexed on pillow. Must be well hydrated with IV fluids to alleviate hypotension. Postoperative: Usually quick recovery but kept flat 6 to 8 h as precaution against spinal headache. Watch for postural hypotension when walks.	Any coughing, pushing, or unusual movement during first few minutes may force anesthetic up spinal fluid to cause higher anesthesia.
Spinal	Just prior to cesarean section or difficult delivery	Insertion of needle at 4th lumbar through dura and into spinal fluid. Blocks to 6th to 8th thoracic.	Patient in side-lying position, neck and knees flexed. Usually obliterates contractions, so forceps and fundal pressure may be necessary for vaginal delivery.	Hypotension is most common complication. Other adverse effects: (1) back pain from muscle trauma; (2) postpuncture headache from loss of spinal fluid and stretching of meninges; patient kept flat until hydration by IV fluids restores CSF; (3) postural hypotension when first ambulatory (4) inability to void; (5) very rare, respiratory effect from medication rising in cord to affect nerves to thorax.

General Anesthesia

A variety of agents are used for general anesthesia and are administered either by inhalation or intravenous injection (Table 6-6). Within minutes, fetal levels approach maternal ones, and the dose plus time interval becomes increasingly critical, for the longer any general anesthetic is administered, the more likely it is for depression to occur in the newborn.

General inhalational anesthesia carries a risk of maternal complications as well. There is more rapid uptake because of the physiologic changes of pregnancy; vomiting and aspiration continue to be a danger, especially since digestion and stomach emptying are naturally slowed during labor, with fluids still present in spite of long periods without intake. Once muscle relaxation has been obtained, vena cava compression by the full uterus can precipitate severe hypotension. In every case, the patient must be positioned on the delivery table with a lateral tilt of the abdomen, for such hypotension causes both maternal and fetal hypoxia.

Studies by Brackbill et al. (1974) have demonstrated lasting effects on neurobehavioral responses of infants after birth under general anesthesia. The dose- and time-dependent relationship of all anesthetics and analgesics must always be recognized. Every effort must be made to reduce the need for such medications and to govern carefully the amounts and duration of exposure when analgesia/anesthesia is necessary for the parturient.

DRUGS TO DELAY PRETERM LABOR

In order to reduce the mortality in prematurely born infants, research has been directed toward inhibiting preterm labor. No agent appears to be effective once labor has entered the active phase. Therefore, studies concentrate on the latent period when dilation of 0–5 cm and most cervical effacement take place. Three major types of agents are currently being investigated. With a few exceptions, these drugs are not released for general use. Therefore, the pregnant woman should be fully informed of risks and benefits prior to institution of therapy in a research setting.

Table 6-6 General Anesthetics

Anesthetic	Absorption, Fate, Excretion	Effect	Comments
INHALATION ANESTHETICS			
Diethyl ether, ether	Absorbed through pulmonary epithelium. Slow induction but well marked planes of anesthesia. Eliminated unchanged by lungs with very small amount metabolized (<10%).	Depresses CNS at all levels with excellent muscle relaxation. Stimulates secretions and increases respiratory rate, heart rate. Supraventricular arrhythmias may occur. Decreases renal function. *Toxicity*: with overdose—respiratory arrest.	Irritating to respiratory tract; patient may gag, cough, and have laryngospasm. Extra secretions from upper respiratory tract. Usually given with preoperative atropine. Watch urine output. Artificial ventilation removes ether from system and restores respirations. Postoperative: Nausea and vomiting common after ether anesthesia persisting into recovery period.
Halothane (Fluothane)	Administered with nitrous oxide to obtain quicker analgesia and hasten anesthesia. 80% pulmonary exchange with 20% excreted through urine; however, may be stored in body tissue for long periods, and metabolites may have some toxicity.	Produces stage IV anesthesia without oxygen loss. Causes mild cerebral vasodilation and also causes arterial hypotension because of generalized vasodilation. Alterations in cardiac rhythm may occur. *Toxicity*: acute hypotension. Fetal toxicity occurs with prolonged anesthesia. Ventricular arrhythmias may occur if catecholamines are injected.	Most commonly used anesthetic except for obstetric patients. Nonirritating to respiratory tract. Causes bronchiolar dilation, therefore useful with asthmatic patients. Since has smooth muscle dilation effect, strongly inhibits uterine tonus, and reduces responses to oxytocics. Rarely used in obstetrics. Used when uterine relaxation is desired effect. Not used with cardiac, renal, or liver disease. Profound hypotension must be prevented. Must be used with adjunct

Table 6-6 General Anesthetics (Continued)

Anesthetic	Absorption, Fate, Excretion	Effect	Comments
			medication and neuromuscular blockers because does not cause adequate muscle relaxation. Postoperative: Shivering may occur to increase body temperature. Provide blankets. Nausea and vomiting rare in recovery. Watch for hypotension. Observe for delayed awakening. Observe for extra bleeding. Check fundal contraction after delivery.
Fluoroxene (Fluoromar)	Similar to halothane but less potent. Does not appear to adversely affect infant if given less than 10 min before delivery.	Excites sympathetic activity, produces cardiac stability. Does not cause vasodilation.	Flammable but not explosive. Can be used when patient is in hemorrhagic shock, or central, peripheral circulatory failure. After 10 min, look for depression of infant.
Methoxyflurane (Penthrane)	Extensively metabolized and excreted slowly. Used with nitrous oxide and muscle relaxants or barbiturates.	Most potent inhalation agent, with good muscle relaxation, but because of slow induction (up to 20 min), other agents are added. Depresses respirations and causes mild hypotension and sometimes bradycardia. Some question of toxicity of metabolites and long-	Nausea and vomiting infrequent, non-irritating to respiratory tract. Does not cause laryngospasm. Tolerated well by asthmatics. Special care with obstetric patients on the time–dose interval because 70% of maternal level is in fetal system by 10 to 15 min. Some very low Apgar scores

Drug	Metabolism/Excretion	Effects	Comments/Nursing Implications
		lasting neurobehavioral effect on infants. Delirium during induction not uncommon.	after prolonged administration. In very low doses, has been used for inhalational analgesia throughout active labor, without apparent adverse effect on Apgar score. Postoperative: Very slow recovery since slowly metabolized.
Enflurane (Enthrane)	Very little metabolism, 85% expired; therefore less danger of toxic metabolites than halothane.	Anesthesia similar to that obtained with halothane with some respiratory depression. Arterial hypotension common. Sensitizes myocardium to catecholamines, and if used with them, may cause ventricular extrasystoles. Temporary depression of kidney, liver function.	Nonflammable, chemically stable. Occasional seizurelike EEG patterns noted plus involuntary movements. Newly introduced anesthetic (1973). Information incomplete about fetal response. Postoperative: Observe for hypotension. Check urine output. Observe for involuntary muscle movements.
Nitrous oxide	Low solubility in blood. Excreted unchanged through lungs, small amount through skin.	Cannot produce deep planes of anesthesia; therefore, used most often with IV barbiturates and supplemented with other agents. In subanesthetic doses, provides extensive analgesia, especially useful during 2nd stage labor. Does not provide muscular relaxation.	Nonflammable, but supports a flame. Caution must be taken to prevent hypoxia. Few side effects with normal doses, but nausea and vomiting may occur. Nonirritating to respiratory tract. Postoperative: Quick recovery depending on adjunct medication.
Cyclopropane	Must be given with anticholinergic preoperatively. Absorbed and eliminated through	Can produce any desired level of anesthesia, with muscular relaxation. Some respiratory depres-	Flammable and explosive. Rapid induction of 2 to 3 min. Minimal irritation to respiratory tract, but

Table 6-6 General Anesthetics (*Continued*)

Anesthetic	Absorption, Fate, Excretion	Effect	Comments
	lungs. Recovery very rapid, with only traces left by 3 h after delivery.	sion but spontaneous respirations can be maintained during anesthesia. Some increase in blood pressure due to increased peripheral resistance. Stimulation of sympathetic nerves to myocardium; cardiac rate slows. Arrhythmias may occur if catecholamines are added during administration. Smooth muscle constriction is expected and reduced flow to renal and hepatic tissue. Incidence and magnitude of fetal depression is directly related to depth and duration of cyclopropane administration.	some salivation unless given atropine-like preoperatively. Laryngospasm possible, sometimes delirium. Not used for asthmatics. Increased blood flow to skin and muscles; therefore, some extra bleeding at wound may occur. Enhances intestinal muscle tone and maintains uterine tone. Postoperative: Nausea and vomiting frequent during recovery. Some recovery delirium unless narcotic administered IV prior to termination of anesthesia. Prepare to give narcotic in half dose soon in recovery room. Hypotension and headache fairly common. Observe wound for oozing. Check urine output.

INTRAVENOUS ANESTHETICS

Anesthetic	Absorption, Fate, Excretion	Effect	Comments
Thio barbiturates: thiopental (Pentohal), thiamylal (Surital)	Penetrates all body tissues, so initial high effect on brain diminished quickly as drug diffuses and distributes to fat and lean tissue. Final elimination after many hours. Crosses placenta rapidly but does	Very short acting; blocks brain stem core. Does not provide analgesia until higher doses administered. Usually used for induction hypnosis accompanied by inhalational anesthetics.	Laryngospasm, bronchospasm may occur, especially in asthmatics. Cold clammy skin due to peripheral vasoconstriction may be seen. Depresses respirations, reduces cardiac output, but increases total periph-

Drug	Administration	Action	Effects
	not depress infant unless dose larger than 6.3 mg/kg is used and total dose over 250–300 mg.		eral resistance. Depresses aortic and carotid chemoreceptors as well as respiratory center. Postoperative: Recovery may include restlessness because of sensing pain. Shivering may occur due to hypothermia. Vomiting is minimal.
Ketamine hydrochloride (Ketaject, Ketalar)	Given IV, IM; may be used for rapid induction followed by nitrous oxide for anesthesia.	Causes "dissociative" anesthesia. Patient is awake and without respiratory depression. Elevates heart rate 10 to 25% and cardiac output, has antiarrhythmic effect. Traverse placenta rapidly so that if 5 to 10 min elapse, infant is depressed and newborn is *hypertonic*, so that resuscitation is difficult.	Valuable for procedures about the head and neck. Analgesia and anesthesia good, but muscle relaxation is poor. Cough reflex is depressed however, and aspiration has occurred. Postoperative: Nausea and vomiting infrequent. Prolonged recovery period sometimes with bad dreams. In some patients, these dream episodes recur for days or weeks. Usually not used in delivery situations.
Nonbarbiturates (neuroleptic-narcotic combinations): dioperidol (Inapsine) plus fenanyl citrate (Sublimaze) as Innovar	Intravenous injection over a period of 5 to 10 min. Administered with atropine as preoperative medication and accompanied by nitrous oxide if anesthesia desired. Also can be administered IM as a preoperative preparation for difficult procedures.	3 to 5 min later, anesthetic effect evident. Produces mild to moderate arteriolar hypotension and bradycardia. Respiratory depression may occur.	Too rapid injection causes chest-wall spasm. Given alone without nitrous oxide, provides a state of psychic indifference to difficult procedures. Patient remains awake. Postoperative: Nausea and vomiting. Grogginess may persist for 24 h.

Selected Beta₂-Receptor Stimulants

Beta₂-receptor stimulants have been approved for use with asthmatics. Each has shown effective action, relieving bronchospasm when inhaled as a powder or aerosol. However, inhibition of myometrial contractions occurs best when intravenous infusions are used to initiate response. Then, doses are lowered and drugs administered either by intramuscular or oral routes.

Adverse Effects Major adverse effects of these drugs when administered for asthma are discussed in Chapter 5. When given by continuous intravenous infusion, these drugs may initiate postural hypotension, nausea, vomiting, dizziness, trembling, nervousness, and weakness. Tachycardia (average increase of 30 beats per minute) and some degree of hypotension (decrease of 10–15 mmHg) may occur. Vital signs should stabilize as treatment continues and infusion flow is regulated to achieve desired reductions in contraction frequency and intensity. If hypotension becomes severe, uterine perfusion will be reduced, and fetal bradycardia will reflect the increasing fetal hypoxia.

Nursing Implications

1. Because of hypotensive responses, position the patient in the left lateral decubitus position while she is receiving the drug. Monitor vital signs frequently, especially in the initial period. Less frequent intervals are sufficient after stabilization.

2. Continuous monitoring of uterine responses is necessary until pattern slows and patient is placed on intramuscular or oral doses.

3. Be prepared to assist patient because of initial reactions of vomiting, nervousness, weakness. Maintain bed rest.

Isoxsuprine (Vasodilan) Isoxsuprine is accepted as an effective agent to inhibit uterine contractions. Titration is necessary to prevent hypotension and fetal distress. Glucose levels may be increased, and infants should be observed for hypoglycemia in the nursery.

DOSAGE By means of infusion, a dose of 0.25–0.5 mg per minute is given. After stabilization of contraction patterns, 5–20 mg may be given, either IM or PO, q 3 to 6 h for 3 to 10 days.

Ritodrine (Premar) Still under investigation, ritodrine has proved effective if treatment is initiated before 4 cm dilatation. Titration is necessary. Close monitoring and careful patient positioning is important, since hypotension does occur. The patient may be discharged on oral medication.

Fenoterol (Berotec), Metaproterenol (Alupent, Metaprel), Salbutamol (Ventalin), Terbutaline (Brincanyl) These effective antispasmodic agents appear to have less cardiovascular effect than other beta₂-receptor stimulants. Fetal and long-term effects on the infant are still being studied, and the drugs are not widely available.

Ethanol Ethyl alcohol has been used to delay preterm labor with moderate success (70 percent). Action appears to be by the inhibition of oxytocin release from the hypothalamus. It does not appear to affect injected oxytocin (Fuchs, 1967). Labor can be best delayed if treatment is begun before significant cervical dilation has occurred.

Transfer across the placenta is prompt, with fetal levels rapidly equalling maternal levels. Alcohol is metabolized by the liver (maternal rate—7 g/h) and although the fetus can metabolize alcohol, the $T_{1/2}$ is twice that of the mother. The newborn who is born shortly after alcohol therapy will demonstrate drug effect, which will then last for a longer period than in its mother. The very young infant may be further compromised by immature hepatic function.

Adverse Effects In order to inhibit contractions, blood levels of 0.09 to 0.16 percent have been deemed necessary. The patient will demonstrate signs and symptoms of mild to moderate intoxication: slurred speech, headache, sedation, flushed face, elevated pulse, lack of control, mood swings (talking, crying). Especially in the initial period, vomiting with possible aspiration is a very serious problem. For this reason, some physicians order an antiemetic as therapy begins. Urinary incontinence may occur because of increased diuresis, the patient being unable to cooperate at times.

Interactions are to be expected with analgesics, sedatives, antianxiety agents, and anesthetics (potentiation). Moderation of dosages is necessary if the patient progresses into active labor. Numerous other interactions occur, and tables should be consulted, especially if the patient has been receiving anticoagulants, diuretics, and insulin (severe hypoglycemia).

Fetal Alcohol Syndrome   Some women will be concerned about alcohol and potential damage to the fetus. The fetal alcohol syndrome is described well by Mulvihill and Yeager (1976) and Jones and Smith (1975) as a specific pattern of malformations including prenatal and postnatal growth retardation, mental retardation, small head size, and minor abnormalities of eye, face, heart, joints, and external genitalia. The inquiring patient can be assured that the effect of alcohol for inhibition of preterm labor is safe, given the usual guidelines. These extreme adverse effects occurred when the mother had been a severe, chronic alcoholic of several years' duration. In two studies, 26 and 43 percent of the infants were so affected, directly in proportion to the degree of alcohol ingestion (Heinonen et al., 1977).

Newborn Adverse Effects   Signs of elevated blood levels in the newborn infant may include CNS depression with hypotonia, hiccups, hypothermia, hypoglycemia, and changes in acid-base balance. In addition, the chronic use of alcohol by the mother may induce hepatic microsomal activity and affect metabolism of drugs in the infant (see Chapter 7).

Dosage   Using a 9.5% ethyl alcohol solution, 15 ml/kg per hour for 2 h is given IV by an electric infusion pump. The dose is then reduced to 1.5 ml/kg per hour for the next 6 h (some continue it for 10 h). The infusion is stopped if labor progresses more than 4 cm or if membranes rupture.

Nursing Implications

1. Close observation is of primary importance, with safety maintained.

2. Expect nausea and vomiting. Tracheal suction and emesis basin should be easily available. The patient should be kept NPO, and mouth care should be administered as necessary.

3. Expect diuresis and perhaps incontinence. Pad bed. Offer bedpan.

4. Maintain patient in bed, in side-lying position if possible. Continue bed rest for 24 hours after treatment.

5. Monitor response to drug and heart rate elevation in mother and fetus. Contraction rate should decrease below 3 per 10 minutes, and intensity should diminish.

6. Continue close observation when patient is transferred back to antepartum unit, because labor may begin to intensify again as alcohol is excreted.

7. Recovery period may take up to 12 hours. Patient may have signs and symptoms of a "hangover." Administer comfort measures, ice compress to head, diet modifications, etc.

Antiprostaglandins

Agents which inhibit prostaglandin production (aspirin, indomethacin) are being studied for inhibition of myometrial contractility. A retrospective study showed that aspirin in large doses (>3250 mg/day) taken by patients with arthritic or collagen diseases appeared to delay the onset of labor by at least 2 days and increase the duration of labor by more than 5 hours over the time periods noted in carefully matched controls (Lewis and Schulman, 1973).

Zuckerman et al. (1974) have demonstrated indomethacin effectiveness in doses of 100 mg rectally, followed by 25 mg orally every 6 hours up to a total of 200–1100 mg. No adverse effects have been noted in infants in their study after 2 years of follow-up.

Adverse Effects Adverse effects of indomethacin used in long-term treatment as an anti-inflammatory, antirheumatic agent are numerous. However, maternal side effects with dosages such as those above include only headache, dizziness, hypersensitivity, nausea, and GI bleeding. To date, these agents, although apparently effective, are not approved because of still unknown effects on fetal circulation. It is feared that antiprostaglandins may induce premature closure of ductus arteriosus, since they have been used for this purpose in the neonatal period (see Chapter 9).

DRUGS USED TO STIMULATE UTERINE CONTRACTIONS

A number of drugs exhibit oxytocic activity, but only a few are clinically useful: oxytocin, ergot alkaloids, and prostaglandins. Oxytocin, normally secreted throughout pregnancy, is blocked by high progesterone levels, but the uterus becomes increasingly responsive as the time of labor approaches. Ergot alkaloids cause nonphysiologic contractions and are never used prior to delivery. Prostaglandins exert action throughout pregnancy and one, *Prostin F2 alpha* is being used for induction of midterm abortion.

Ergot Alkaloids

Ergonovine Maleate (Ergotrate) and Methylergonovine Maleate (Methergine) Both drugs cause firm, extended contractions of the uterus. There is an initial sustained tetanic contraction and then a series of minor relaxations and vigorous contractions extending over 3 or more hours after injection. Their use, therefore, is only for postpartum hemmorhage, subinvolution, and postabortion bleeding.

ADVERSE EFFECTS Vasoconstrictive responses underlie adverse effects of nausea and vomiting (especially with intravenous route), hypertension, and in excessive doses, peripheral vasoconstriction. Diaphoresis, dizziness, headache, palpitation, tinnitus, dyspnea, and temporary chest pain can occur. When spinal or epidural anesthesia, and oxytocic induction or stimulation of labor have been used, or if vasopressors have been given, hypertension may be serious. Chlorpromazine, 15 mg, appears to be an effective antidote. Occasionally, patients may have hypersensitive reactions. The drugs should not routinely be given intravenously because of this possibility of inducing sudden hypertension and cerebrovascular accidents. (If essential, they must be given slowly over 60 seconds with continuous blood pressure readings.) Finally, ergot alkaloids may suppress lactation.

DOSAGE 0.2 mg (1 ml) IM q 6 h until hemorrhage is controlled. IV (slowly); may repeat in 2 to 4 h if necessary. 0.2 mg PO bid, qid usually for 24 h (maximum, 1 wk).

NURSING IMPLICATIONS
1. In the delivery room, be sure of timing of dose—just after placental separation if given intravenously (effect immediate), or in some cases, ordered with delivery of anterior shoulder when given intramuscularly (effect 2 to 5 min).

2. Do not give just before infant feeding (bottle), as mother becomes uncomfortable. Often administered with analgesic.

3. Not recommended for lactating mother unless hemorrhaging. Give infant formula for one feeding after ergotrate dose. Symptoms of excess amount in infant are vomiting, diarrhea, cardiovascular changes.

4. Check blood pressure and history of hypertension before administering. Follow vital signs after dose as well.

5. Refrigerate parenteral medication, and protect from light. If solution is yellow, discard.

Prostaglandins

First identified in semen, prostaglandins (17 have been identified) have been subsequently found in many body tissues. Since they appear in higher than normal levels during labor and in amniotic fluid, their role in initiating or sustaining labor is being intensively studied. Many therapeutic and adverse effects result from contraction of smooth muscle (especially PGF_2). Since these substances are so widely distributed, and their effects so numerous, they are still under study. Clinical use is limited to research centers.

Certain prostaglandins appear to be effective in inducing midtrimester abortion, whereas oxytocin is ineffective at that time (16 to 20 weeks). Oral PGE_2 has been used for induction of labor as well as intravenous PGF_2, but neither drug is yet released for routine labor induction. Contractions are physiologic and parallel oxytocin-induced contractions, but hypertonus appears somewhat more likely (Anderson and Schooley, 1975). It may take at least an hour for the effect to wear off (Beasley, 1971) in contrast to the short half-life of oxytocin. Since contractions of umbilical and placental vessels have also been noted, using prostaglandins for labor induction may place a borderline fetus into further jeopardy.

Dinoprost Tromethamine (Prostin F2 Alpha) PGF_2 may be the drug of choice for midterm abortion, causing fewer problems than hypertonic saline and a shorter period until abortion. All routes of administration except intra-amniotic have had unacceptable levels of adverse effects, especially nausea, vomiting, and diarrhea (smooth muscle contraction). The low dose given into amniotic fluid has been effective with mean installation-to-abortion interval between 8 and 20 hours (*AMA Drug Evaluations*). However, the drug's use is still under investigation.

ADVERSE EFFECTS   Gastrointestinal upsets: nausea and vomiting and diarrhea are common (50 percent) especially after oral doses. High doses also cause tachycardia, flushing, and fever. Sometimes severe bronchospasm occurs (contraindicated in asthmatics), and chest pain, hiccups, and dysuria have been noted. Laceration of the cervix, retention of placenta, and hemorrhage are major complications but may be less common than with the hypertonic saline method. Accidental intravenous administration into maternal uterine blood vessels after amniocentesis results in severe hypotension, shock, severe cramping, vomiting, and diarrhea (duration 15 to 30 minutes). Corrective therapy must be quickly available.

DOSAGE All routes under investigation. Intra-amniotic: After tap of fluid, 40 mg dinoprost injection slowly with test dose of 1 ml injected over 1 to 2 min. Then, 10–20 mg repeated in 6 h if progress has not been made.

Extra-Amniotic: 14–16 Foley catheter with 30 ml balloon inserted through cervix into lower uterine segment. 0.5 mg test dose followed by several repeated instillations of 0.75–1.0 mg until abortion occurs.

NURSING IMPLICATIONS
1. Be sure patient is instructed about procedure and follow-up.

2. Usually, intramuscular antiemetic administered prior to and during labor period.

3. Results are more rapid than with hypertonic saline. Be alert for progress of cervical dilation.

4. Be prepared for adverse effect of severe hypotension. Check vital signs frequently just after test dose and completion of procedure.

Oxytocin (Pitocin, Syntocinon)

Oxytocin selectively affects uterine muscle and myoepithelial tissues of the mammary glands (milk ejection). A very short half-life of 1 to 3 minutes is a safeguard in therapy, since once an intravenous injection is stopped, metabolism occurs quickly, and the effect is diminished to a safe level. "Oxytocinase," which appears to deactivate oxytocin, is found in placental and uterine tissues in higher levels during the labor period. Oxytocin is used to induce or stimulate labor in the latter part of pregnancy but is ineffective in the first and second trimesters because of high levels of circulating progesterone. After delivery, it is used to control hemorrhage. Its short half-life must then be taken into account, for when an infusion is discontinued, the effect is rapidly diminished. Recently, oxytocin has been utilized for a "trial run" of labor, the oxytocin challenge test.

Oxytocin Challenge Test   Prior to the due date, a high-risk mother is given a trial infusion of low-dose oxytocin in 5% dextrose in water infusion to determine fetal response to mild labor contractions. For a period of 30 minutes, after three contractions per 10 minutes have been induced (total nine contractions), signs of fetal intolerance to pressure and normally reduced uteroplacental flow is noted on the monitor. If late decelerations occur, it is inferred that the fetus is in a borderline condition and would not tolerate the stress of labor. Results of this test are always considered with estriol levels and L/S ratios before a conclusion is drawn about the course of action.

Induction   Under normal circumstances, most women need no stimulus to begin labor. Induction is used when a problem indicates that the normal body processes need to be augmented. Induction (the use of agents to bring on the onset of labor) and stimulation (the use of agents to increase the speed and intensity of labor) should both require a situation that demands intervention in the body timing.

Under ordinary circumstances, the blocks to uterine contractility are extremely effective. The processes during prelabor which normally take several weeks prior to the beginning of regular contractions and dilation must be effected within a few hours during induction. These changes are movement of the head into the pelvic inlet to engagement station, stretching of the lower uterine segment and upper vaginal wall, and softening (ripening) of the cervix.

If induction is begun before the cervix is ready, there will be a time lag before true labor begins. An oxytocin infusion may be administered for 8 to 12 hours and then discontinued so that the patient can sleep. The following morning, marked changes may be seen in the progressive cervical effacement. Contractions during this period are painless and yet effective.

If induction is used after the cervix is ready, the nurse must understand that the patient goes through the same "work of labor," only over a shorter span of time. Thus the total pressure needed (measured in Montevideo units) to dilate the cervix completely and to cause the descent and expulsion of the fetus is the same as for spontaneous labor, but the contractions may be more intense, more frequent, and longer in duration. The individual sensitivity to oxytocin changes from phase to phase of labor and from woman to woman, so that the dosage must be adjusted by her response to the infusion.

ADVERSE EFFECTS   The chief adverse effect is uterine hypertonus during labor, which if uncorrected, results in uterine rupture, cervical or perineal tears, and in rare cases, amniotic fluid embolism. Damage to the fetus results from impaired uteroplacental blood flow (hypoxia) and from the extreme pressure (intracranial hemorrhage). With large doses such as might be given for abortion (>20 mU per minute) a mild antidiuretic effect of oxytocin may result in water intoxication.

Oxytocin in large doses may have an opposite, transient effect of relaxing smooth muscle, thus precipitating transient hypotension, especially decreasing diastolic pressure. This period is followed by a sustained rise in blood pressure. Finally anaphylactoid reactions have occurred. Interactions with other drugs include diminished effect in the presence of vasodilating drugs, smooth muscle relaxants, and a potentiating effect with other oxytocics. Some questions of elevated bilirubin levels in newborns after oxytocin induction have not been completely answered (Drew and Kitchner, 1977).

DOSAGE   Oxytocin, IM, IV 10 U/1 ml = 10,000 mU, always diluted in 500–100 ml of 5% dextrose in water solution for IV use and administered via an electric infusion pump, so that the *average* dose for induction is as follows:

Initially: 0.2–0.4 mU per minute as a test dose, with rate increased at intervals until three to four moderately strong contractions occur in a 10-min interval. Rate is stabilized during the latent phase of labor. Then when the phase of maximum slope begins, the rate should be set at no more than 7 mU/min. Infusion is stopped if good labor contractions are sustained without oxytocin.

Postpartum injection IV: 0.6–1.8 U diluted in 3–5 ml normal saline given slowly IV. Avoid bolus (*AMA Drug Evaluations*).

Postpartum hemorrhage: 10 U/500 ml 5% dextrose in water at 125 ml per hour—(40 mU per minute or 2.4 U per hour). 10 U may also be given IM.

Oxytocin citrate—buccal tablets: 200 U per tablet. One sublingually q 30 min until desired effect (unpredictable absorption, much inactivated by gastric trypsin, therefore uncommonly used).

NURSING IMPLICATIONS

1. Very few patients can tolerate oxytocin-augmented contractions. Usually, some analgesia will be needed.

2. Oxytocin sensitivity varies from person to person and from phase to phase of labor. The patient may indicate her progress in labor by a change in her response to oxytocin.

3. The setup, observation, and maintenance of a problem-free infusion fall within nursing measures, but the obstetrician is responsible for beginning the intravenous infusion and for adjusting dosage (which includes remaining with the patient for a sufficient period after each change in rate or dosage to ensure a problem-free administration). The physician must be within call for unexpected problems.

4. An infusion pump is the preferred means of controlling the rate of flow; tubing is inserted as a piggyback addition to an infusion of 5% dextrose in water solution.

5. Labor may be substantially shortened and may move toward delivery more rapidly than expected. Therefore, close observation is mandatory.

6. Because labor is speeded up, there will be more pressure on the head (presenting part), less recovery time between contractions, and greater possibility of fetal distress. Therefore, fetal heart tones must be regularly observed. [Hon (1969) recommends a minimum of every 10 min.] External or internal monitoring of each patient is highly recommended.

7. The nurse should shut off the infusion at the first indication of a hypertonic or tetanic contraction and notify physician. The nurse must never flush the intravenous tubing or manipulate a poorly running intravenous infusion in such a way as to inject larger doses of oxytocin into the vein.

BIBLIOGRAPHY

American Hospital Formulary Service: "Current Drug Therapy—Barbiturates," *American Journal of Hospital Pharmacy*, **33**:333, April 1976.

Anderson, G.G., and G.L. Schooley: "Comparison of Uterine Contractions in Spontaneous and Oxytocin—or PGF$_2$—Induced Labor" *Obstetrics and Gynecology*, **45**:284–86, March 1975.

Barden, T.P.: "Premature Labor, Its Management and Therapy," *Journal of Reproductive Medicine*, 9(3):113, September 1972.

Barton, Dennis M.: "Obstetrical Anesthesia," Mead Johnson Symposium, June 1974.

Beasley, J.M.: "The Induction of Labor with Prostaglandins," *Research in Prostaglandins*, 1(2):1, 1971.

*Brackbill, Y., J. Kane, R.L. Maniello, and D. Abramson: "Obstetric Meperidine Usage and Assessment of Neonatal Status," *Anesthesiology*, **40**:116, February 1974.

Cooper, J.M., Sorronoff, and R.J., Bolognese: "Oxytocin Challenge Test in Monitoring High-Risk Pregnancies," *Obstetrics and Gynecology*, **45**:27–33, January 1975.

Cree, J.E., J. Meyer, and D.M. Haeley: "Diazepam in Labor: Its Metabolism and Effect On The Clinical Condition and Thermogenesis of the Newborn," *British Medical Journal*, 4:251, 1973.

*Denotes particularly pertinent references.

Dancis, J. (ed.): *Perinatal Pharmacology*, Raven Press, New York, 1974.

Fuchs, Fritz: "Effect of Alcohol on Threatened Premature Labor," *American Journal of Obstetrics and Gynecology*, 99:627, 1967.

Drew, J.H., and W.H. Kitchner: "The Effect of Maternally Administered Drugs on Bilirubin Concentrations in the Newborn Infant," *Journal of Pediatrics*, 89(4):657, 1977.

Goodman, L.S., and A. Gilman (eds.): *The Pharmacological Basis of Therapeutics*, 5th ed., MacMillan; New York, 1975, pp. 397–401.

Gottshalk, W. (ed.): "Anesthesia in Obstetrics," *Clinical Obstetrics and Gynecology*, 17(2):139–287, June 1974.

Grad, R.K., and J. Woodside: "Obstetrical Analgesia and Anesthesia," *American Journal of Nursing*, 77:241, February 1977.

Greenblatt, D.J., and R.I. Shader: "The Clinical Choice of Sedative-Hypnotics," *Annals of Internal Medicine*, 77:91, 1972.

———, and ———: "Benzodiazepines," *New England Journal of Medicine*, 291(23):1011, 1974.

Halbert, D.R., L.M. Demers, and D.E. Darnell-Jones: "Dysmenorrhea and Prostaglandins," *Obstetrical and Gynecological Survey*, 31(1):77, 1976.

*Heinonen, O.P., D. Slone, and S. Shapiro: *Birth Defects and Drugs in Pregnancy*, PSG Publishing, Littleton, Mass., 1977.

Hon, Edward R.: An Introduction to Fetal Heart Monitoring, Harty Press, New Haven, 1969.

Hyo, J.C.: "Arresting Premature Labor," *American Journal of Nursing*, 76(5):810 May 1976.

Jones, K.L., and D.W. Smith: "The Fetal Alcohol Syndrome," *Teratology*, 12:1, 1975.

Lewis, R.B., and J.D. Schulman: "Influence of Acetylsalicylic Acid on the Duration of Human Gestation and Labor," *Lancet*, 2:1159, 1973.

Mandelli, M., et al.: "Placental Transfer of Diazepam and Its Disposition in the Newborn," *Clinical Pharmacology and Therapeutics*, 17:564, 1975.

*McDonald, J.S.: "Preanesthetic and Intrapartal Medications," *Clinical Obstetrics and Gynecology*, 20(2):447, June 1977.

Milkovich L., and B.J. Van Den Berg: "Effects of Prenatal Meprobamate and Chlordiazepoxide Hydrochloride on Human Embryonic and Fetal Development," *New England Journal of Medicine*, 291:1286, December 12, 1974.

Mulvihill, J.J., and A.M. Yeager: "Fetal Alcohol Syndrome," *Teratology*, 13:345, 1976.

Scanlon, J.W., W.U. Brown, J.B. Weiss, and M.H. Alper: "Neurobehavioral Responses of Newborn Infants After Maternal Epidural Anesthesia," *Anesthesiology*, 40:121, February 1974.

Schinder, S.M. (ed.) and F. Moya; "Post Graduate Seminar of Anesthesiology," *The Anesthesiologist, Mother and Newborn*, Williams & Wilkins, Baltimore, 1974.

Standley, K., A.B. Soule III, S.A. Copans, and N.S. Duchowney: "Local-Regional Anesthesia During Childbirth: Effect on Newborn Behaviors," *Science*, 186:635, June 1974.

*Tepperman, H.M., S.N. Beydoun, and R.W. Abdul-Karim: "Drugs Affecting Myometrial Contractility in Pregnancy," *Clinical Obstetrics and Gynecology*, 20(2):423–445, June 1977.

Thornburg, J.E., and K.E. Moore: "Pharmacologically Induced Modifications of Behavioral and Neurochemical Development," in B.L. Mirkin (ed.), *Perinatal Pharmacology and Therapeutics*, Academic Press, New York, 1976, Chap 4, p. 331.

Zuckerman, H., U. Reiss, and I. Rubenstein: "Inhibition of Human Preterm Labor by Indomethacin," *Obstetrics and Gynecology*, 44:787, December 1974.

7

Drugs and the Newborn

Elizabeth J. Dickason
Elaine Muller Morris

For the human infant the period of growth should be regarded
as a continuum of development during which body functions
mature at varying rates. In considering drug administration
to the newborn infant, individual differences resulting from
genetic makeup, nutritional status, and state of recovery from
the birth process should be considered in addition to gestational maturity. Furthermore, although the preterm infant
is, in many ways, physiologically different from the full-term
infant, both mature rapidly after the first postnatal days of
adjustment. These changes, as well as the very rapid growth
rate seen in the neonatal and infancy periods, make drug
effects somewhat variable and unpredictable. Newborn infants, therefore need extremely careful observation of signs
and symptoms related to drug effect, both beneficial and
adverse.

Drug dosage for newborn infants cannot be determined by
the usual rules for children and are often based upon preliminary data applied to incompletely understood physiology.
Each infant should be considered individually, assessing its
current physiologic status before drug administration. The
following discussion should assist the nurse in understanding
why infants respond differently clinically and why dosages

The authors gratefully acknowledge discussions with, and advice
freely given by, Dr. S. Ganapathy concerning this chapter.

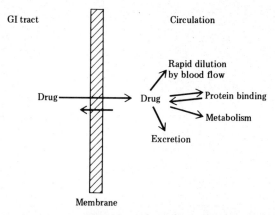

Figure 7-1   Drug distribution after oral administration. (*After R. Bressler and P. Walson, "Drug Absorption, Distribution, Metabolism and Excretion," Symposium on Perinatal and Developmental Medicine, Mead Johnson, June 1975, p. 4.*)

often vary between infants and within periods in a given infant's development.

ABSORPTION

Absorption of Oral Medication

Absorption from the GI tract involves drug transfer across the membranes (layers of lipoprotein cells) lining the stomach and intestines. Fat-soluble molecules penetrate easily through these membranes by diffusion. Smaller water-soluble molecules move with water through the microscopic pores in the membranes, while larger water-soluble molecules must be transported by proteins in the membrane, linked for this membrane passage, and then unlinked on the other side. Once across the membrane, the drug molecule moves into the plasma and is transported to its site of action (Fig. 7–1).

Although there is a lack of specific information about absorption of drugs from the newborn GI tract, several general physiologic factors are thought to be of significance in the neonatal period.

1. At birth the gastric contents are highly alkaline as a result of the presence of swallowed amniotic fluid. The stomach rapidly begins excreting hydrochloric acid, and its contents become progressively more acidic. This lower newborn gastric pH results in increased absorption of acidic drugs in the stomach as compared with the small intestine.

2. In the term infant, rapid gastric emptying allows some acidic drugs to be passed into the intestine before the absorption process is completed. However, slower transit time through the bowel may allow a longer period for contact of drug molecule with membranes.

3. Specialized transport mechanisms in the intestine may be absent or deficient, depending on gestational maturity. Absence of these developmental mechanisms may hinder movement of those drugs which do not cross into plasma by simple diffusion, e.g., riboflavin, which is absorbed less readily by the preterm infant.

4. Finally, drugs which require partial metabolic alteration in the intestinal tract for absorption may be inadequately broken down as a result of deficiences of enzymes, bile salts, and/or intestinal flora (Giacoia and Gorodisher, 1975). These deficiencies, most prominent in the preterm infant, often result in reduced absorption of fat soluble drugs. It should be noted, however, that maturation of these functions may proceed at different rates and vary from baby to baby.

All these variables must be considered when the oral route of drug administration is chosen. Since many of these variables are not completely studied in sick or small infants, the oral route is not usually the method of choice for drug administration for these infants.

Dermatomucosal Medication

Specially prepared medications placed on skin or mucous membrane are usually absorbed rapidly, since the thin immature stratum corneum is much more permeable to lipid-soluble substances in infancy than later in childhood (Solomon and Esterly, 1971). Extreme caution with topical medications is thus warranted, especially in the preterm infant, whose skin acts like a highly porous membrane.

Central nervous system changes resulting from the use of hexachlorophene demonstrate severe toxicity resulting from systemic absorption of an agent formerly thought to be "benign." Studies showed that infants washed daily with a 3% hexachlorophene solution and then rinsed developed varying plasma levels. Despite elevated blood levels, serious toxic effects were noted only when hexachlorophene was left on the skin, e.g., as a lotion or in diaper powder (Lockhart, 1972), or when infants weighed under 1400 g, necessitating nursery care for prolonged periods. The infants' increased surface area to body weight ratio, permeable skin, and inadequate elimination of hexachlorophene probably all contributed to increased blood levels of the agent.

Conclusive evidence of toxicity was obtained in well-designed experiments in which baby rhesus monkeys were subjected to washing, thorough rinsing and drying several times daily over a period of 28 days and developed central nervous system vacuolization (cystic lesions of cerebellum, brain stem, and spinal nerves) (Lockhart, 1972).

Parenteral Medication

The precautions related to solubility of parenteral drugs identified in Chapter 2 also apply to the infant. Further variations in absorption will occur in the infant under conditions causing vasodilation or vasoconstriction. For example, phototherapy for hyperbilirubinemia causes marked peripheral vasodilation, which may increase absorption of medication from skin and muscle sites (Wu et al., 1974).

Conditions causing vasoconstriction (cold stress, hypotension, asphyxia, infection) or poor peripheral circulation to an extremity (edema, birth injury, repeated venipunctures) will delay absorption time. The small muscle mass available for injection in the neonate requires careful rotation of sites to minimize tissue injury, since injection into muscle tissue will cause some irritation with a degree of inflammatory response.

Table 7–1 Percentages of Body Water for Infants and Adults

	Body Water	Fatty Tissue
Preterm infant	85%	1%
Term infant	70%	15%
Adult	15 to 20%	Variable

The intravenous route of administration bypasses problems of absorption and should be used for compromised infants whose peripheral circulation may be impaired. Control of intravenous infusion can be precise, making this route preferable during a critical period of neonatal distress. For specific techniques and problems affecting routes of administration, see Methods of Administration, page 248. More specific information on rates of absorption and modifying factors in the newborn awaits further studies.

DISTRIBUTION

Drug distribution in the newborn differs from the adult (Yaffee and Stern, 1976) primarily because infants have relatively more body water than adults and smaller amounts of fatty tissue (see Table 7–1).

Although one might expect that these major differences would change drug concentrations in fatty tissue as well as interstitial and cellular fluids, few confirmatory studies on these effects have been published. Drug excretion may also be affected, since water turnover in the infant is so much more rapid in the premature and term neonate.

Drug molecules are conveyed in the plasma to their sites of action, metabolism or excretion. The newborn's relatively small amount of circulating fluid in the vascular compartment (80 ml/kg average) will influence drug transport in states of dehydration or hemodilution, as well as with compartmental fluid shifts, as in edema. In addition, the plethoric newborn with a high hematocrit reading may demonstrate differences in drug plasma concentration when the dose of drug is absorbed into a diminished plasma volume.

Tissue Binding

Tissue binding is a mechanism by which a drug is removed from the circulation and stored for variable periods of time. The bound drug may be released slowly to the circulation as free drug to be metabolized and excreted. This reservoir for drugs may exist in any tissue of the body but is most commonly found in fatty tissue. It seems reasonable that the preterm infant, possessing scanty fat and low muscle mass, has reduced tissue-binding ability. Therefore, adverse effects could be produced from resulting higher levels of circulating free drug.

Protein Binding

Drugs may also be dissolved in serum water or linked loosely with blood erythrocytes, globulins, lipoproteins, or albumin. Most bound drugs are linked up to an albumin molecule by ionic bonds which may easily be reversed.

Unbound drug + albumin = drug − albumin complex

Binding of a drug will be limited by the available number of albumin molecules (Koch-Weser and Sellers, 1976), the specific protein-binding sites available for that drug, the presence of other molecules competing for those same protein-binding sites, and conditions which may alter pH and thus binding affinity.

Protein binding is a mechanism for intravascular storage of drug molecules so that they are unable to move to receptor sites or across body membranes. Binding is usually easily reversible, and an equilibrium is maintained by releasing bound drug when a quantity of free drug is "used up" by being metabolized and excreted. Drugs which become highly bound may have 80 to 98 percent of the drug dose attached to serum albumin. An initial larger dose ("loading") or repeated doses may be needed to achieve the minimum effective concentration of free drug at its designated site of action. With highly bound drugs, there may be slow release from binding sites and a persistent drug effect after medication has been discontinued.

The reduced amount of albumin in the newborn serum compared to the adult leads to quantitative differences in protein binding. Drugs that would ordinarily be protein-bound might bind to tissue sites as a result of a lack of available plasma protein. Maternal endogenous substances, such as steroids, may occupy more binding sites in the first few post-natal days, further reducing available protein molecules. This lowered availability is reflected in the reduced binding of most drugs administered to the newborn, although a few drugs may attain adult ratios of bound/free drug.

Competition for Binding Sites

Newborn serum albumin appears to bind drugs with the same capacity as adult albumin. Elevated bilirubin levels may change bound/free drug ratios. Recent studies have found that in some instances, the bilirubin molecule will displace other protein-bound substances, e.g., phenytoin (Krasner and Yaffee, 1975).

Conversely, other drugs, such as sulfa, furosemide, sodium benzoate, and sodium salicylate, may effectively compete with bilirubin for albumin-binding sites. In vitro studies, using concentrations much higher than normally used clinically, showed that sodium benzoate produced a 30 percent reduction in bilirubin binding and sodium salicylate, a 20 percent reduction (Krasner and Yaffee, 1975, p. 364). Both substances could create adverse effects when present in newborn serum, since bilirubin, when displaced from albumin, enters the circulation and may then be free to cross the blood-brain barrier to deposit in lipoid cells of the brain.

Blood-Brain Barrier

The layer of lipoprotein cells that forms the walls of the brain capillaries and the adjacent glial membranes make up the *blood-brain barrier* (BBB), separating plasma from the extracellular fluid of the brain. Because this membrane has no pores through which water-soluble substances may move, only fat-soluble drugs may traverse the barrier into brain tissue. Drugs which are ionized and non-lipid-soluble may also enter the extracellular fluid compartment, however, under conditions of anoxia, trauma, or inflammation, conditions which alter its pH.

The BBB has major clinical relevance in relation to bilirubin deposition in the brain. When serum bilirubin levels rise, the non-protein-bound fraction of unconjugated bilirubin may, under certain conditions, traverse this barrier and be taken up predominantly by the basal ganglia of the brain. Hyperbilirubinemic encephalopathy (kernicterus) was formerly thought to occur at serum bilirubin levels exceeding 16–18 mg/100 ml. It is now understood, however, that preterm infants, especially those stressed by such conditions as infection, hypoxia, acidosis, or hypoglycemia, may suffer kernicteric brain damage at much lower levels of serum bilirubin.

Placental Barrier

The role of the placenta as a membrane "barrier" to xenobiotics is of critical importance in understanding drug influence on the newborn. The placental barrier, made up of lipoprotein tissue with some pores allowing small water-soluble molecules to enter, acts in most ways like other body membranes separating body compartments. Rapid transfer of lipid-soluble, nonionized molecules occurs in either direction, as well as active transfer by protein-linkage of larger water-soluble molecules which cannot move through the pores. Equilibrium of the drug on both sides of the placental barrier will usually be reached within an hour of maternal oral intake and within a few minutes of parenteral injection. In light of the rapid transfer of most molecules, the placenta cannot be thought of as a "barrier" to any substance except maternal and infant blood cells, molecules of molecular weight over 1000, and substances which are very highly tissue-bound or protein-bound in the mother.

Transfer across the placenta is favored by electrochemical differences between maternal and fetal circulations and follows the principles identified in Chapter 1. Cord blood pH is normally 0.10–0.15 pH units below maternal pH and, under conditions of fetal stress, may be reduced further. When this happens, drugs which "prefer" a more acidic pH may accumulate on the fetal side of the placenta rather than in the mother's circulation across the placental membrane.

An example of how this pH *gradient* fosters drug retention in the fetus is found in the salicylate response in infants of mothers who had ingested aspirin within 20 minutes of delivery (Levy, 1974). The maternal/fetal plasma concentrations were very different in three out of four subjects. Mothers had a range of 2.0–26.0 μg/ml and infants a range of 8.3–30.8 μg/ml. Metabolism differed as well, for the newborns eliminated half the salicylate dose by 4.5 to 11.5 hours, compared with an average of 3 hours for the mothers, and salicylate was still found in infants' urine for 3 days after birth (Levy and Gaurettson, 1974).

BIOTRANSFORMATION

Enzymatic processes in the liver metabolize most drugs to other substances, some of which may be more active or more toxic than the parent drug. These metabolites must be water-soluble and capable of renal filtration to be excreted in the urine. If any of the steps of the metabolic cycle are absent or incomplete, a drug will not be "processed" completely, leaving metabolites still circulating in the body fluids.

Many drugs undergoing *biotransformation* in the liver are excreted in the bile. If adequate bile salts and requisite intestinal flora are present, these metabolites may be further reduced in the small intestine. Products which are incompletely metabolized, however, may be reabsorbed across the intestinal membrane and be recycled through the liver. This internal recycling constitutes the *enterohepatic cycle*, which may greatly influence excretion of drugs and, therefore, serum or tissue levels.

Most of these enzymatic reactions take place in the microsomal portion of the liver, although some metabolism can also occur in the plasma, kidneys, and GI tract. These enzymatic reactions, occurring in one or two phases, change the drug molecule to a form which can be excreted. Phase I, nonsynthetic, reactions change a parent drug to metabolic products, which are weakly ionized and less fat-soluble. These products are less able to bind to carrier protein, to cross membranes, or to be reabsorbed across the tubular membranes of the kidney. Nonsynthetic reactions result from processes of oxidation, reduction, or hydrolysis. If drugs need phase I alone, metabolism may not be much delayed, since these processes appear to function as well in the young infant as in the adult (with the exception of some hydroxylation and oxidation reactions) (Cohen and Ganapathy, 1976).

Phase II–synthetic reactions, like phase I reactions, continue to convert nonionized drugs into ionized less fat-soluble ones which can be excreted into the bile or urine. These reactions include glucuronide conjugation, an essential step in the metabolism of bilirubin in the newborn. Studies of bilirubin metabolism have indicated that glucuronidation is deficient for the first few days of life. Therefore, if a drug is known to require conjugation (or any other phase II reactions), it should be given to the preterm infant or newborn only with recognition that partially changed substances may be more active than the parent drug, increasing the possibility of adverse effects if present in high concentrations or circulating for extended periods. Examples of drugs with markedly delayed metabolism apparently contributing to adverse effects seen in the young infant are diazepam and chloramphenicol (Cohen and Ganapathy, 1976, p. 181).

Induction of Enzymes

Enzymes residing in the microsomal portion of the liver may be induced (stimulated) or inhibited by as many as 200 different chemicals (Geleherter, 1976). Very few of these agents are deliberately given therapeutically to young infants. Induction appears to result from increased production of the enzymes, making larger amounts available for drug metabolism. The affected drugs are thus changed more quickly into their final metabolites. Conversely, inhibition of a specific enzyme would generally lead to higher serum levels of those drugs affected by that enzyme. The principle of induction

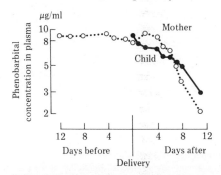

Phenobarbital 150 mg PO daily

Figure 7-2 Concentration of phenobarbitol in maternal and infant plasma following prenatal treatment of the mother for toxemic symptoms. (After L. O. Boreus et al., "Clinical Pharmacology of Phenobarbital in the Neonatal Period," in P. L. Morselli (ed.), Basic Therapeutic Aspects of Perinatal Pharmacology, Raven Press, New York, 1975.)

has been used therapeutically to treat hyperbilirubinemia in preterm infants. When phenobarbital, an effective enzyme inducer, is given at least 5 days before delivery to the mother and continued in her newborn infant, it speeds metabolism and excretion of many substances in the newborn, including bilirubin (Geleherter, 1976). (See Fig. 7-2.) It is important to note, however, that the enzyme-induction effect is not specific for bilirubin, so that other medications and natural products may be affected by the same enzyme. Although enzyme induction may not be involved, the enhanced production of surfactant in the immature infant has been produced by maternal corticosteroid (betamethasone) administration. Experimental evidence suggests that administration of this agent 24 hours prior to delivery will reduce the incidence of hyaline membrane disease. The mechanism of action is thought to be stimulation of the surfactant by the corticosteriod (Korones, 1976, p. 161).

Half-Life   The metabolic rate of a drug can be measured by its half-life $(T_{1/2})$, the time in which half the drug is eliminated. The effect

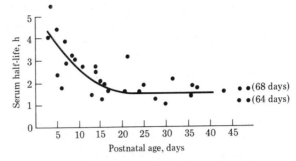

Figure 7-3 Correlations of ampicillin half-life with postnatal age. (From P. Walson, "Absorption and Distribution of Antibiotics in the Developing Child," Symposium on Perinatal and Developmental Medicine, Mead Johnson, June 1975, p. 80.)

of immaturity on drug metabolism and excretion can be seen in Fig. 7-3, which illustrates the change in ampicillin half-life resulting from maturation during neonatal and early infancy periods. As maturation proceeds, the half-life of a drug decreases and slowly assumes adult values. A drug's half-life can serve as an index of metabolism and excretion, permitting anticipation of necessary adjustments in drug dosage.

Enterohepatic Cycle

Many drugs which are incompletely metabolized may be recycled from the intestine to the liver instead of being excreted. Bilirubin, a natural product of heme catabolism can provide a suitable model. Bilirubin is excreted from the liver in the form of *bilirubin diglucuronide* and is normally reduced to *urobilinogen* by intestinal flora in the adult. In the newborn the absence of specific flora and the abundance of β-glucuronidase converts the diglucuronide metabolite to fat-soluble bilirubin, which is reabsorbed and recycled to the liver.

This enterohepatic cycle is also operative in drugs which undergo similar pathways of conjugation and excretion. It is generally believed that appropriate intestinal flora are established by 3 to 4 days after birth. Combined with increasing maturity of metabolism, this should result in decreased serum levels of such affected substances. Therefore, the nurse should note the presence of jaundice as well as the stool pattern while these drugs are being administered.

EXCRETION

Although excretion through skin and the gastrointestinal and respiratory routes may account for a small portion of drug disposition, renal clearance forms the major excretory route. Renal handling of drugs depends on three processes: glomerular filtration, tubular reabsorption, and tubular secretion. Each of these three functions is affected by gestational and postnatal maturation. At birth the term newborn can achieve a filtration rate of 30 to 40 percent and tubular secretion of 20 to 30 percent of adult values. This quantitative impairment is even more striking in the preterm infant. Renal function develops rapidly, however, so that by the term infant's seventh day of life, glomerular filtration has increased to 50 percent of the adult rate, and by 6 months to 1 year, this function may be considered to be "mature."

Urinary concentrating ability depends on tubular reabsorption of water, electrolytes, and un-ionized lipid-soluble molecules from the renal filtrate. "Mature" ability to concentrate urine is generally achieved by 2 months of age in the preterm infant and somewhat earlier in the term infant (Nelson, 1973).

Secretion or reabsorption of weak acids and bases varies with the urine/plasma pH gradient; alterations in that ratio will affect rates of excretion. For example, when urine or plasma pH changes, basic compounds will move from an alkaline into an acidic medium. Conversely, acidic drugs become more concentrated in an alkaline medium, affecting excretion and reabsorption in the same way. Thus, pathologic states accompanied by acidosis or alkalosis may change rates of drug excretion. Studies to quantitate these effects, especially in the neonatal period, are incomplete at this time.

The kinetics of drug binding to serum proteins and tissue

also affect the excretory process. When the "free" fraction of a circulating drug is eliminated by active transport or filtration, more molecules are instantly freed from the "bound" state to maintain drug equilibrium in the circulation. Thus, renal status and drug kinetics tightly interrelate in the process of excretion.

Application of these maturational kinetics dictates the appropriate clinical use of kanamycin. Yaffee found that a baby of less than 48 hours of age excreted 20 percent of a known dose of kanamycin in 12 hours, but by 1 week of life it excreted 60 percent or more of the dose during the same time period. Kanamycin is therefore usually administered every 12 hours up to 1 week of age, but more frequently as maturational changes occur.

CALCULATION OF DOSAGE

The term *correct dosage* refers to the smallest quantity of drug capable of effecting the desired clinical response without producing undesirable side effects. Numerous physiologic and pharmacologic variables make it difficult for the physician to determine correct dosage with complete accuracy for each individual infant. It becomes necessary, therefore, to rely on the clinically established dosage range for each drug as a starting point. Knowledge of the processes involved in absorption, distribution, metabolism, and elimination of drugs and the alterations imposed upon these processes by disease and immaturity is essential. A full understanding of normal patterns of growth and development assist the health professional to determine the optimal drug dosage for an individual infant.

The *initial dose* of medication is determined in part by the *average dose* based on pharmacokinetic studies. Subsequent doses are referred to as *maintenance doses* and will frequently vary from the initial dose based on the response of the infant to the medication. The *official dose* of a drug is that dose listed in the United States Pharmacopeia (USP) and the National Formulary (NF). *Minimal dose* refers to the least amount of drug which can be expected to produce a therapeutic effect; this dosage hopefully becomes the maintenance dose for the infant. *Maximal dose* refers to the greatest dose which has been tolerated during clinical trials without the appearance of toxic symptoms; these trials however, are usually conducted on an adult population. Between these two extremes lies the *therapeutic dose*, which is tailored to the needs of the individual infant and determined, in part, by such factors as age, physiological state, and the presence of disease.

Methods of Drug Dosage Calculation

Several rules have been formulated to aid in determining drug dosages for infants and children. The two formulas most frequently used in infancy are outlined below:

Fried's Rule (for Children Less Than 1 Year of Age)

$$\frac{\text{Age in months}}{150} \times \text{adult dose} = \text{approximate infant's dose}$$

Body Surface Area (BSA)   This is another method often used to determine drug dosage for infants and children but is least accurate for newborns. Charts are available to determine body surface area in square meters in relation to weight and height. Knowledge of the average adult dose of the drug to be given is essential to both methods.

$$\frac{\text{Child's surface area } (m^2)}{1.75} \times \text{adult dose} = \text{child's dose}$$

or   Surface area $(m^2) \times 60$ = percent of adult dose

Example 1   The average adult dose of meperidine is 100 mg. The child's BSA has been determined to be 0.5 m^2. How much meperidine should the child receive?

$$\frac{0.5 \times 100 \text{ mg}}{1.75} = 28.57 \text{ mg } (29 \text{ mg})$$

For sample problems in infant doses, see p. 314.

The many variables related to the neonate dictate that none of the above can be used without consideration of:

- Age

- Weight

- Organ maturity

- Fluid and electrolyte balance

- Physiochemical properties of the drug

- Physiological state of the infant

- Presence of specific disease states

At the present time, dosage based on weight most frequently determines infant dosage, with modification by the above variables. Because it is often difficult to determine the therapeutic dosage of a given drug for any *individual* infant, it is essential that the nurse be extremely knowledgeable as to both desired and adverse effects of drugs administered to infants in neonatal and pediatric units. Only by careful monitoring of the infant and accurate recording and reporting of observations to the physician can the therapeutic dose for a given infant be accurately determined.

ADMINISTRATION OF DRUGS

The route of drug administration chosen by the physician will depend on several factors. The physiologic condition of the infant, the desired rate of absorption, the physiochemical properties of the drug, and its site of therapeutic action are representative of factors which influence the choice of route of drug administration.

Administration of medication to infants and young children can be made easier if nurses utilize their knowledge of developmental tasks and behaviors in establishing guidelines. Developmental norms relating to motor skills, feeding behavior, and social and language skills provide the most significant implications for administration of oral medication for this age group (Ormond and Caulfield, 1976).

Oral Administration

Infants with intact and coordinated sucking and swallowing reflexes can generally be medicated by the oral route. Usually, infants who have nasogastric tubes in place can also be given oral medication. The optimal time to offer medication by the oral route is prior to a feeding, since the infant will presumably be hungry and feed avidly at this time. However, medications such as Mycostatin, used for control of oral moniliasis (thrush) would be less effective if given prior to a feeding since topical contact with the lesions of thrush is desired.

After placing a bib on the infant, the child should be held in a sitting position, or the head and shoulders of the infant should be raised if sitting is contraindicated. This will reduce the incidence of aspiration of medication into the lungs should the infant gag or cough. The medication should be administered slowly from the tip of a small spoon, a rubber-tipped dropper, or a plastic medicine dropper. Following administration of the oral medication, the infant should be placed in a side-lying position with the head slightly elevated. If the medication is regurgitated, the time and approximate amount should be noted and the physician immediately notified.

Intramuscular Administration

The young infant has less fear regarding injections than the preschool child. Because of lack of experience and poorly developed cognitive functioning, the infant is unable to recall the discomfort of previously administered injections. Levy (1960) attributed the absence of anticipatory crying in young infants receiving injections to lack of memory of pain or discomfort from previous injections. This applied to infants age 5 months or less. Between 12 and 17 months of age, he noted a sharp rise in anticipatory crying.

Infants in this age group require special consideration. The manner in which the first injection is given and the child's response is important, since the child's attitude toward future injections may be dependent upon it. When possible, a second member of the health team should assist by restraining and distracting the child during the procedure.

Following the injection, the child will often cry because of the pain and discomfort experienced. The nurse should offer support and encouragement but allow the child a brief period in which to express these negative feelings.

Although the deltoid area may be used for amounts under 1 ml which are easily soluble and quickly absorbed, the anterior aspect of the midlateral thigh is the site of choice for intramuscular injection in infants and young children. The vastus lateralis and the rectus femoris muscles are anterolateral to the femur, with major nerves or blood vessles posterior to the femur. Injury has been noted if the injection is outside of an area bounded by midline on the anterior surface of the thigh to a midlateral line on the side of the thigh, "center seam to side seam" (Johnson and Rapton, 1965). The thigh is divided into thirds from patella to trochanter, and only the middle third utilized. The upper border of this middle portion can be used if the needle is inserted at a 45° angle pointed toward the knee (Blake et al., 1970, p. 561).

The length and gauge of the needle used should be determined by the size of the infant's muscle mass and the viscosity of the medication. The length of the needle must be chosen with care—just long enough to deposit the medication in the belly of the muscle. Injury to the femur is avoided by maintaining correct angle and depth of insertion (see Fig. 7-4).

The injection should be prepared in the medication room rather than at the infant's bedside. After identifying the infant and exposing the area to be injected, restrain the infant as necessary. Swab the injection site with an antiseptic and insert the needle as quickly and carefully as possible; be sure to aspirate, then inject the fluid slowly. Remove the needle and replace its cover. Following the injection, allow the infant to move its legs freely, as this will speed absorption. Before leaving the patient, the nurse should spend a few minutes comforting the child and observing for untoward reaction to the medication.

Modified Z-Track Technique for Infants and Young Children   It is advisable to administer intramuscular injections via the Z-track

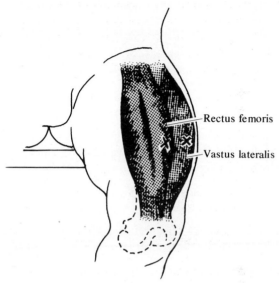

Rectus femoris

Vastus lateralis

Figure 7-4 Midanterolateral thigh: site of choice for intramuscular injections for infant.

technique whenever the injectable material is irritating to local tissue. (This method is not used for newborns because of lack of fatty tissue.) Modifications must be made for the anterior aspect of midlateral thigh. The needle size varies, depending on the size of infant or child and should be long enough to ensure delivery of medication into belly of muscle. The infant is placed in a supine position with restraint by an assistant if necessary.

1. Attach needle 1 to syringe and draw up prescribed quantity of medication.

2. Add 0.2 cm of air to syringe.

3. Remove needle 1 and replace with needle 2. (This will ensure that no medication is present on the needle to cause irritation to subcutaneous tissues as the injection is given.)

4. Place palm of hand directly over the infant's knee, firmly enough to restrain movement. Nurse's thumb should be level with the infant's midthigh.

5. Displace infant's skin *laterally* with thumb.

6. Spread middle and index fingers *laterally*, forming a "V".

7. Inject into *anterior aspect of midlateral thigh* at 45° angle with point of needle directed toward infant's knee (90° in larger infant).

8. Aspirate using thumb of same hand holding syringe.

9. Inject medication *slowly*. Injection of 0.2 ml of air will help seal medication in place and will clear needle, thus preventing leakage along injection pathway as needle is withdrawn.

10. Wait *10* seconds after injecting before withdrawing needle from injection site.

11. *Do not* massage injection site. Allow infant to kick freely, as this will increase absorption rate of medication.

12. Comfort infant and observe closely for untoward reaction to medication.

Intravenous Administration

The administration of fluids and most medications by the intravenous route is safe and effective provided certain precautions are taken. Concentrated solutions should not be used because of the danger of thrombophlebitis and tissue necrosis at and around the injection site. Rates of infusion must be monitored closely to prevent circulatory overload, which could lead to serious cardiac compromise.

Peripheral intravenous sites most frequently used for infants and young children are the veins of the dorsum of the hands and feet, the anticubital area, and the scalp. In the latter, a small portion of the head must be shaved and the infant secured in a comfortable position before the needle is inserted. Once the intravenous infusion is in place, the infant must be restrained to maintain the integrity of the intravenous flow. The physician should be notified immediately if difficulty is encountered in setting or maintaining the prescribed flow rate, if infiltration into the subcutaneous space is suspected, or if marked changes are noted in the infant's condition or behavior.

Hypodermoclysis

Although improved intravenous techniques have reduced the need for subcutaneous infusion (hypodermoclysis), the latter technique is occasionally used to supply additional fluids to infants. This method is limited by the following factors: only small amounts can be administered without compromising blood flow to overlying skin; adjacent tissue may be damaged from certain infusates; and absorption may be variable as a result of poor cirulation to peripheral areas. After cleansing the skin with an antiseptic solution, fluid is placed between the skin and muscle layers of the chosen area, usually the lateral aspect of the anterior portion of the thigh or the interscapular area. The sterile needle should be bent so that entry is parallel to the skin. Colladion may be applied to the site to prevent leakage when the needle is withdrawn.

BIBLIOGRAPHY

Blake, F., F. Howel, and E. Walchtes: *Nursing Care of Children*, J.B. Lippincott, Philadelphia, 1970.

*Cohen, S.N., and S.K. Ganapathy: "Drugs in the Fetus and Newborn Infant," *Clinics in Endocrinology and Metabolism* 5(1):179, March 1976.

Geleherter, T.D.: "Enzyme Induction," *New England Journal of Medicine* 214(11):589, March 11, 1976.

Giacoia, G.P., and R. Gorodisher: "Pharmacologic Principles in Neonatal Drug Therapy," *Clinics in Perinatology* 2(1):131, March 1975.

*Johnson, E.W., and A.D. Rapton: "A Study of Intragluteal Injections," *Archives of Physical Medicine*, 46:167, 1965.

Jusko, W.J., et al.: "Pharmaco Kinetic Principles of Pediatric Pharmacology," *Pediatric Clinics of North America*, 19:84, 1972.

Koch-Weser, J., and E. M. Sellers: "Binding of Drugs to Serum Albumin," *New England Journal of Medicine* 294(6):311, 1976.

*Denotes particularly pertinent reference.

Korones, S.B.: *High-Risk Newborn Infants*, C.V. Mosby, St. Louis, 1976.

Krasner, J., and S.J. Yaffee: "Drug-Protein Binding in the Neonate," in P.L. Morselli (ed.), *Basic and Therapeutic Aspects of Perinatal Pharmacology*, Raven Press New York, 1975, p. 364.

Levy, D. M.: "The Infants' Earliest Memory of Inoculation," *Journal of Genetic Psychology*, 96:3, 1960.

Levy, G., and L.K. Gaurettson: "Kinetics of Salycilate Elimination by Newborn Infants of Mothers Who Ingested Aspirin Before Delivery," *Pediatrics* 53:201, 1974.

*Lockhart, J.D.: "How Toxic Is Hexachloraphene?" *Pediatrics* 50:229, 1972 (review).

Mirkin, B.L.: "Biological Maturation and Drug Disposition," *Perinatal Pharmacology*, Mead Johnson Symposium 5, June 1974, p. 37.

————, and S. Singh: "Placental Transfer of Pharmacologically Active Molecules," in B.L. Mirkin (ed.), *Perinatal Pharmacology and Therapeutics*, Academic Press, New York, 1976, p. 36.

Nelson, W.A. (ed.): *Textbook of Pediatrics*, W.N. Saunders, Philadelphia, 1973.

*Ormond, E.A.R., and C. Caulfield: "A Practical Guide to Giving Oral Medication to Young Children," *The American Journal of Maternal and Child Nursing*, pp. 320–322, September-October, 1976.

Shirkey, H. C.: *Pediatric Dosage Handbook*, American Pharmaceutical Association, Washington, D.C., 1973.

Solomon, L.M., and N.B. Esterly: "Neonatal Dermatology, I. The Newborn Skin," *Journal of Pediatrics*, 77:889, 1971.

*Watson, J.: "Research and Literature on Childrens Response to Injection." *Journal of Pediatric Nursing*, 2(1):7; January 1975.

Wu, P.Y.K., et al.: "Changes in Blood Flow in the Skin and Muscle with Phototherapy," *Pediatric Resident*, 8:257, 1974.

Yaffee S.J., and S. Sterns: "Clinical Implication of Perinatal Pharmacology," in B.L. Mirkin (ed.), *Perinatal Pharmacology and Therapeutics*, Academic Press, New York, 1976, pp. 383, 385, 410.

Problems with Drugs During Newborn Transition to Extrauterine Life

Stephen R. Kandall

RESUSCITATION OF THE NEWBORN

Since labor and delivery comprise a set of events which are complex and dramatic, it is remarkable that approximately 90 percent of neonates make a smooth transition from intrauterine to extrauterine life. The remaining 10 percent of newborns, however, require resuscitative assistance to ensure that they begin life with their best chance for excellent neurobehavioral outcome. Physicians and nurses responsible for neonatal resuscitation must be highly trained, constantly available to the delivery room, and supported by equipment and medications which can be employed instantly. This state of readiness has been aided by recent advances in fetal medicine, which now make it possible to predict fetal distress in many cases. Obstetricians now designate certain pregnancies as "high risk" on the basis of past obstetric history, intercurrent medical problems, assessment of the current gestation, and progress of the current labor. During pregnancy, expanded use of ultrasound techniques, serum and urine estriol determination, oxytocin challenge tests, assays of placental hormones, and amnioscopy, among other techniques, have led to critical refinement of the "high-risk" state. During labor, more judicious use of premedication and anesthesia, as well as increased dependence on cesarean section in certain situations, has become an important obstetric principle. Development of techniques to record and assess continuous fetal heart rate patterns and to objectively determine the biochemical well-being (pH) of the fetus are thought to be responsible for reducing perinatal mortality in recent years.

Despite these significant advances, however, fetal distress may develop with little or no warning, resulting in the birth of a compromised infant suddenly in need of full perinatal support. Because of this, all deliveries should take place under medically controlled circumstances. Although out-of-hospital deliveries are gaining in popularity, the facilities usually lack the equipment and personnel needed in an acute emergency.

Within the hospital setting, an effective resuscitation must be predicated on preparedness and a knowledge of the pathophysiology of neonatal asphyxia. Best results are obtained with specially trained personnel working with standardized equipment and with medications prepared from a set protocol. These precautions should minimize confusion and allow all involved personnel to focus their attention on the needs of the baby.

Although a discussion of asphyxia should be sought in a complete text, one should be aware that areas of major neonatal adaptation are of concern in the compromised newborn. Those areas are (1) pulmonary, (2) cardiovascular, (3) acid-base, (4) metabolic, and (5) thermoregulatory.

Pulmonary Considerations

Successful neonatal respiratory adaptation depends on three basic factors: anatomic differentiation of the alveolar units to allow gas exchange, stability of alveoli conferred by surface-active materials, and integrity of central control of respiration. Pulmonary insufficiency may therefore result from a great variety of conditions, including prematurity, pulmonary problems (aspiration, pneumonia, pneumothorax, congenital anomalies, etc.), asphyxia, and excessive maternal analgesia and anesthesia, among others.

Major factors responsible for the onset and maintenance

of neonatal respiration include tactile and thermal stimuli, input from systemic arterial chemoreceptors, and clearing of fetal fluid. In the great majority of infants, therefore, respiratory support need only consist of gentle suctioning and stimulation and, at times, provision of supplemental oxygen for a short period. In more seriously compromised infants, ventilation with a bag and mask or endotracheal intubation and positive pressure ventilation may be necessary. In aspiration syndromes (meconium, amniotic fluid, blood), immediate tracheal lavage has significantly improved neonatal outcome.

The most important drug used to support neonatal ventilation is *naloxone hydrochloride (Narcan)*. This agent is a narcotic antagonist which lacks the morphinelike properties of other narcotic antagonists. Naloxone counteracts the respiratory and central nervous system depression induced by narcotics used for obstetric analgesia. Because of its specific action and lack of side effects, naloxone has completely replaced nalorphine hydrochloride (Naline) in neonatal resuscitation.

Naloxone is usually administered in a dosage of 0.01 mg/kg, either intravenously, intramuscularly, or subcutaneously. The first route is preferable when peripheral perfusion may be impaired. The neonatal form of naloxone is prepared in a 2 ml vial, with each milliliter containing 0.02 mg, so that a complete vial may be given to term infants. One-half the dose may be used in smaller neonates. Response to intravenous naloxone should occur within 1 minute and slightly longer after intramuscular or subcutaneous administration. If no effect is seen, the dose can be repeated intravenously. Naloxone is rapidly metabolized to the glucuronide form and excreted in the urine.

It is critical to remember that neonatal depression may result wholly or in part from pathologic processes or nonopiate drugs even when narcotic analgesia is employed. If an infant is depressed, therefore, a full resuscitation should be carried out while the naloxone is being administered, rather than administering the naloxone alone and awaiting a hoped-for response.

Many obstetricians have adopted the practice of administering naloxone to mothers who have received narcotic analgesia in the hopes of delivering babies who do not show effects of narcotic depression. Since placental transfer of naloxone is unpredictable, one must be extremely vigilant in this group of infants. All infants who receive naloxone either transplacentally or directly after birth merit close observation, since rapid metabolism of naloxone with persistence of narcotic levels may lead to secondary narcotic-induced depression in the infant as late as 6 to 8 hours after delivery.

Administration of naloxone may also lead to rapid onset of narcotic-withdrawal symptoms in infants born to women with *chronic narcotic-dependence* (heroin, methadone, etc.). Extreme caution should thus be exercised in passively addicted newborns should administration of naloxone prove necessary.

Acetylcysteine (Mucomyst) may be useful in solubilizing intra-airway meconium in meconium aspiration syndrome. By "opening" disulfide bridges, acetylcysteine reduces the viscosity of pulmonary secretions and thus may aid in pulmonary care. Acetylcysteine is prepared as a 20% solution, which should be reduced before use to a 2% solution by mixing the following in a 10 ml syringe: 1 ml of acetylcysteine, 1.5 ml of sodium bicarbonate, and 7.5 ml of sterile water. Instillations of 0.25 ml of this solution, followed by gentle suctioning, should continue until the pulmonary return is clear. *If this solution is not already prepared, one should not delay; initiate intubation and lavage with normal saline.* Since the acetylcysteine itself may be irritating to airways, its use should be discontinued when pulmonary return is clear and subsequent lavage performed with sterile saline.

Cardiovascular Considerations

Complex cardiovascular changes which occur in the transitional period include reduction in pulmonary vascular resistance, closure of the ductus arteriosus, closure of the foramen ovale, closure of the ductus venosus, and obliteration of the umbilical placental circulation. These changes are necessary for maintenance of pulmonary blood flow, systemic cardiac output, and peripheral perfusion in the neonate. Any or all of these critical adaptations may be impaired in perinatal asphyxia as a result of hypovolemia, impairment of cardiac contractibility, and reduction of pulmonary blood flow. Systemic hypoperfusion, manifested clinically by pallor, poor capillary filling, reduced pulses, hypotonia, and alterations in systemic blood pressure, may also result from other causes, such as infection, hemorrhage, and central nervous system insult. Whatever the cause, aggressive treatment is indicated under careful physiologic monitoring (clinical observation, arterial blood pressure, venous pressure, if possible). Reduction in pulmonary blood flow, such as in "persistence of fetal circulation," usually presents with severe hypoxemia.

Expanders of Intravascular Volume   Expansion of the intravascular space may be accomplished with a suitable replacement solution, such as plasma protein fraction (human), 5 percent (Plasmanate), blood, saline, or dextrose in water. If objective physiologic monitoring is unavailable, an initial dose of any volume expander should approximate 10 ml/kg. It is critical to stress, however, that *administration of such fluid should continue until peripheral perfusion has been restored.* This normalization may require infusion of up to 50 ml/kg of fluid in the first hours of life. Some of this volume correction may be achieved with diluted sodium bicarbonate if acidemia and hypovolemia are treated concurrently (see Acid-Base Correction).

Maintenance of Cardiac Output   Infants with significant bradycardia who do not show immediate response to ventilation should receive closed-chest cardiac massage. Persistent bradycardia should be treated with intravenous epinephrine in a dosage of 0.1 ml/kg of a 1/10,000 aqueous solution. Less commonly, an intravenous infusion of isoproterenol at a rate of 0.1–0.5 μg/kg per minute is employed. Since depletion of cardiac glycogen stores usually accompanies asphyxia of this degree, 3–5 ml/kg of 20% dextrose in water should be administered during the resuscitation.

Reduction of Pulmonary Vascular Resistance   The use of tolazoline hydrochloride (Priscoline) should be considered in the face of severe persistent hypoxemia thought to result from a marked increase in pulmonary vascular resistance. Examples include persistence of fetal circulation, severe meconium aspiration, and rarely, respiratory distress syndrome. When used to reduce pulmonary vascular resistance, tolazoline should be administered into a peripheral vein at a dosage of 2 mg/kg initially, followed by a continual infusion of 1 mg/kg per hour. In all cases, therapy is aimed at maintenance of systemic arterial oxygen tensions over 30 mmHg and normalization of the pH.

Cardiac Failure   The use of digoxin and furosemide (Lasix) in the immediate transitional period is generally reserved for conditions such as severe erythroblastosis fetalis when associated with hypervolemia and cardiac decompensation. In those circumstances, intravenous administration of all resuscitative drugs is advisable.

Acid-Base Correction

Although labor is normally an asphyxiating process associated with a reduction in fetal pH, it is usually not necessary to support neonatal adaptive corrections in acid-base balance. True fetal acidemia is usually defined as a fall in fetal or umbilical cord pH to levels below 7.25. More severe pH derangements may result in pulmonary artery constriction, interference with surfactant activity, compromise of cardiac function, and eventually cessation of cellular metabolic activity. Neurobehavioral outcome has been correlated with 5 minute Apgar scores and arterial pH at 30 minutes of age, stressing the need for rapid diagnosis and treatment of neonatal acidemia. Although obstetric suspicions of fetal distress, presence of low Apgar scores, and the findings of pallor, hypotonia, and poor perfusion in the newborn may strongly suggest acidemia, arterial blood gas determination must be performed *immediately* to objectively assess the degree of neonatal compromise.

As previously noted, neonatal hypovolemia and acidemia often coexist. Expansion of intravascular volume may result in clinical improvement by increasing peripheral blood flow and tissue perfusion. The infant's pH must be carefully monitored, since metabolic acids may move from the peripheral into the central circulation and require buffering.

Although some improvement can be expected with volume expansion, most neonatologists prefer to administer a base directly to correct acidemia. The most extensively used buffer is *sodium bicarbonate*, usually prepared as a 7.5 to 8.4% solution. Before administering sodium bicarbonate, one would ideally like to know the results of arterial blood gases and calculate the "base deficit" (that portion of the acidemia attributable to metabolic rather than respiratory causes). Administration of bicarbonate would then follow the formula:

$$\text{Bicarbonate (meq)} = \text{bicarbonate space (0.6)} \times \text{weight} \times \text{base deficit}$$

Example   A 2-kg infant with a base deficit of 15 meq would therefore be treated with 0.6 times 2 times 15, or 18 meq of bicarbonate to achieve full correction of pH to 7.4.

Since the neonate has some adaptive capacity of its own, *correction is aimed at one-half the base deficit* to avoid "overshooting" the pH and causing an alkalosis. In the case cited, therefore, one would administer 9 meq of bicarbonate intravenously and reassess the infant both clinically and with arterial blood gases.

In the management of the asphyxiated newborn in the delivery room, immediate knowledge of arterial blood gases is not always feasible. If the infant is severely compromised, treatment with bicarbonate must be largely empiric, based on the physician's clinical assessment of the degree of acidemia. Dosages of bicarbonate should range from 2 meq/kg in "mild" acidemia to almost 10 meq/kg in severely asphyxiated infants. To some extent, bicarbonate dosage may be titrated to the clinical response of the infant, e.g., changes in color, tone, and heart rate. Regardless of the total dosage, however, the rate of intravenous administration should not exceed 1 meq/kg per minute; more rapid administration may be associated with hypernatremia and intracranial hemorrhage.

Most solutions of bicarbonate in common use are hyperosmolar, e.g., an 8.4% solution containing 1 meq/ml contains 2000 mosmol/L. It is, therefore, strongly recommended that the bicarbonate be diluted by one-third or one-fourth with 5% glucose before administration. Since volume expansion is usually desirable, this dilution is generally very well tolerated by the acidemic newborn.

In some hospitals, *tromethamine* [THAM, TRIS, tris(hydroxymethyl)aminomethane] is used in place of sodium bicarbonate. This agent, an organic amine buffer with a pH of 8.6, actively binds hydrogen ions and promotes an osmotic diuresis. Tromethamine is rapidly excreted by the kidney.

Carbohydrate Administration

Although the initial response to an asphyxial stress is hyperglycemia, rapid depletion of carbohydrate stores may occur if the stress is severe. This is especially true when acute stress compounds a chronic fetal stress associated with reduction in glycogen stores, e.g., intrauterine growth retardation and postmaturity. In severe asphyxia, depletion of cardiac glycogen may reduce cardiac output. These considerations form the basis of glucose administration to some infants in the delivery room.

The usual amount of dextrose employed is 3–5 ml/kg of 20% dextrose, or an equivalent higher volume of 10 to 15% dextrose. More hypertonic solutions of dextrose may cause vascular sloughing. This is especially relevant when resuscitative medications are injected via the umbilical vein, portal circulation, and vena cava.

Since asphyxia may deplete glycogen stores and dextrose infusion may cause release of insulin, one should monitor all resuscitated infants for hypoglycemia.

Thermoregulation

Full discussion of thermoregulation in the newborn is beyond the scope of this section. One should remember, however, that newborn infants, especially those born prematurely, are *extremely* vulnerable to hypothermic stress. Losses from conduction, convection, radiation, and evaporation must be assiduously controlled in the delivery room. Easily applied delivery room measures include avoidance of cold temperatures and excessive air currents, rapid drying of the infant, and provision of an effective radiant heat source for the infant.

Hypothermia may lead to poor respiratory adaptation, acidosis, hypoxemia, and hypoglycemia and thus affect all of our previous areas of concern.

TRANSITIONAL DRUGS AND NEWBORN EFFECTS

Analgesics

The agents most commonly employed for obstetric analgesia are meperidine (Demerol) and morphine. Excessive dosages of these agents, or appropriate dosages in susceptible newborns, may produce central nervous system and respiratory depression. The route of administration of these analgesics (intravenous or intramuscular) will determine their absorption, placental passage, and onset and duration of fetal and neonatal effects. Use of these agents will diminish or may even eliminate beat-to-beat variability of the fetal heart, thus reducing the importance of this clinical parameter of fetal well-being.

The most obvious neonatal effects of maternal analgesia—depression of respiration and central nervous system response—may require resuscitative intervention. Even in those infants who appear to breathe normally, recent studies have demonstrated blunting of the CO_2 response curve. Generally, infants showing analgesic sedation effects will have normal heart rates and color initially, although failure to establish adequate ventilation will lead to deterioration of these parameters. Intervention may vary from gentle stimulation and suctioning to endotracheal intubation and assisted ventilations for varying periods of time. Insufflation of the lungs with air or oxygen will often lead to initiation of respiration and increase in tone. Naloxone hydrochloride (Narcan) is extremely valuable in counteracting narcotic-induced depression in the newborn.

Apart from these dramatic effects, maternal analgesia may produce more subtle alterations in the newbon examination. Studies have documented changes in neonatal neurobehavioral adaptation following maternal analgesia, but the impact of these changes on ultimate outcome is not known. It should be emphasized, however, that more obvious depressant effects attributed to these agents may represent only the "tip of the iceberg," in terms of adverse neonatal influences.

Anesthetics

It is generally accepted that most forms of anesthesia administered to the mother rapidly cross the placenta and exert a narcotic effect on the infant. As with maternal analgesia, physical and behavioral consequences in the infant range from subtle alterations in neural adaptation to overt respiratory and neurologic depression. As just discussed, ventilatory support should be immediately available in the delivery room. Infants who are less obviously affected should also be observed for a number of hours after birth to ensure a normal transition to extrauterine life.

Antidiabetic Agents

Many classifications have been devised to categorize states of abnormal carbohydrate metabolism during pregnancy. Each of these classifications, although varying slightly, divides patients into groups based on severity of the maternal disease process. Mild, or class A diabetes, refers to women with "gestational diabetes," showing abnormal carbohydrate metabolism only during pregnancy. Increasing severity of maternal diabetes (classes B through E, and R) denotes the need for specific antidiabetic drug therapy and more advanced diabetes, with neuropathy, nephropathy, retinopathy, etc. In an average obstetric population, the great majority of "diabetic" women will fall into the class A category.

Oral hypoglycemic agents have been implicated in congenital defects, fetal deaths, and higher rates of neonatal hypoglycemia. Insulin has therefore emerged as the preferred pharmacologic agent in control of maternal diabetes. Control of the disease process is a critical determinant of neonatal outcome in terms of both morbidity and mortality. It is generally accepted that maternal hyperglycemia, which leads to fetal hyperglycemia and fetal hyperinsulinism, causes most of the "diabetic" problems in affected infants. Provocative preliminary evidence also suggests that strict control of maternal diabetes may sharply reduce this morbidity and mortality in the neonatal period.

The following problems should be anticipated in all infants born to diabetic mothers, regardless of the severity of their disease and of medication taken for diabetic control.

Sudden Fetal Death   The specter of sudden unexplained fetal death after 36 weeks' gestation has haunted obstetricians for many years and has resulted in the planned early delivery of many "diabetic" infants. Newer means of monitoring high-risk pregnancies, such as estriol determinations and serial ultrasound measurements, may identify some at-risk fetuses, but others die suddenly in spite of reassuring laboratory studies. The mechanism of this fetal death is not known. Therefore, the obstetrician must, in each case, balance the dangers of sudden fetal death against the known risks associated with prematurity.

Pulmonary Problems   Despite some controversy, it is generally felt that maternal diabetes predisposes the neonate to hyaline membrane disease. This remains true even after correction for prematurity and cesarean section delivery, which are predisposing factors by themselves. Unfortunately, determination of surfactant activity in amniotic fluid has proven to be an unreliable prognosticator of hyaline membrane disease in the presence of maternal diabetes. This complicates the obstetric decision-making process still further.

"Diabetic" infants may also develop transient tachypnea

of the newborn, with respiratory rates reaching 100 to 140 breaths per minute. This is often associated with generalized organomegaly and a radiologic picture of pulmonary over-circulation and cardiomegaly. Aside from mild respiratory alkalosis, the tachypnea is generally well tolerated. One must be absolutely certain, however, that the tachypnea is not a reflection of other pulmonary disorders, congenital heart disease, hypoglycemia, etc.

Macrosomia   It has long been recognized that women with abnormal carbohydrate metabolism tend to deliver infants that are large for gestational age. This phenomenon is believed to result from the fetal growth-promoting effects of insulin, produced by the fetus in response to hyperglycemia. This macrosomia must be taken into consideration when estimation of fetal size is used as a guide for elective preterm delivery. It should be remembered, however, that insulin-dependent women with advanced diabetes complicated by vascular disease usually deliver infants who are small for their gestational age. These infants may be quite runted and are subject to the complications of intrauterine growth retardation, including chronic hypoxia, meconium aspiration, and hypoglycemia.

Traumatic Injuries   Large infant size may result in traumatic injuries suffered during delivery, especially vaginal delivery. "Diabetic" infants should therefore be carefully examined at the time of delivery, with special attention paid to fractures of the skull and clavicles, brachial plexus injuries, pneumothorax, extensive bruising, spinal cord injury, and hemorrhage into the liver, adrenals, and duodenum.

Hypoglycemia   Hypoglycemia is the most common metabolic problem encountered in "diabetic" infants. This condition results from fetal hyperinsulinism and acute interruption of fetal glucose supply (cord clamping). Hypoglycemia usually occurs within the first 48 hours of life, but only about half the infants born to diabetic mothers will develop this condition. Symptoms may be extremely nonspecific and may include apathy, pallor, tremors, convulsions, cyanosis, and vomiting. Many infants who develop biochemical hypoglycemia (less than 30 mg/100 ml in the term infant) will be asymptomatic. Since hypoglycemia has been correlated with neurobehavioral problems, all "diabetic" infants should be monitored carefully with Dextrostix or glucose determinations every hour for the first 8 hours and then preprandially during the next 2 days.

Treatment consists of early feeding of sterile water or dextrose followed by formula or breast milk feedings under clinical and biochemical monitoring. Should hypoglycemia develop, treatment with intravenous dextrose will control blood glucose levels in most infants, although stabilization with glucagon, epinephrine, or steroids may occasionally be necessary.

Hypocalcemia   Many infants of diabetic mothers also develop hypocalcemia within the first 3 days of life. This is reportedly caused by a functional maternal hyperparathyroidism during pregnancy, resulting in transient suppression of fetal and neonatal parathyroid function. Symptoms of hypocalcemia may be easily confused with those of hypoglycemia; serum calcium levels should therefore be monitored during the first few days of life.

Hyperbilirubinemia   Large-for-gestational-age infants, especially "diabetic" infants, may develop unconjugated hyperbilirubinemia exceeding physiologic levels. The mechanism underlying this bilirubin elevation is not known. Since many "diabetic" infants are born prematurely, with an increased risk of kernicterus, it is important to monitor serum bilirubin levels once jaundice becomes clinically evident.

Renal Vein Thrombosis and Hyperviscosity   "Diabetic" infants may rarely develop hematuria, proteinuria, and a flank mass, characteristic of renal vein thrombosis. This condition may be related to a syndrome of polycythemia and hyperviscosity. Hematocrit readings, used as a general index of viscosity, should therefore be determined within the first few hours of life. Generally, a central hematocrit reading of 70 percent or higher is associated with an increased thrombotic tendency. Polycythemia may be treated with vigorous hydration or by partial exchange transfusion with Plasmanate or albuminated saline to reduce the central hematocrit reading below 60 percent.

Congenital Anomalies Infants born to diabetic mothers show a slightly increased incidence of congenital anomalies compared to the general population. Specific anomalies, such as transposition of the great vessels and sacral agenesis with congenital lower limb amputations, appear to be more specific in this group of infants.

Magnesium Sulfate

Magnesium sulfate has been successfully used in the treatment of toxemic states during late gestation. Therapeutic doses of this agent are generally well tolerated by the newborn infant, despite elevations of cord magnesium levels to three to four times normal. Excessive doses, however, may result in marked neonatal depression, requiring cardiopulmonary support. Careful intravenous infusion of calcium gluconate under continuous ECG monitoring will often reverse magnesium depression. Exchange transfusion constitutes the most specific and direct therapy for magnesium toxicity, but this therapy should only be undertaken by skilled, experienced personnel.

Antithyroid Medication

The fetal thyroid gland functions autonomously and is relatively unaffected by maternal therapy directed at thyroid replacement. On the other hand, the fetal thyroid is quite sensitive to antithyroid medications taken by the mother (iodides, methimazole, propylthiouracil). It should be noted that iodides may be found in medications such as those prescribed for asthma, as a result of which the mother may be unaware of iodide ingestion. Antithyroid preparations readily cross the placenta and may cause hypothyroidism in the neonate with or without obvious goiters. Failure to recognize and treat hypothyroidism early in life may lead to mental retardation. Physical examination of the infant should focus on coarse features, large tongue, large fontanels, umbilical hernia, poor peripheral circulation, hypotonia, etc. In unusual cases, a large thyroid goiter may cause respiratory distress. Temperature instability, hyperbilirubinemia, and constipation may be noted during the infant's hospital stay. Cord blood samples should be sent for T3, T4, and TSH determinations, since these values change dramatically after birth, as the newborn enters a state of biochemical hyperthyroidism for almost a week. Bone age determined radiologically should be retarded in hypothyroid infants. Treatment with thyroid replacement usually gives a satisfactory result.

Antibiotics With few exceptions (sulfa, tetracycline, novobiocin), administration of antibiotics to the mother does not pose a significant hazard to the fetus or newborn. In the consideration of neonatal sepsis, however, the presence of transplacentally passed antibiotics may confuse both clinical signs and bacteriologic studies in the newborn.

Hormones Maternal ingestion during pregnancy of preparations such as testosterone and certain progestational agents may lead to the development of ambiguous genitalia in the newborn. This condition creates a terrible emotional stress for the parents, which must be handled with extreme sensitivity by the medical and nursing staffs. The medical workup for genital ambiguity is quite extensive, involving genetic, endocrine, and radiologic studies. These tests must be begun immediately and the results obtained rapidly in order to help the parents cope with this unfortunate occurrence.

Psychotropic Drugs

Drugs such as diazepam, chlordiazepoxide, and phenothiazines may cause neonatal neurologic depression (hypotonia, poor sucking, listlessness, etc.) and hypothermia. Infants born to mothers receiving these agents should be subjected to careful external thermal regulation to maintain their body temperature. These precautions include prevention of excessive heat loss through evaporation (drying), radiation (radiant heat source), convection (control of air currents), and conduction (warm mattress and blankets). Significant hypothermia may result in acidosis, increased oxygen consumption, cyanosis, pulmonary hemorrhage, and hypoglycemia. As with maternal analgesia and sedation, cardiopulmonary support should be available for the infant should be need arise.

Chronic usage of these agents may cause fetal dependency and neonatal withdrawal.

Sedatives Sedatives employed for maternal relaxation cross the placenta and may exert depressant action on the fetus and newborn. Phenobarbital is the agent most commonly used for maternal sedation. Barbiturates, as well as other sedatives, may produce a range of effects from subtle neurobehavioral changes to overt neurologic depression.

Chronic barbiturate usage, either licit or illicit, may lead to fetal dependency and neonatal withdrawal. Neonatal abstinence from barbiturates may be quite severe. The syndrome usually begins after day 5 and is associated with a higher incidence of neonatal seizures than with methadone or heroin. Treatment with phenobarbital should be instituted as soon as the infant is symptomatic.

Since phenobarbital is a potent inducer of microsomal enzyme systems, this agent influences drug metabolism to a major extent. This property of enzyme induction also explains the use of phenobarbital in the management of hyperbilirubinemia. This clinical application, however, should be restricted to a few specific conditions, such as partial deficiency of glucuronyl transferase (Arias syndrome), in which phenobarbital may result in marked reduction in levels of unconjugated bilirubin.

NEONATAL DRUG WITHDRAWAL

Since most drugs taken by the mother during pregnancy cross the placental barrier into the fetal circulation, it is not surprising that these agents may produce well-defined fetal and neonatal effects. The group of drugs, encompassing narcotics and other agents with addicting potential, when taken by the mother, poses a unique set of problems for the newborn infant. Fetal dependency and neonatal withdrawal has now been recognized following chronic maternal use of alcohol, amphetamines, barbiturates, codeine, diazepam (Valium), ethchlorvynol (Placidyl), glutethimide (Doriden), heroin, meperidine (Demerol), methadone, morphine, pentacozine (Talwin), and propoxyphene hydrochloride (Darvon). Although in some cases, these drugs are prescribed by the physician with proper clinical indications, in other cases, they are used illicitly by the pregnant patient. It is also well known that "polydrug abuse," use of multiple controlled substances, is extremely common during pregnancy in the drug-using population. Most published data, however, have been accumulated on the perinatal effects of heroin and methadone.

Recognition of the Drug User

When neonatal drug withdrawal is suspected, it is not always possible to elicit a history of maternal drug usage. If use of injectable narcotics is suspected, the mother should be carefully examined for needle marks, scars, skin ulcerations, and tattoos. A past history of hepatitis, endocarditis, phlebitis, and the like should prompt a careful investigation of drug intake. Detection of oral use of controlled substances is extremely difficult. The widespread growth of methadone maintenance has lessened the problem of concealment of an active drug history. Urine assay for drug metabolites, despite its limitations, should be obtained on every known or suspected drug-using mother and her infant. Although thin-layer chromatography is extensively used for urine drug screening, more sensitive methods, such as gas chromatography, radioimmunoassay, or spectral analysis, should be used to confirm positive results.

Fetal Effects

Methadone maintenance provides the opportunity to ensure proper prenatal care for the pregnant patient. Maternal heroin usage leads to increased fetal wastage and neonatal death rates; methadone maintenance is felt to reduce this mortality. Methadone corrects in a dose-related fashion the fetal growth retardation associated with heroin use. Maternal use of heroin, with or without other illicit drugs, causes an increased incidence of fetal meconium passage prior to delivery, which, in association with fetal asphyxia, may cause meconium aspiration. Methadone usage is not associated with an increased rate of fetal meconium passage. Apgar scores are usually normal in drug-dependent newborns. Heroin has been reported to reduce the incidence of hyaline membrane disease in preterm infants, as well as reducing the incidence of neonatal hyperbilirubinemia by stimulation of the hepatic microsomal enzymes responsible for bilirubin conjugation. Although syndromes of congenital anomalies have been reported for alcohol and barbiturates, drugs with addicting potential have generally not been associated with a well-defined teratogeny.

Neonatal Withdrawal

Neonatal withdrawal symptoms are usually divided into four major types as listed below:

1. Central nervous system: irritability, excessive crying, poor coordination of sucking and swallowing, tremors, and convulsions. Seizures are reported to occur in about 1 to 2 percent of babies born to heroin-using mothers and in about 6 to 10 percent of infants born to methadone-using mothers. Convulsions tend to be of the tonic-clonic or myoclonic variety, may occur even when the infant is under treatment for withdrawal, and are often quite difficult to control pharmacologically.

2. Gastrointestinal tract: vomiting and diarrhea, which may progress to dehydration if treatment is not instituted.

3. Respiratory tract: tachypnea and hyperpnea, resulting in respiratory alkalosis; in more advanced stages of withdrawal, cyanosis and terminal apnea may be seen.

4. Autonomic nervous system: sneezing, lacrimation, yawning, hyperpyrexia.

Although the latter group is the most specific, *none* of the listed symptoms is diagnostic of neonatal drug withdrawal. Therefore, symptomatic infants should always be considered suspect for conditions such as infection, metabolic imbalance (hypoglycemia, hypocalcemia, hyponatremia, etc.), and thyrotoxicosis, which may mimic drug withdrawal.

Approximately 80 percent of neonates born to drug-dependent mothers will show signs of withdrawal after birth. Controversy exists as to whether time of onset or severity of neonatal symptoms can be correlated either to the amount of maternal drug ingested or to the time of the last maternal drug administration. Heroin-related symptoms usually are apparent within 72 hours after birth, but methadone-related symptoms are more variable in onset and progression. This is probably related to the differences in pharmacokinetics between the two drugs. Heroin is short acting and not stored in tissues to any appreciable extent. Methadone, on the other hand, is longer acting, stored bound to protein in tissues such as lung, liver, kidney, and spleen, and requires hepatic N demethylation and cyclization prior to excretion in bile and urine. Withdrawal from phenobarbital usually appears after 5 to 7 days of life and is often quite severe, with a high incidence of neonatal seizures. Extended observation of the barbiturate-dependent and methadone-dependent infant is therefore of extreme importance.

Although most individual symptoms appear with equal frequency, neonatal withdrawal from methadone is felt to be more severe than from heroin, based on the need for pharmacologic therapy, time of treatment required, and dosage of specific medication needed.

Treatment   Treatment of the infant exhibiting withdrawal signs should be both general and specific. Extremely close observation of the infant should be carried out in a unit with a high nurse/infant ratio. Onset, progression, and severity of symptoms, as well as vital signs and strict intake and output should be recorded. Once specific treatment has been started, clinical response of the infant to that treatment must be assessed at frequent intervals. Although infants in withdrawal may show improvement when they are swaddled prone in a quiet, dimly lit room, this regimen reduces the nurse's ability to carefully observe the infant's symptoms, especially tremors, convulsions, and diarrhea. Ample fluids should be provided when the infant shows increased water loss (diarrhea, vomiting, sweating, hyperpnea), and caloric supplementation is advised when the infant shows hyperirritability and increased motor movements.

Pharmacologic treatment of the passively addicted infant involves the use of either an opiate or a nonspecific sedative. Most workers agree that intrauterine opiate dependency should be treated in the newborn with another opiate, preferably camphorated tincture of opium (paregoric). If the mother admits to polydrug abuse, or if symptoms are felt to be nonopiate related, treatment may be started with a sedative either alone or in combination with paregoric. Since some infants may not become symptomatic or show only mild withdrawal, treatment should not be started until symptoms have progressed to the "moderate" stage, as judged by an experienced observer.

OPIATES   Paregoric has the advantage of oral administration, but persistent vomiting may limit its usefulness. Excessive doses may result in constipation. Treatment is usually begun at a dose of 0.2–0.3 ml every 3 hours; the dose is raised by 0.05 ml at each administration until symptoms are controlled. After 5 to 7 days of clinical stabilization, the dose is carefully lowered by 0.05 ml every 2 to 3 days, while the infant is under close observation for acute exacerbations of withdrawal. One must be careful not to confuse paregoric with pure tincture of opium, which is approximately 40 times as potent as paregoric. Experience with use of methadone to treat neonatal withdrawal is quite limited and is not presently recommended.

NONSPECIFIC SEDATIVES   Phenobarbital is usually administered in a dosage of 5–10 mg/kg per day, first intramuscularly until the infant is clinically stable and then orally. Tapering of the dosage should proceed stepwise every 1 to 2 days. High doses of phenobarbital may cause lethargy and poor feeding, as well as respiratory depression. Diazepam (Valium) is administered intramuscularly every 8 hours in a dose of 1–2 mg, depending on severity. Once the infant is stable, the dosage can be lowered stepwise until it reaches 0.5 mg every 8 hours. Treatment intervals are then increased to every 12 hours and then to every 24 hours. Diazepam may cause respiratory depression, and breakthrough symptoms have also been observed. Chlorpromazine (Thorazine) is administered in a dosage of 2–3 mg/kg per day in four divided doses. Treatment is started intramuscularly and continued orally once the infant is stable. Lowering of medication dosage can usually be effected every 1 to 2 days. Treatment with any of the above four agents should be quite effective, and mortality resulting from acute withdrawal, once reported to be very high, should approach zero.

9

Neonatal and Infant Drugs in Common Use

Elaine Muller Morris

ANTIMICROBIAL AND CHEMOTHERAPEUTIC AGENTS

Although adverse reactions to antimicrobial agents in the neonate can occur, symptoms of anaphylactic shock (i.e., pallor, severe dyspnea) and circulatory collapse are rare. Rash, auditory and renal impairment, and gastrointestinal symptoms are observed more frequently. Overgrowth of organisms resistant to the microbial agent is frequently a problem with neonates and young children.

Penicillins

Penicillin, discovered by Fleming in 1928, remains an effective and widely used antibiotic agent. The expanded group of natural and semisynthetic penicillins are bactericidal to a wide range of organisms but are far more effective against gram-positive than gram-negative bacteria. Penicillins act by inhibiting synthesis of cell walls of susceptible organisms. Absorption following oral administration in the neonate is variable and therefore should be discouraged. Absorption following parenteral administration is rapid and complete. Distribution throughout the body is wide, and although penetration into the cerebrospinal fluid may be limited, higher CSF levels are achieved when the meninges are inflamed. Excretion occurs primarily through the kidneys.

Three factors limit the clinical usefulness of the penicillin group of antimicrobials. The natural penicillins are unstable in acid environments, are ineffective against bacteria which produce enzymes (penicillinases) capable of destroying penicillin, and have limited effectiveness against gram-negative organisms. Although adverse or toxic effects are rare following administration of the penicillins to neonates, skin rashes or renal problems may complicate treatment. Occasional neuromuscular irritability in the premature infant has been observed in the presence of high CSF levels of penicillin. Serious allergic reactions are more commonly seen in older children following repeated doses of the drug. However, close observation is necessary for signs of allergic reaction, and emergency equipment and drugs should be readily available in the clinical area for the treatment of acute anaphylactic shock.

The penicillins are not metabolized and are therefore primarily excreted in the urine in a biologically active form. The kidney therefore regulates, to a great extent, the serum levels of the drug. The presence of disease and the maturity of the renal system must be considered by the physician when determining the correct dosage for the individual neonate. Renal clearance of penicillins has been found to be markedly diminished, even in full-term infants free of renal disease.

Aminoglycosides

This group of antimicrobial agents is widely used in the treatment of infections during the neonatal and early childhood periods. This group includes, in order of clinical importance, kanamycin, gentamycin, streptomycin, neomycin, tobramycin, and spectinomycin. Aminoglycosides are bactericidal mainly against gram-negative organisms, and one of these agents is usually included in the initial treatment of suspected or proven neonatal bacterial infections.

Aminoglycosides should be administered parenterally, since they are poorly absorbed from the GI tract. Distribution is wide, but levels of drug in the CSF may be inadequate to treat meningitis. The major route of excretion is the renal system.

The most serious toxicities caused by drugs of the aminoglycoside group include injury to the eighth cranial nerve, which results in deafness, and renal damage reflected in proteinuria and azotemia. Renal damage can be reversed if symptoms are discovered early and usage of the drug discontinued.

Cephalosporins

Similar in chemical structure to the penicillins, these agents are capable of resisting hydrolysis by penicillinase and have a broader spectrum of activity than most penicillins. Cephalothin (Keflin) is the most commonly used drug in this group. It is not well absorbed from the GI tract and therefore should be given parenterally. Cephalexin (Keflex), another commonly used cephalosporin, is very well absorbed from the GI tract and is frequently administered orally.

While not the drug of choice in any specific disease, cephalosporins have proved valuable in the treatment of neonatal infections caused by strains of *Escherichia coli* resistant to ampicillin and kanamycin. Similar to the penicillins, excretion is primarily renal, and therefore dosage must be carefully calculated for neonates with impaired renal function and for premature infants.

Polymixins

The polymixins represent a small group of antimicrobial agents. Only two, polymyxin B sulfate and polyxin E, are currently in use. The others have been discarded as a result of excessive nephrotoxicity following usage.

Polymixin E (Colistin) is recommended for use in newborn infants only in the treatment of infections proven resistant to other antibiotics. Its major applicability lies in the treatment of *Pseudomonas* infections. This agent should not be administered intravenously or intrathecally. Renal function should be monitored closely during the course of treatment, which should not exceed 7 days.

Chloramphenicol

Chloramphenicol (*Chloromycetin*) is a potent antimicrobial agent effective against a wide range of gram-negative and gram-positive organisms and rickettsiae. However, except in cases of gram-negative meningitis, it is not usually the drug of choice in the treatment of neonatal infections because of serious adverse reactions. Neonates may demonstrate toxicity by manifesting signs and symptoms of the gray syndrome (due to deficient glucuronidation and deficient excretion). These include hypothermia, rapid irregular respirations, vasomotor collapse, diarrhea, and pallor. This agent, therefore, is reserved for the treatment of serious infections which have failed to respond to other antibacterial agents.

CARDIAC AGENTS

Congestive heart failure and paroxysmal supraventricular tachycardia in the newborn are most commonly treated with digitalis preparations. *Digoxin*, the digitalis preparation of choice during the neonatal period, is well absorbed, acts rapidly, and is excreted quickly except in cases of hepatic or renal immaturity. Because of the possibility of increased myocardial sensitivity to this agent during the newborn period, the recommended dosage for newborns differs slightly from that of older infants.

Recently, indomethacin (Indocin) and, to a lesser extent, aspirin have been used effectively in the pharmacologic closure of a patent ductus arteriosus in some infants. Indomethacin is believed to act through inhibition of prostaglandins, and this treatment with indomethacin has reportedly resulted in a reduced need for surgical closure of the ductus arteriosus (Friedman et al., 1976; Heymann et al., 1976).

Propranolol (Inderal), lidocaine (Xylocaine), and procainamide (Pronestyl) are cardiac depressants occasionally used in the treatment of neonatal cardiac arrhythmias. Careful observation of the infant following administration of these agents is essential. Changes in the rate, rhythm, or quality of the heart sounds should be immediately reported to the physician. Resuscitation equipment and emergency drugs should be readily available should severe cardiac depression or cardiac arrest result.

DIURETICS

Diuretics agents increase the flow of urine and sodium loss from the body. In neonates they are used primarily in suspected acute renal failure and congestive heart failure in conjunction with digoxin therapy.

Furosemide (Lasix) is a potent diuretic administered to neonates. Its rapid action is observed, about 5 minutes after intravenous administration. The primary site of action of Lasix is believed to be the ascending limb of Henle's loop. Although side effects are few, this agent can inhibit protein binding and therefore should not be given to jaundiced newborns during the first week of life.

The thiazide diuretics, e.g., Diuril, are also believed to displace bilirubin from albumin-binding sites. This limits their usefulness during the immediate newborn period. The thiazide diuretics are also known to be photosensitizing and may cause adverse reactions among infants receiving phototherapy treatment.

ANTITUBERCULOSIS THERAPY

Isoniazid (INH) is a highly effective antituberculosis agent, used in the treatment of active tuberculosis and in the presence of a positive tuberculin test in infants. Those infants who have not received BCG vaccine and who are considered likely to be exposed may receive INH prophylactically. Treatment continues for an extended period, up to a year in some cases. Side effects are rare in young infants.

IMMUNIZATIONS

The recommended schedule for active immunization in healthy infants and children is listed in Table 9-1. It is vital that the infant receive these immunizations at the appropriate time. Parents should be advised that frequently fever and irritability develop 12 to 24 hours after immunizations. Only healthy children should receive immunizations, and any immunologic deficiency states, immunosuppressive drug therapy, or allergies to ingredients are contraindications to vaccinations.

Table 9-1   Recommended Schedule for Active Immunization of Normal Infants and Children

Age	Vaccines
2 mo	DTP,[a] TOPV[b]
4 mo	DTP, TOPV
6 mo	DTP, TOPV[c]
1 yr	Tuberculin test[d]
15 mo	Measles-rubella,[e] mumps[e]
1½ yr	DTP, TOPV
4–6 yr	DTP, TOPV
14–16 yr	Td[f]

[a] DTP = diphtheria and tetanus toxoids combined with pertussis vaccine.

[b] TOPV = trivalent oral poliovirus vaccine. This recommendation is suitable for breast-fed as well as bottle-fed infants.

[c] A third dose of TOPV is optional but may be given in areas of high endemicity of poliomyelitis.

[d] Frequency of repeated tuberculin tests depends on risk of exposure of the child and on the prevalence of tuberculosis in the population group. For the pediatrician's office or outpatient clinic, an annual or biennial tuberculin test is appropriate unless local circumstances clearly indicate otherwise. The initial test should be done at the time of, or preceding, the measles immunization.

[e] May be given at 15 months as measles-rubella or measles-mumps-rubella combined vaccines.

[f] Td = combined tetanus and diphtheria toxoids (adult type) for those more than 6 years of age, in contrast to diphtheria and tetanus (DT) toxoids which contain a larger amount of diphtheria antigen. Tetanus toxoid at time of injury: for clean, minor wounds, no booster dose is needed by a fully immunized child unless more than 10 years have elapsed since the last dose; for contaminated wounds, a booster dose should be given if more than 5 years have elapsed since the last dose.

Source: American Academy of Pediatrics, Report of the Committee on Infectious Diseases, 1977.

Table 9-2 Neonatal and Infant Drugs in Common Use

Analgesics and Antipyretics

Acetaminophen (Tylenol, Tempra Tenlap, Liquiprin)

Indications: Pyrexia, pain
Dosage: Under 1 yr—60 mg PO q 4 to 6 h
Adverse Reactions: Generally none in recommended doses.
Nursing Implications: Monitor vital signs carefully.

Anthelmintics

Pyrimethamine (Daraprim)

Indications: Congenital toxoplasmosis
Dosage: 1–2 mg/kg per day PO for 3 d, then 1 mg/kg per day for 4 wk (do not exceed 25 mg per day)
Adverse Reactions: GI upsets, CNS stimulation; dermatitis, folic acid deficiency
Nursing Implications: Observe for anorexia, vomiting, CNS stimulation. Medicate at feeding time to reduce incidence of vomiting. Hematologic studies should be done periodically during course of therapy, since folic acid levels may fall during treatment.

Antibiotics and Chemotherapeutics

NATURAL PENICILLINS
Penicillin G (benzathine penicillin G, crystalline, aqueous)

Indications: Treatment of neonatal infections caused by gram-positive (nonpenicillinase-producing) organisms including hemolytic streptococci, "sensitive" staphylococci, pneumococci, and spirochetes.
Dosage: 100,000–200,000 U/kg per day IV, IM, PO administered in equal doses every 8 to 12 h. Can be given PO, but only one-third absorbed.
Adverse Reactions: Rare cause of neuromuscular irritability in premature infants. Allergic reactions, skin eruptions, and anaphylactic shock. Overgrowth of penicillin-resistant organisms: *Pseudomonas*, *Candida*, *Proteus*. Drug is incompatible with acid solutions, B-complex vitamins, amphotericin B, chloramphenicol, vancomycin, metaraminol, phenylephrine, tetracyclines.

Table 9-2 Neonatal and Infant Drugs in Common Use (*Continued*)

	Antibiotics and Chemotherapeutics
	Nursing Implications: Observe for allergic reaction, CNS irritability, signs and symptoms of thrush, and loose stools. Monitor vital signs. Observe IM site for swelling, irritation.
SEMISYNTHETIC PENICILLINS Ampicillin (Polycillin, Ominipen)	*Indications*: Treatment of infections caused by gram-positive organisms, except penicillin-resistant staphylococci and some gram-negative organisms. Effective against *Shigella*, *Salmonella*, streptococci and some *Proteus* organisms. Used frequently in treatment of suspected neonatal sepsis. *Dosage*: 50–150 mg/kg per day IM, IV, PO in equal doses every 8 to 12 h. Dosage may be increased to 200–400 mg/kg per day for meningitis. *Adverse Reactions*: Elevation of transaminase, rashes, eosinophilia, neuromuscular irritability, sensitization, and loose stools. *Nursing Implications*: Observe for allergic reaction, CNS irritability, signs and symptoms of thrush, and loose stools. Monitor vital signs.
Methicillin (Staphcillin) Oxacillin (Prostaphlin) Natcillin (Unipen)	*Indications*: Treatment of infections caused by penicillin-resistant staphylococci and some gram-negative organisms. *Dosage*: Methicillin 100–200 mg/kg per day IM, IV; inactivated if given PO. Oxacillin 50–200 mg/kg per day PO, IM, IV, in three to four divided doses. Natcillin 50–200 mg/kg per day PO, IM, IV, in three to four divided doses. *Adverse Reactions*: Nephrotoxic, albuminura, vomiting, sterile abscesses at IM sites, sensitization. Generally safe in newborn period when administered recommended dosage. *Nursing Implications*: Observe for hematuria; monitor intake and output. Do not mix with other drugs in same syringe. Once reconstituted, discard after 2 days if stored at room temperature, and after 4 days if refrigerated. Incompatible with acid solutions and vitamin B complex.
Carbenicillin (Geopen Pyopen)	*Indications*: Treatment of severe systemic infections caused by gram-negative bacteria, *Proteus*, *Pseudomonas*, and certain *E. coli*. Used primarily to treat urinary infections.

Dosage: 225–400 mg/kg per day IM or IV. Dosage varies with severity of infection and organism involved.

Adverse Reactions: Hypersensitivity reaction, pruritus, urticaria, drug fever, anaphylactic reaction.

Nursing Implications: Monitor vital signs; observe for signs and symptoms of hypersensitivity. Medication is not absorbed orally.

AMINOGLYCOSIDES

Kanamycin (Kantrex)

Indications: Treatment of neonatal infections caused by gram-negative organisms E. coli, Klebsiella, Proteus, and excluding Pseudomonas.

Dosage: Small prematures—7.5 mg/kg per day IM in two equal doses. Large prematures—10–15 mg/kg per day IM in two equal doses. Full-term—15 mg/kg per day IM in two equal doses. Total dose of 20–30 mg/kg. May also be given in three equally divided doses. Maximum total kanamycin dosage should not exceed 500 mg/kg. Intrathecal dosage—1 mg per day for 3 d.

Adverse Reactions: Renal, irreversible hearing loss, CNS damage and overgrowth of nonsensitive organisms, especially Candida (monilia).

Nursing Implications: Store in a cool place, do not mix with other antibacterial agents. Administer IM always and carefully rotate sites. Monitor intake and output. Poor hydration increases incidence of renal toxicity and is an indication for reducing dosage or discontinuing use of drug. Observe for irritability and skin reactions.

Gentamycin (Garamycin)

Indications: Treatment of infections caused by gram-negative bacilli, E. coli, Klebsiella, Pseudomonas, Proteus, and most S. aureus and strains resistant to ampicillin and kanamycin.

Dosage: 5–7.5 mg/kg per day. Infants less than 1 wk old—5 mg/kg per day in two divided doses. Infants more than 1 wk old—7.5 mg/kg per day in three divided doses. Prematures—medicate every 12 h. Full-term—medicate every 8h IM, IV.

Adverse Reactions: Nephrotoxicity, auditory damage, photosensitivity, pruritus, overgrowth of nonsusceptible organisms

Nursing Implications: Absorbed poorly when given by mouth. Monitor intake and output,

Table 9-2 Neonatal and Infant Drugs in Common Use (*Continued*)

	Antibiotics and Chemotherapeutics
	observe for CNS irritability, bacterial overgrowth (thrush), and diarrhea. Avoid direct and indirect sunlight. Do not mix with other drugs; inactivated by carbenicillin.
Neomycin (Mycifradin Neobiotic)	*Indications*: Treatment of enterocolitis and diarrhea caused by *E. coli.* Used to "sterilize" bowel in preparation for surgery. *Dosage*: Prematures and full-term infants—50 mg/kg per day PO divided into four doses, or 4 mg/kg per day IM divided into four doses. Bowel preparation—40/mg/kg per day PO divided into six doses. *Adverse Reactions*: Nephrotoxicity, ototoxicity, diarrhea, bacterial overgrowth of nonsusceptible organisms. *Nursing Implications*: Monitor intake and output. Observe for overgrowth of nonsusceptible organisms, indicated by thrush, foul-smelling stools. Low-residue diet during bowel preparation; expect increase in stools because of laxative effect of drug (greenish, *odorless*, and very soft).
Streptomycin	*Indications*: Treatment of disseminated tuberculosis, frequently given with INH. *Dosage*: 20 mg/kg IM q 12 h. *Adverse Reactions*: Nephrotoxicity, CNS damage to eighth nerve (auditory), cardiovascular collapse when excessive dosages are given. Must be used with care in presence of renal insufficiency, prematurity. *Nursing Implications*: Monitor intake and output; observe for CNS depression. Administer via Z-track technique for older infant. Observe injection site for signs of inflammation.
CHEMOTHERAPEUTICS	
Chloramphenicol (Chloromycetin)	*Indications*: Treatment of some severe infections caused by gram-negative and some gram-positive organisms including *Salmonella typhi, H. influenza*, and *Klebsiella.* *Dosage*: Prematures and newborns—25–50 mg/kg per day IV, IM, q 6 h. Older infants—50–75 mg/kg per day PO. *Adverse Reactions*: Gray syndrome, aplastic anemia, optic nerve dysfunction.

Nursing Implications: Observe for CNS depression, lethargy, stupor, coma, flaccidity, respiratory depression. Observe for symptoms of the gray syndrome: hypothermia, rapid irregular respirations, diarrhea, and pallor. Observe skin for petechiae and ecchymoses as early signs of blood dyscrasias. Monitor intake and output.

CEPHALOSPORINS

Cephalothin (Keflin)

Indications: Treatment of infections caused by both gram-positive and gram-negative organisms, including *E. coli, Klebsiella, Proteus*.

Dosage: 50–100 mg/kg per day IM divided into four to six doses.

Adverse Reaction: Nephrotoxicity.

Nursing Implications: Monitor intake and output. Older infant—administer via Z-track technique; very painful IM—rotate sites. When solution is kept at room temperature, discard after 6 hours, and when refrigerated, discard after 48 hours. Incompatible with calcium gluconate, calcium chloride, polymyxin B, erythromycin, and tetracycline. Coombs' and glucose test may register false-positives while receiving medication.

POLYMYXINS

Colistin sulfate (Polymyxin E, Colymycin)

Indications: Treatment of gram-negative infections including *Pseudomonas*. Used to sterilize bowel prior to surgery.

Dosage: Bacterial enterocolitis—3–5 mg/kg per day PO divided into three doses.
Systemic infections—5 mg/kg per day IM divided into two to four doses.

Adverse Reactions: Nephrotoxic, neurotoxic. Nitrogen retention, albuminuria, microbial overgrowth.

Nursing Implications: Medication is not absorbed orally but has an antibacterial effect on the lumen of the bowel and is then excreted with the stool. When given IM, observe for hematuria, flushing, poor coordination, thrush. Monitor intake and output, administer via Z-track technique to older infants.

Polymyxin B (Aerosporin)

Indications: Treatment of *Pseudomonas* infections and infections resistant to other antimicrobial drugs. Used *infrequently* in newborn period.

Dosage: 3.5–5 mg/kg per IM, IV, in two to three divided doses q 8 to 12 h.

Adverse Reactions: Nephrotoxic, may cause irreversible neurotoxicity. Nitrogen retention, microbial overgrowth, albuminuria.

Table 9-2   Neonatal and Infant Drugs in Common Use (*Continued*)

	Antibiotics and Chemotherapeutics
	Nursing Implications: Monitor intake and output, observe for hematuria, thrush, flushing, poor coordination. Administer via Z-track technique to older infant; painful when given IM.
ANTIFUNGAL AGENTS Nystatin (Mycostatin)	*Indications*: Treatment of cutaneous and mucocutaneous mycotic infections caused by C. albicans. *Dosage*: 400,000 U per day PO divided into four doses. *Adverse Reactions*: Almost none. *Nursing Implications*: The tongue should be swabbed with sterile water prior to administration. Medication should be given between or after feedings.
ANTITUBERCULOUS AGENTS Bacillus Calmette-Guérin (BCG) vaccine	*Indications*: Infant with negative tuberculin tests who are at high risk of contracting tuberculosis. *Dosage*: 0.05–0.1 ml of freshly prepared vaccine administered intradermally. *Adverse Reactions*: Almost none. *Nursing Implications*: Keep vaccination site clear and dry. Observe for signs of infection at vaccination site.
Isoniazid (INH)	*Indications*: Treatment of tuberculous meningitis. Prophylactically following conversion of tuberculin test without manifestation of disease or administration of BCG. Infants who are deemed to be "at risk" may also receive drug prophylactically. *Dosage*: 15–20 mg/kg per day PO divided into two to three doses. Usual period of therapy is 1 y. Often given with streptomycin. *Adverse Reactions*: Rare in newborns when correct dosage is given. CNS stimulation, liver damage. May intensify epilepsy. *Nursing Implications*: Observe for CNS irritability, hypersensitivity reaction, skin rashes, anorexia, constipation, jaundice, urticaria. Vitamin B$_6$ sometimes given prophylactically to prevent neurotoxic effects of drug.

SULFONAMIDES

Sulfadiazine

Indications: Treatment of systemic infections caused by susceptible organisms: group A streptococci, pneumococci, *Neisseria meningitis, N. gonorrhea,* and *E. coli.* Used primarily in the treatment of urinary tract infections in older children. Sulfonamides are not commonly used in the newborn period because of competition with bilirubin in protein binding, thereby increasing risk of kernicterus.

Dosage: Initial—Half of maintenance dose as calculated for 24-h period. PO.

Maintenance—150 mg/kg per day (maximum 6 g per day) PO divided in four to six doses.

Adverse Reactions: Vomiting, diarrhea, headache, lethargy rash, crystalluria.

Nursing Implications: Provide adequate fluid, monitor intake and output carefully.

Anticonvulsants

Phenobarbital (Luminal)
Phenobarbital sodium (Sodium Luminal)

Indications: Prevention and control of seizures in narcotic and phenobarbital withdrawal. Also for sedation.

Dosage: Withdrawal regime sedation—5–10 mg/kg per day, IM, IV, PO, or rectally, divided in three doses, depending on severity of condition. Then taper doses every 1 to 2 days, depending on response.

Anticonvulsant dose—15–20 mg/kg per day as loading dose; 6–8 mg/kg per day as maintenance dose.

Adverse Reactions: Respiratory, circulatory depression, urinary suppression, poor feeding.

Nursing Implications: Monitor vital signs, observe closely for symptoms of respiratory distress, pallor, and cyanosis. Do not confuse phenobarbital (Luminal) with phenobarbital sodium, as they are *not* the same drug. Luminal cannot be given IM or IV, while Sodium Luminal can.

Diazepam (Valium)

Indications: Acute control of seizures, sedation, treatment of drug withdrawal.

Dosage: Sedation—0.1–0.8 mg/kg per day IV, IM, PO, divided in three to four doses.

Withdrawal regime—0.5–2.0 mg IM q 8 h, depending on severity of condition.

Acute seizure control—0.5–2 mg IV, depending on severity of condition.

Adverse Reactions: Excessive drowsiness, ataxia, tremors, cardiac and respiratory depression, hypotension when given rapidly IV.

Table 9-2 Neonatal and Infant Drugs in Common Use (*Continued*)

	Anticonvulsants
	Nursing Implications: Monitor vital signs closely for changes in cardiac rate or rhythm, decreased respiratory rate. Observe for drowsiness. Do not dilute drug or add to parenteral fluids. Drug should not be used for chronic control of seizures.
Phenytoin sodium (Dilantin Sodium—IV, IM use) Phenytoin (Dilantin—PO use only)	*Indications*: Control of seizures, treatment of supraventricular arrhythmias. *Dosage*: Initial—8–10 mg/kg IV, repeated and increased up to 15–20 mg/kg during first 24 h. Maintenance—3–8 mg/kg IM q 24 h in three divided doses. Then phenytoin PO when stable. *Adverse Reactions*: Increased CNS irritability, rashes, nausea and vomiting. *Nursing Implications*: Monitor vital signs. Observe for nervousness, tremors, skin eruptions, vomiting when drug is given PO. Color of urine may change to pink or red-brown.
Paraldehyde	*Indications*: Control of seizures. *Dosage*: Sedation—0.15 ml/kg PO with juice q 4 to 5 h. May be given rectally with equal parts of vegetable oil or via suppository. Hypnotic and anticonvulsant dose—Double sedative dose and administer PO or rectally. *Adverse Reactions*: Respiratory and cardiac depression. *Nursing Implications*: Monitor vital signs carefully. Report changes in either rate or rhythm of pulse or respirations. Avoid use of plastic syringes, store medication in a dark bottle. Observe for increased bronchial secretions following administration of drug and position infant on it's side.
Camphorated tincture of opium (paregoric)	*Indications*: Withdrawal of infant from opiate addiction. *Dosage*: Initial—0.2–0.5 ml PO q 3 h. May be raised by 0.05 ml each further dose until symptoms controlled. Maintenance—After 5 to 7 days' stability, then tapered. *Adverse Reactions*: Constipation, respiratory depression, nausea, vomiting, urinary retention. Nursing Implications: Observe for signs of inadequate dosage when dose is being increased or tapered. Observe for lethargy, respiratory depression. Monitor intake and output. Elevate head and place in side-lying position after administration.

Bronchiodilators

Aminophylline (85% theophylline)

Indications: Physiological apnea in premature infants, bronchospasm.

Dosage: Initial—6 mg/kg PO, IM, IV, or rectally. Maintenance—2 mg/kg q 12 h.

Adverse Reactions: CNS stimulation convulsions. Increased gastric secretions and urinary excretion. Hypotension, cardiac collapse.

Nursing Implications: Monitor vital signs, especially pulse and respirations. Administer via Z-track technique when giving IM—extremely painful. Rectum should be free of feces prior to insertion of rectal suppository. When giving PO, administer with feeding to reduce gastric discomfort. IM and IV preparation may not be used interchangeably.

Calcium Salts

Calcium gluconate (10% calcium)

Indications: Treatment of hypocalcemia and hypocalcemic seizures. Often added to blood for exchange transfusion—1 ml 10% calcium gluconate per 100 ml of blood.

Dosage: 0.5–1.0 g/kg per 24 h PO in three to four divided doses. 0.1–0.2 g/kg, *slow IV*, for hypocalcemic seizures. Stop if bradycardia occurs. Do not add to IV solution containing $NaHCO_3$.

Calcium lactate (13% calcium)

Indications: Treatment of hypocalcemia (serum calcium below 8 mg/100 ml).

Dosage: 0.5 g/kg per 24 h PO in three to four divided doses. Dilute.

Calcium chloride (27% calcium)

Indications: Treatment of hypocalcemia.

Dosage: Newborn—0.3 g/kg per 24 h of a 2% solution PO in four divided doses. Infant—1–2 g per 24 h. Dilute; can be added to formula in four divided doses.

Adverse Reactions: Bradycardia, necrosis of tissue at IV site due to leakage from vein. Incidence of toxicity increases if drug is given parenterally with digitalis compounds.

Nursing Implications: Monitor vital signs, check IV site frequently for signs of infiltrations. Administer orally after meals—absorption is increased in the presence of vitamin D, lactose, bile salts, protein, and aluminum hydroxide gel. Calcium chloride is acidifying; treatment with this agent should be limited to 2 to 3 days.

Table 9-2   Neonatal and Infant Drugs in Common Use (*Continued*)

	Cardiac Agents
Digoxin (Lanoxin)	*Indications*: Treatment of congestive heart failure, supraventricular tachycardia, and premature extrasystoles. *Dosage*: Prematures and full-term infants—Digitalizing dose, 0.03–0.05 mg/kg IM, IV, PO. Maintenance dose, one-tenth to one-fifth of digitalizing dose. Infants age 2 wk to 2 yr—Digitalizing dose, 0.06–0.08 mg/kg PO, and 0.04–0.06 mg/kg IV, IM. Maintenance dose, one-fifth to one-third of digitalizing dose PO, and one-tenth to one-fifth of digitalizing dose IV or IM. Digitalization may be accomplished in the following manner: One-half of digitalizing dose stat, one-fourth of digitalizing dose in 6 h, one-fourth of digitalizing dose 6 h later. Same formula can be utilized to digitalize over a 24-h period by increasing intervals from 6 h to 8. *Adverse Reactions*: Low pulse, diarrhea, irritability. *Nursing Implications*: Infant's pulse and dosage should be checked by two members of the health team prior to administration of drug as an added safety precaution. Pulse should also be checked at regular intervals during the day. If pulse is below 90, notify physician and obtain an order before administering medication. Observe for increased irritability and diarrhea. Do not confuse digoxin (Lanoxin) with digitoxin, which is approximately *1000 times more potent.*
Acetylsalicylic acid (aspirin)	*Indications*: To constrict patent ductus arteriosus. *Dosage*: 20 mg/kg PO q 6 h for four doses. *Adverse Reactions*: GI irritation, jaundice; drug displaces bilirubin during process of protein binding. Interference with coagulation may occur. *Nursing Implications*: Administer following a feeding via feeding tube. Flush tube with sterile water following administration of medication. Observe closely for signs and symptoms of GI disturbance. Place in side-lying position to facilitate drainage should infant regurgitate. Monitor vital signs.

Indomethacin (Indocin)

Indications: To constrict patent ductus arteriosus.

Dosage: 0.2–0.3 mg/kg PO, rectally. Can be repeated q 12 to 24 h for two to three doses.

Adverse Reactions: GI irritability, lethargy, bone marrow depression, and interference with renal functioning.

Nursing Implications: Administer PO following a feeding tube. Flush tube with sterile water following administration of medication. Observe closely for signs and symptoms of GI disturbance. Place in side-lying position to facilitate drainage should infant regurgitate. Monitor vital signs.

Propranolol (Inderal)

Indications: Supraventricular arrhythmia, anoxic spells as in severe tetralogy.

Dosage: 0.5–1.0 mg/kg PO or IV q 4 to 6 h.

Adverse Reactions: Cardiac failure due to blocking of sympathetic stimulation. Bradycardia, asystole, hypotension.

Nursing Implications: Monitor vital signs closely. Observe for vomiting, diarrhea, and lethargy. Any changes in rate, rhythm, and quality of heart sounds must be reported immediately to physician.

Lidocaine (Xylocaine)

Indications: Ventricular arrhythmias.

Dosage: 1.5–2.0 mg/kg IV.

Adverse Reactions: Hypotension, cardiac failure.

Nursing Implications: Observe for CNS irritability, nausea, vomiting. Monitor vital signs. Report changes in rate, rhythm, or quality of heart sounds to physician immediately.

Procainamide (Pronestyl Hydrochloride)

Indications: Ventricular and supraventricular arrhythmias.

Dosage: 50 mg/kg per day PO in four to six divided doses. 2 mg/kg single dose IV at rate not faster than 0.5–1 mg/kg per minute.

Adverse Reactions: Hypotension, hypersensitivity, fever, chills, urticaria.

Nursing Implications: Monitor vital signs closely; observe for untoward cardiac response and lethargy. Discard parenteral solution if darker than light amber. If giving IV, resuscitation drugs and equipment should be readily available and infant monitored with ECG and blood pressure q 1 min.

Table 9-2 Neonatal and Infant Drugs in Common Use (*Continued*)

	Diuretics
Chlorothiazide (Diuril)	*Indications*: Cardiac and pulmonary congestion, edema. *Dosage*: 20–40 mg/kg per 24 h PO in two divided doses.
Furosemide (Lasix)	*Indications*: Acute control of cardiac failure, edema. *Dosage*: 1–3 mg/kg per day IM, IV. *Adverse Reactions*: Electrolyte imbalance, lethargy, vomiting, anorexia, constipation or diarrhea, low-salt syndrome, hypochloremic alkalosis, hypokalemia, hyperglycemia, glycosuria, elevated blood ammonia, skin rash, thrombocytopenic purpura, aplastic anemia, and leukopenia occur with both Diuril and Lasix. *Nursing Implications*: Monitor intake and output. Observe for lethargy, hypotension, oliguria, tachycardia, and GI upsets. Daily weights should be recorded. Administer via Z track when giving Lasix IM.
	Hormones, Enzymes, and Steroids
Pancreatic enzymes (Cotazym, Viokase, Pancreatin, Pancrelipase)	*Indications*: Treatment of malabsorption syndromes. *Dosage*: 0.3–0.5 g PO. Dosage is determined by quality and quantity of stool, generally given with each feeding. *Adverse Reactions*: Allergic reaction in presence of pork sensitivity in older children 12 to 18 mo. *Nursing Implications*: Should be administered with meals.
Glucogon	*Indications*: Treatment of insulin reaction and certain types of hypoglycemia. *Dosage*: 300 µg/kg stat, then 100 µg/kg q 3 h until glucose homeostasis is established. *Adverse Reactions*: Hyperglycemia following overdose. *Nursing Implications*: Observe for tremors, convulsions, and apnea. Neonatal hypoglycemia may be asymptomatic. Highest incidence noted among infants of diabetic mothers, premature infants, those small for gestational age, and those under severe neonatal stress.

Insulin

Indications: Neonatal diabetes or severe hyperglycemia.
Dosage: 1–2 U/kg initially IM, IV; 0.5 U/kg q 1 to 3 h prn.
Adverse Reactions: Hypoglycemia following overdose.
Nursing Implications: Observe for signs of hypoglycemia, lethargy, pallor, sweating, rising pulse rate, decrease in body temperature, convulsions.

Dexamethasone (Decadron)

Indications: Treatment of cerebral edema and meconium aspiration.
Dosage: 0.2–0.4 mg/kg IM, IV q 8 h.
Adverse Reactions: Hypokalemia, hypertension, edema, moon facies, lethargy, hyperglycemic effect, vomiting, petechiae, purpura, decreased resistance to infection.
Nursing Implications: Strict asepsis must be observed while rendering nursing care to infant because of reduced defenses against infection. Observe for signs of hyperglycemia, monitor intake and output, and record daily a.m. weights.

Desoxycorticosterone acetate (Doca, Dortate, Decortin, Percorten)

Indications: Adrenal insufficiency.
Dosage: 1–5 mg per 24 h IM.
Adverse Reactions: Increased blood volume, edema, elevation of blood pressure, cardiac failure, and low potassium syndrome, lethargy, ECG changes.
Nursing Implications: Observe for irritability; weigh daily. Monitor vital signs closely; administer via Z-track technique.

Sedatives and Other Agents

Meperidine (Demerol)

Indications: Treatment of tachycardia, sedation.
Dosage: 6 mg/kg per 24 h PO, IM, in six divided doses.
Adverse Reactions: Respiratory depression, urinary retention, hypotension.
Nursing Implications: Administer via Z-track technique—pain and local tissue irritation can occur at injection site. When giving via elixir, mix with water to avoid topical anesthetic effect on mucous membranes. Monitor vital signs, observe for tremors and uncoordinated movements. Record intake and output.

Table 9-2   Neonatal and Infant Drugs in Common Use (*Continued*)

Sedatives and Other Agents

Atropine sulfate

Indications: Preanesthetic agent; bradycardia from vagal hyperactivity.

Dosage: 0.01 mg/kg dose IM; may be repeated q 2 to 4 h.

Adverse Reactions: Tachycardia, hyperpyrexia, erythema, dilated pupils, urinary retention.

Nursing Implications: Record intake and output. Observe closely for lethargy; monitor vital signs.

Chlorpromazine (Thorazine)

Indications: Sedation and treatment of narcotic withdrawal.

Dosage: 2 mg/kg per 24 h PO in four to six divided doses.

Drug withdrawal regime—2–3 mg/kg in four divided doses. IM, then PO when stable.

Adverse Reactions: Lethargy, tremors, sweating, pyrexia, pallor, tachycardia, skin reactions, urinary retention.

Nursing Implications: Record intake and output; monitor vital signs. Do not mix with other medication in the same syringe. Administer via Z-track technique and rotate sites.

Vitamins and Minerals*

Vitamin K (Phytonadione) (AquaMephyton—IM, IV, SC use; Konakion—IM use only)

Indications: Fat-soluble vitamin K, used to correct hemorrhage due to hypoprothrombinemia. Normal levels of prothrombin are depressed in first 5 days of newborn period until intestinal bacteria and milk are present in intestine.

Dosage: Prophylactic—0.5–2 mg IM immediately after birth. 1–2 mg IM daily prn.

Adverse Effects: Hyperbilirubinemia has been reported in newborns, especially preterm infants when doses are five to ten times usual, but less incidence than with other forms of vitamin K.

Nursing Implications: May administer IM in deltoid or midanterolateral sites. Observe site for inflammation. Observe infant for hyperbilirubinemia or evidence of low prothrombin time. Protect medication from light.

*See Table 9-3 for additional vitamin and mineral requirements.

Table 9-3 Vitamin and Mineral Requirements and Preparations for Infants

	RDA	Preparation	Effects of Deficiency
VITAMINS			
A	1500 IU	Vi-Daylin (A, D, C)	Nyctolopia, photophobia, faulty epiphyseal bone formation, defective tooth enamel, retarded growth
D	400 IU	Tri-Vi-Sol (A, D, C)	Infantile tetany, rickets, osteomalacia, poor growth
C (ascorbic acid)	25–30 mg (newborns) 100 mg (prematures)	Vitron C (C only)	Scurvy, increased susceptibility to infection, hemorrhagic manifestations, poor wound healing
E (tocopherol)	15–25 U	Aquasol E elixir	Vitamin E deficiency, anemia
B_1 (thiamin)	0.4 mg		Beriberi
B_2 (riboflavin)	0.6 mg		Photophobia, blurred vision, burning and itching of eyes, poor growth
B_6 (pyridoxine)	0.2–0.3 mg	Poly-Vi-Sol (A, D, C, also) Vi-Syneral	Irritability, convulsions, hypochromic anemia Pellagra
Niacin	6 mg		
Folic acid	0.2–0.5 mg		Megaloblastic anemia usually secondary to malabsorption disease or ascorbic acid deficiency
B_{12}	2 μg		
K*			Blood-clotting deficit
MINERALS			
Iron	6 mg	Feosol Fergon	Anemia
Calcium	0.6–0.8 g	Calcium gluconate Calcium lactate Calcium chloride	Convulsions, poor bone formation, rickets, impaired growth

*Manufactured in GI tract only after milk intake adequate. RDA not known.

Table 9-4 Other Drugs Used During the Period of Infancy

Category	Drug	Indication
Ophthalmic preparations	Silver nitrate 1% followed by NS flush	Prevention and control of ophthalmia neonatorum caused by gonococcus organisms
	Tetracycline	Eye infections caused by susceptible organisms
	Tearisol	Applied to eyes in conjunction with bilirubin lamp treatments
Topical antibiotics and chemotherapeutics	Bacitracin ointment	Bacterial infections of the skin or mucous membranes caused by susceptible organisms
	Neomycin ointment	
	Polysporin ointment	
	Tetracycline ointment	
Total or supplementary parenteral alimentation	Amino acid solution (Fre Amine) Protein hydrolysate (Amigen) Dextrose Trace metals Electrolytes IN&RA lipid	Infants unable to eat, digest, or absorb nutrients for a prolonged period may be placed on parenteral alimentation
Resuscitation	Sodium bicarbonate	Correction of metabolic acidosis
	Tham (tromethamine)	Correction of metabolic acidosis; buffer
	Dextrose	Hypoglycemia
	Plasmanate	Expansion of intravascular volume
	Whole blood	
	Albumin (serum)	Correct hypoalbuminemia
	Narcan	CNS and respiratory depression 2° narcotic administered to mother during labor
	Mucomist	Viscid bronchial secretions, especially after meconium aspiration
	Epinephrine (adrenalin)	Cardiac, circulatory depression

Table 9-5 Special Infant Formulas

Formula	Content	Comments
MILK-BASE FORMULAS		
Similac with Iron	12 mg Fe/L added	Iron supplementation, anemia
Enfamil with Iron		
Bramil with Iron	8 mg Fe/L	
Modilac	10 mg Fe/L	
Similac PM 60/40		Low-solute load 7 meq Na/L
		Used for infants requiring lower protein, mineral, and salt levels than cow's milk—premature infants, cardiac disease
Lofenalac	Corn base for carbohydrates, fats	Dietary management of infants with phenylketonuria
	Low level of phenylalanine	
MILK PROTEIN-SENSITIVE FORMULA		
Soy-Bee (Sobee)	Hypoallergic formula, soybean base	Dietary management of infants allergic to cow's milk protein or lactose
Prosobee		
Soyalac		
Mull-Soy liquid		
Isomil	Lactose-free soy bean base	Infant sensitivity to protein found in cow's milk
		Lactose-free feeding
NONSOY (MILK-FREE) FORMULAS		
Meat base	Plus tapioca starch, sesame, or corn oil	Milk-sensitive infants
Lambase		Needs added carbohydrates plus iron and vitamin C and D supplements
Dale's goat's milk		

299

Table 9-5 Special Infant Formulas (*Continued*)

Formula	Content	Comments
FORMULAS FOR FAT MALABSORPTION		
Probana powder		Celiac disease
		Cystic fibrosis, steatorrhea
		Supplement with vitamins E, K, and C and iron
Portagen		Steatorrhea, biliary atresia
Alacta		Poor fat tolerance or absorption
		Supplement with vitamins A, D, and C and iron
CARBOHYDRATE MALABSORPTION		
Nutramigen		For galactosemia, hydrolysate of casein
Cho-free		Carbohydrate-free soy protein
ELECTROLYTE SOLUTIONS		
Pregestemil		Elemental formula used in GI upsets
Vivonex		Elemental formula

BIBLIOGRAPHY

Axline, S.G., and H.J. Simon: "Clinical Pharmacology of Antimicrobials in Premature Infants: I. Kanamycin, Streptomycin and Neomycin," in *Antimicrobial Agents and Chemotherapy*, American Society for Microbiology, Ann Arbor, 1964.

————, S.J. Yaffe, and H.J. Simon: "Clinical Pharmacology of Antimicrobials in Premature Infants: II. Ampicillin, Methicillin, Oxacillin, Neomycin, and Colistin," *Pediatrics*, **39**: 97, 1967.

Bergersen, B.: *Pharmacology in Nursing*, C. V. Mosby, St. Louis, 1976, pp. 458, 465.

Cohen, M.D. et al.: "Pharmacology of Some Oral Penicillins in the Newborn," *Archives of Disease in Childhood*, **50**: 230, 1975.

*Cohen, S., and S. Ganapathy: "Drugs in the Fetus and Newborn Infant," *Clinics in Endocrinology and Metabolism* **5**(1):175, March 1976.

*Drew, J.H., and W.H. Kitchner: "The Effect of Maternally Administered Drugs on Bilirubin Concentrations in the Newborn Infant," *Journal of Pediatrics*, **89**(4):657-61, 1977.

*Finnegan, P., and B.A. Macnew: "Care of the Addicted Infant," *American Journal of Nursing*, **74**(4):685–693, 1974.

Friedman, W.F. et al.: "Pharmacologic Closure of Patent Ductus Arteriosus in the Premature Infant," *New England Journal of Medicine*, **295**:26, 1976.

Garattini, S., P.L. Morselli, and F. Sereni: *Basic and Therapeutic Aspects of Perinatal Pharmacology*, Raven Press, New York, 1975.

*Giacola, G.P.: "Pharmacologic Principles in Neonatal Drug Therapy," *Clinics in Perinatology*, **2**(1):125–138, May 1975.

Heymann, M.A. et al.: "Closure of Ductus Arteriosus in Premature Infants by Inhibition of Prostaglandin Synthesis," *New England Journal of Medicine*, **295**:530, 1976.

Krazner, A. et al.: "Drug-Protein Binding," *New York Academy of Science*, **226**:101–104, 1973.

*Denotes particularly pertinent references.

McCracken, G., H. Eichenwald, and J. Nelson: "Antimicrobial Therapy in Theory and Practice, II. Clinical Approach to Antimicrobial Therapy," *Journal of Pediatrics*, **75**:923, 1969.

McCraken, G.H.: "Pharmacologic Basis for Antimicrobial Therapy in Newborn Infants," *Clinics in Perinatology*, **2**(1):139–161, May 1975.

Peppringer, C.E.: "Phenobarbital Levels in Neonates," *Clinics in Perinatology*, **2**(1):118–115, May 1975

Rane, A.: Drug Metabolism in Human Fetus and Newborn, *Pediatric Clinics of North America*, **19**:37–49, 1972.

Shirkey, H. C.: *Pediatric Dosage Handbook*, American Pharmaceutical Association, Washington, D.C., 1973.

Appendix A
Systems of Measurement

METRIC SYSTEM

The units of the metric system are based on the decimal system. Both decimal fractions and arabic numerals are used. Numbers precede any abbreviation or symbol, and a zero is always placed before the decimal point to ensure accuracy. A decimal fraction is a decimal number indicating a denominator of 10 or a power (multiple) of 10. The numerator is expressed, and the denominator is indicated by the placement of the decimal point.

	Tenths	Hundredths	Thousandths	Ten-thousandths
0.	1	2	3	4
	Place			

$\frac{1}{10}$ = 0.1 = one tenth
$\frac{12}{100}$ = 0.12 = twelve hundredths
$\frac{4}{1000}$ = 0.004 = four thousandths
$\frac{8}{10,000}$ = 0.0008 = eight ten-thousandths

Units of measure in the metric system are labeled with prefixes indicating placement of the decimal point. These prefixes are Latin in origin.

mega $= 10^6$ $= 1,000,000.$
kilo $= 10^3$ $= 1,000.$
hecto $= 10^2$ $= 100.$
deka $= 10^1$ $= 10.$

---

deci $= 10^{-1}$ $= 0.1$
centi $= 10^{-2}$ $= 0.01$
milli $= 10^{-3}$ $= 0.001$
micro $= 10^{-6}$ $= 0.000,001$
nano $= 10^{-9}$ $= 0.000,000,001$

The metric system provides units of measure for length, volume and weight. Those used most commonly in nursing are listed below.

Length	Volume	Weight
millimeter, mm	milliliter, ml	milligram, mg
centimeter, cm	cubic centimeter, cc	centigram, cg
meter, m	liter, L	gram, g (gm)
		kilogram, kg

Increasingly, small units of weight are being used. A *microgram*, which is $\frac{1}{1000}$ of a milligram and is abbreviated as either μg or mcg, and a *nanogram*, which is $\frac{1}{1000}$ of a microgram and is abbreviated ng, are used particularly in measuring body chemistry levels.

Equivalents can easily be seen by referring to prefix meanings; for example,

1 kg $= 1000$ g (gm)   1 L $= 1000$ ml (cc)
1 g $= 1000$ mg   1 m $= 1000$ mm
1 mg $= 1000$ μg (mcg)   1 cm $= 100$ mm
1 μg $= 1000$ ng

APOTHECARIES' SYSTEM

The apothecaries' system is a system of weights and measures widely used until recently in the United States. The basic unit of weight is the *grain* (gr), originally the weight of a grain of wheat. The basic unit of fluid measure is the *minim* (𝕞),the quantity of water weighing the same as one grain of wheat.

Lowercase roman numerals are used to express whole numbers, and fractions are used to express numbers less than 1. The symbol ss may be used for one-half. Abbreviations and symbols precede the numbers: for example, gr v.

Weight	Volume
grain, gr	minim, 𝕞
dram, ℨ	fluidram, f ℨ
ounce, ℥	fluidounce, f ℥
pound, lb	pint, pt
	quart, qt
	gallon, gal

HOUSEHOLD SYSTEM

The household system is the least accurate measure. It is considered safe for administering medication in the home but should not be used when more accurate measures are available.

Table A-1   Equivalent Measurements

Metric	Apothecaries'	Household
VOLUME		
1 ml	𝕞 xv	15 gtt
4 ml	f ℨ i	1 tsp
30 ml	f ℥ i	2 tbsp
180 ml	f ℥ vi	1 teacup

Table A-1   Equivalent Measurements (*Continued*)

Metric	Apothecaries'	Household
VOLUME		
240 ml	f℥ viii	1 glass
500 ml	pt i	
1000 ml	qt i	
WEIGHT		
1 g	gr xv (15.43)	
0.06 g (60 mg)	gr i	
0.001 g (1 mg)	gr 1/60 (0.01543)	
0.4536 kg (453.6 g)	gr v̄mm (7000)	1 lb
1 kg		2.2 lb
LENGTH		
1 mm		0.039 in
1 cm		0.3937 in
1 m		39.37 in
1 km (kilometer)		0.621 mile (5/8 mile)
2.54 cm		1 in
30.48 cm (0.3048 m)		1 ft

CALCULATION OF DOSAGE

Ratio and Proportion

The development of a consistent method is an important consideration in computing dosage. By using ratio and proportion the nurse can compute the amount of available drug that is needed to administer the amount of drug ordered by the physician. A ratio is a comparison between two quantities and can be expressed as a fraction, a percent, or a decimal. For example:

Ratio	20/100
Fraction	$\frac{1}{5}$
Percent	20%
Decimal	0.2

A proportion consists of two ratios that are equal to each other. The first and fourth terms of a proportion are called the *extremes*, and the second and third terms are called the *means*.

Means
$$1 : 2 = 2 : 4$$
Extremes

In a proportion the product of the means is equal to the product of the extremes. The number 2 multiplied by 2 equals 4 (product of the means), and 4 multiplied by 1 equals 4 (product of the extremes).

The terms of the ratios in a proportion must correspond in value; therefore, both sides of the proportion must be labeled in the same units of measure. The first and the third term, and the second and the fourth term, must be the same units of measure. For example:

First term   Second term   Third term   Fourth term
Milligrams : milliliters = milligrams : milliliters

If we substitute x at the second term position, then to find the value of x, find the product of the means and the product of the extremes:

$$1 : x = 2 : 4$$
$$2x = 4$$

Undo the number next to the x by dividing both sides of the equation by that number, since $2x$ means 2 times x.

$$\frac{2x}{2} = \frac{4}{2}$$
$$x = 2$$

Dimensional Analysis

Dimensional analysis is a method that is used by engineers and physicists and can be applied to solve dosage problems.

Dosage problems require changing what is ordered in one unit to the amount in another unit which should be administered in the available medication. The original quantity should be multiplied by 1 in the form of a fraction whose numerator and denominator are equivalent to each other. For example: 1 ft = 12 in, so

$$\frac{1\,\text{ft}}{12\,\text{in}} = \frac{12\,\text{in}}{1\,\text{ft}} = 1$$

If we wish to change 36 in to feet, we multiply 36 in × (1 ft/12 in). Notice that the unit inches in the numerator and denominator cancel, as well as 12 into 36.

$$\overset{3}{\cancel{36\,\text{in}}} \times \frac{1\,\text{ft}}{\cancel{12\,\text{in}}} = 3\,\text{ft}.$$

If on the other hand, we wish to change 2 ft to inches, we invert the fraction to multiply

$$2\,\text{ft} \times \frac{12\,\text{in}}{1\,\text{ft}} = 24\,\text{in}$$

The end product should be the unknown x (quantity desired) in the correct unit. Dimensional analysis requires the person to know equivalents from the measurement systems and how to multiply fractions.

In setting up the problem, list what is ordered over a digit of 1. Next, multiply by any transfer equivalents (milligrams to grams, grains to milligrams, hours to minutes, etc.). Third, multiply by what is available (milligrams in milliliters, grams in tablets, etc.). For example:

Ordered: 50 mg

How many milligrams should be given if the following is available?

Available: 25 mg/1 ml (25 mg = 1 ml)

Equation: $\dfrac{50\,\text{mg}}{1} \times \dfrac{1\,\text{ml}}{25\,\text{mg}} = x$

$\dfrac{50\,\cancel{\text{mg}}}{1} \times \dfrac{1\,\text{ml}}{25\,\cancel{\text{mg}}} = 2\,\text{ml}$

Note that what is known has been *inverted* so that the factor of milligrams can be cancelled, since what is the unknown is the number of milliliters to be administered.

[The following examples are alternatively worked by ratio and proportion (Examples A, B, etc.) and by dimensional analysis (Examples A', B', etc.).]

Example A   *Ordered:*   Crysticillin 300,000 U IM
               Available: Crysticillin 600,000 U/1.2 ml (multiple dose vial)
               Problem: Determine the number of milliliters containing 300,000 U of drug

Step 1   Set up a proportion to determine the number of milliliters containing 300,000 U of drug

        Units : milliliters = units : milliliters

Step 2   Start with a ratio of two known values—available medication—as labeled:

        Units : milliliters
      600,000 : 1.2

Step 3   Complete the proportion. Set up a ratio with x designating the number of milliliters containing 300,000 U.

        Units:milliliters = units:milliliters
        600,000:1.2 = 300,000:x

        Divide both sides by 600,000 and cancel the zeros.

$$\frac{\cancel{600,000}x}{\cancel{600,000}} = \frac{3\cancel{60,000}}{6\cancel{00,000}}$$

$$x = 0.6 \text{ ml}$$

Answer: 300,000 U in 0.6 ml

Example A'   *Ordered*:   Crysticillin 300,000 U IM
               Available: Crysticillin 600,000 U in 1.2 ml

Step 1   Place ordered dose first over 1.

$$\frac{300,000\text{ U}}{1}$$

Step 2   Multiply times available dose, placed in a fraction so as to cancel U in numerator. x then equals leftover factor in milliliters. (Cancel zeros, too!)

$$\frac{\cancel{300,000}\,\text{U}}{1}\times\frac{1.2\text{ ml}}{\underset{2}{\cancel{600,000}\,\text{U}}}=x$$

$$\frac{1.2\text{ ml}}{2}=x$$

Answer: x = 0.6 ml, which contains 300,000 U

Example B   *Ordered*:   Ampicillin 0.5 g IM
            Available: Ampicillin 1 g vial of dry powder
            Manufacturer's
            directions: Dilute with 3.5 ml of sterile water for injection to provide 250 mg/1 ml.

Step 1   The available medication, when diluted, will be labeled 250 mg/ml. The physician's order is in grams (0.5 g). First, convert the physician's order (0.5 g) to milligrams, since the terms of the ratios in a proportion must be in the same units of measure.

Step 2   Set up a proportion to convert grams to milligrams.

           Milligrams : grams = milligrams : grams

           Start with a ratio of two known values. The known value is the appropriate equivalent 1000 mg = 1 g. Complete the proportion. Set up a ratio with x designating the number of milligrams that is equal to 0.5 g.

           Milligrams: grams = milligrams:grams
                    1000 : 1 = x : 0.5
                         x = 500 mg

           Answer: 0.5 g = 500 mg

Step 3   Set up a proportion to determine the number of milliliters containing 500 mg of drug.

Milligrams : milliliters = milligrams : milliliters

Complete the proportion. Set up a ratio with x designating the number of milliliters containing 500 mg of drug.

$$\text{Milligrams:milliliters} = \text{milligrams:milliliters}$$
$$250:1 = 500:x$$
$$\frac{250x}{250} = \frac{500}{250}$$
$$x = 2 \text{ ml}$$

Answer: 0.5 g (500 mg) in 2 ml

Example B   *Ordered*:   Ampicillin 0.5 g IM
Available: Ampicillin 1 g as a dry powder
Directions: Dilute 1 g with 3.5 ml water to provide 250 mg/ml.

Step 1   Ordered   Transfer   Available
$$\frac{0.5\,\text{g}}{1} \times \frac{1000\,\text{mg}}{1\,\text{g}} \times \frac{1\,\text{ml}}{250\,\text{mg}} = x$$

Cancel units and label x with remaining unit.

Step 2 $$\frac{0.5\,\cancel{\text{g}}}{1} \times \frac{1000\,\cancel{\text{mg}}}{1\,\cancel{\text{g}}} \times \frac{1\,\text{ml}}{250\,\cancel{\text{mg}}} = x$$

$$\frac{500\,\text{ml}}{250} = x$$

Answer: $x = 2$ ml, which contains 0.5 g

Intravenous Fluid Flow Rates

The physician's order for intravenous fluids specifies the amount of solution, type of solution, and total infusion time. The nurse is responsible for calculating and maintaining the correct rate of flow. Since all intravenous administration sets are calibrated in varying drops per milliliter, check manufacturers' directions on administration set to be used.

To calculate the rate of flow of intravenous fluids using ratio and proportion:

Step 1   Determine the number of milliliters per hour:

$$\frac{\text{Total milliliters of IV solution}}{\text{Number of hours}} = \text{ml/hour}$$

Step 2   Determine the number of milliliters to be delivered per minute:

$$\frac{\text{ml/hour}}{60 \text{ minutes/hour}} = \text{ml/minute}$$

Step 3   Determine drops per minute to be administered:

ml/minute $\times$ gtt/ml (of given set) = gtt/minute

Example C   *Ordered*:   1000 ml 5% dextrose in water to be administered IV over a 10-hour period

Available: Intravenous administration set delivering 10 gtt/ml

Step 1 $$\frac{1000 \text{ ml}}{10 \text{ hours}} = 100 \text{ ml/hour}$$

Step 2 $$\frac{100 \text{ ml/hour}}{60 \text{ minutes/hour}} = 1.7 \text{ ml/minute}$$

Step 3   1.7 ml/minute $\times$ 10 gtt/ml = 17 gtt/minute

Example C′   Set up equation with ordered dose set up first:

Step 1 $$\frac{1000 \text{ ml}}{10 \text{ hours}}$$

Step 2   Then multiply by transfer fraction of 1 hour/60 minutes:

$$\frac{1000\,\text{ml}}{10\,\text{hours}} \times \frac{1\,\text{hour}}{60\,\text{minutes}}$$

Step 3   The final fraction is the available rate utilized by the administration set, i.e., 10 gtt/ml:

$$\frac{1000\,\cancel{\text{ml}}}{10\,\cancel{\text{hours}}} \times \frac{1\,\cancel{\text{hour}}}{60\,\text{minutes}} \times \frac{10\,\text{gtt}}{1\,\cancel{\text{ml}}} = x$$

Step 4   Cancelling like units leaves x expressed in gtt/minute:

$$\frac{10,\cancel{000}\,\text{gtt}}{6\cancel{00}\,\text{minutes}} = x$$

16.6 gtt/minute $= x$

Answer: $x = 17$ gtt/minute

Calculation of Oxytocin Dosage

Example D   If there are 10 U of oxytocin in 500 ml of 5% dextrose in water, how many *milliunits* (1 U = 1000 mU) of oxytocin are there in 1 ml of this mixture?

Step 1   Units : milliliters = units : milliliters
$$10 : 500 = x : 1$$
$$500\,x = 10$$
$$x = \frac{10}{500}$$
$$x = 0.02\ \text{U}$$

Step 2   Millunits : units = millunits : units
$$1000 : 1 = x : 0.02$$
$$x = 0.02 \times 1000$$
$$x = 20\ \text{mU}$$

Answer: 20 mU in 1 ml

Example D′ $\dfrac{1\,\cancel{\text{ml}}}{1} \times \dfrac{10\,\cancel{\text{U}}}{\cancel{500}\,\cancel{\text{ml}}} \times \dfrac{\overset{2}{\cancel{1000}}\,\text{mU}}{1\,\cancel{\text{U}}} = 20\ \text{mU}$

Example E Then, using the above concentration, if an IV for induction is ordered to run at 7.5 mU/minute, the electric pump should be set at how many milliliters per minute?

$$\text{Milliunits : milliliters} = \text{milliunits : milliliters}$$
$$20 : 1 = 7.5 : x$$
$$20x = 7.5$$
$$x = \frac{7.5}{20}$$
$$x = 0.375 \text{ ml}$$

Answer: 0.375 ml/minute

Example E' $\dfrac{7.5 \, \text{mU}}{1} \times \dfrac{1 \, \text{ml}}{20 \, \text{mU}} = 0.375 \, \text{ml}$

Calculating Infant Doses

Example F *Ordered*: 29 mg meperidine IM
Available: 50 mg in 1 ml ampul

$$\text{Milligrams:milliliters} = \text{milligrams:milliliters}$$
$$50:1 = 29:x$$
$$50x = 29$$
$$x = \frac{29}{50}$$
$$x = 0.58 \text{ ml}$$

(Do not round off child doses under 1 ml. Use a tuberculin syringe measured in hundredths.)

Example F' $\dfrac{29 \, \text{mg}}{1} \times \dfrac{1 \, \text{ml}}{50 \, \text{mg}} = 0.58 \, \text{ml}$

Example G The infant weighs 3180 g. The order reads: give chlorpromazine 2 mg/kg. (Convert grams to kilograms and multiply by dose.)

Step 1   Grams:kilograms = grams:kilograms
$$1000{:}1 = 3180{:}x$$
$$1000x = 3180$$
$$x = \frac{3180}{1000}$$
$$x = 3.18 \text{ kg}$$

Step 2 $3.18 \text{ kg} \times 2 \text{ mg/kg} = 6.36 \text{ mg}$ (total dose)

Available: 5 mg/ml (PO, liquid). (It is necessary to convert the dose to milliliters.)

Step 3   Milligrams:milliliters = milligrams:milliliters
$$5{:}1 = 6.36{:}x$$
$$5x = 6.36$$
$$x = \frac{6.36}{5}$$
$$x = 1.272 \text{ ml}$$

Answer: 1.3 ml. (This has been rounded off since the dose is over 1 ml.)

Example G'   Weight   Transfer   Ordered   Available

$$\frac{3180 \, \cancel{g}}{1} \times \frac{1 \, \cancel{kg}}{1000 \, \cancel{g}} \times \frac{2 \, \cancel{mg}}{1 \, \cancel{kg}} \times \frac{1 \text{ ml}}{5 \, \cancel{mg}} = \frac{6360 \text{ ml}}{5000} = 1.272 \text{ ml} \, (1.3 \text{ ml})$$

(If there is more than one transfer fraction, two separate equations should be set up.)

Calculating Infant Intravenous Flow Rate Using a Micro Dropper

Example H   *Ordered*:   260 ml of 5% dextrose in water to be given over a 12-hour period
                 Available: 60 gtt/ml micro dropper

Step 1   Milliliters:hours = milliliters:hours
$$260{:}12 = x{:}1$$
$$12x = 260$$
$$x = \frac{260}{12}$$
$$x = 21.6 \text{ (in 1 hour)}$$

Step 2   Now reduce to gtts/minute. (See p. 312 for the method followed.)

$$\frac{21.6 \text{ ml/hour}}{60 \text{ minutes/hour}} = 0.36 \text{ ml/minute}$$

Step 3   0.36 ml/minute × 60 gtt/ml = 21.6 gtt/minute

Answer: 22 gtt/minute

Example H' $\dfrac{260 \text{ ml}}{12 \text{ hours}} \times \dfrac{60 \text{ gtt}}{1 \text{ ml}} \times \dfrac{1 \text{ hour}}{60 \text{ minutes}}$

$$= 21.6 \text{ gtt/minute } (22 \text{ gtt/minute})$$

Appendix B
Administration of Parenteral Injections

PREPARATION FOR PARENTERAL INJECTIONS

Needles   Select the smallest possible gauge and the shortest length to deliver the medication to the correct location. The needle will inevitably leave a track in the tissue as it is inserted and will carry into this track any bacteria on the skin surface and any drops of medication at the tip or on the outer wall of the lumen. Because of this, after drawing up medication, use the "double needle technique," i.e., change to a fresh needle when there is any medication which might be injurious to subcutaneous tissue as a result of "tracking" (oily medication, magnesium sulfate, Imferon).

Measurement

Select the syringe according to the volume you expect to use. Always use a tuberculin syringe (measured in hundredths) for doses under 1 ml. When using a vial, always insert air into air space above medication before drawing up liquid. Always check the measurement at eye level with syringe held vertically. The plunger is shaped to account for the medication above the first line on the barrel.

After accurate measurement, draw back 0.1–0.3 ml of air for aqueous solutions, and 0.5 ml of air for oily or suspension and emulsion preparations. Air will be injected last and, clearing the needle, will act as a plug to prevent medication from seeping back up the track of the needle.

Volume The nearer a fluid is to normal body fluid concentration, the less it irritates the tissue. Hypertonic fluids which can be diluted will cause less discomfort.

Never give more than 5 ml of fluid IM in one location to child or adult. Never give more than 1 ml in one location to an infant. Subcutaneous injections for children and adults are usually less than 1 ml.

Asepsis Skin surfaces are always contaminated! Alcohol alone is not able to cleanse the site from many pathogenic agents. Some units are recommending alcohol solution first followed by iodine-containing scrub, allowing each wipe to dry (30 seconds) on the skin before proceeding. Other units do not use cleansing at all (Lewis, 1975). Nursing judgment must be used, with extra care taken when a patient's defenses are compromised. Especially when a patient is incontinent, anaerobic bacteria might be taken into the puncture site. Therefore, in that case, scrub site with soap and water, rinse, dry, and then proceed with prescribed preparation.

Aspiration Never aspirate with the same hand which holds the syringe! One-handed injections are usually unnecessary. An exception to this rule is when using self-medication technique for Z track (Hays, 1976). Use the hand which has held skin taut to aspirate and inject, holding plunger with thumb and first and second fingers. Never use thumb alone on the plunger, since fine control is not possible.

Look at the medication to observe blood return. Draw back slightly on the needle in case it is lodged against the wall of a vessel. If air bubbles are added on aspiration, the needle is loose. When medication is darkly colored, a change in fluid volume is your cue to blood return.

Injection Local trauma is always produced at the site of medication deposit. Prevent additional physical trauma and the pain of sudden separation of muscle fibers or fatty tissue by injecting slowly. Wait a few seconds after injection is completed before removing needle to allow time for medication to "settle" in place. (Wait 10 seconds for Z track.)

Remove needle in a swift, straight reverse dart following exact angle of entry. Apply firm pressure over puncture site for a few seconds. Massage of site is unnecessary. If there is superficial capillary bleeding (common in some patients) apply a Band-Aid. *Always* have a Band-Aid ready for injections for children. For a preschooler, there is a great body concern about bleeding and losing body fluids. To the child the Band-Aid is a symbol of being kept intact.

SELECTION OF SITE

The site is selected by patient condition, ability to be positioned, the volume of medication, and the level of irritation expected in tissue from the type of solution.

Rotate sites, marking on the Kardex when giving a traumatic injection. If necessary, keep a chart at the bedside with site, date and time.

How are the sites chosen? Some understanding of why medications are labeled for intramuscular or subcutaneous injection is necessary for the nurse. There are four basic kinds of preparation (Martin, 1969):

1. Aqueous with quickly soluble ingredients, isotonic or only slightly hypertonic solutions, which are given subcutaneously with minimum injury to tissue. Quickly absorbed into capillaries and into body fluids but more rapidly absorbed in muscular tissue.

2. Aqueous with active ingredients almost insoluble in body fluids, e.g. suspensions, which are sometimes given subcutaneously with slower absorption into lymph stream. May cause pain and be traumatic to tissue. Usually given intramuscularly.

3. Water-insoluble, often oil-based but with soluble ingredients, which given deep intramuscularly, are slowly absorbed, and may cause prolonged soreness at site.

4. Water-insoluble, often oil-based but with almost insoluble ingredients, which are given deep intramuscularly and may cause local fibrosis or necrosis. These are very slowly absorbed.

Subcutaneous Sites

The subcutaneous site can be selected from an area with at least 1 inch of fatty tissue. Since subcutaneous tissue can be injured by acidic, alkaline, and oil-based medications, those medications most recommended for subcutaneous injection are water-based, tissue-soluble, nearly neutral in pH, isotonic in concentration, and nonhemolytic. On rare occasions, drugs in very dilute alcohol or slightly hypertonic solutions may be ordered.

Soluble substances are absorbed by small capillaries and enter into the bloodstream. The more insoluble are picked up by the lymph stream and thus are more slowly distributed. Because of this, subcutaneous medication is generally absorbed *more slowly* than one given intramuscularly, averaging about 30 minutes.

Delay in Absorption   Delay in absorption will be seen with peripheral vasoconstriction (shock, hypotension, cold, hypoxia) edema of tissues, any constricting tournequet, and by the addition of epinephrine or protein and metallic salts to the mixture (insulin).

Increased Absorption   Increased speed of absorption is obtained by the application of a warm compress to the site and by movement of the part or elevation of the extremity into which injection has been made. Rubbing or massaging is unnecessary after a subcutaneous injection.

Triceps Site   The triceps site can be uncomfortable, as the skin is tougher to penetrate than in other sites. Avoid the area where the deltoid and triceps meet, a diagonal indentation in tissue under which runs the brachial artery, vein, and nerves to the lower arm.

Alternate Subcutaneous Sites   The following sites are also useful when patients have to self-inject: The ventrogluteal site in heavier patients, and the fatty tissue of the thigh and abdomen. The tissue over the thoracic back and dorsogluteal area can be used for patients who must lie prone. (See Fig. B-1.) (For insulin and heparin injections, see individual drug listings.)

Technique   Pinch up the fatty tissue, cleanse the area with antiseptic, and using a 25-gauge needle ⅝ inch long (for adult), inject at 90° if more than 1 inch of fat, at 45° if less than 1 inch (see Fig. B-2). Injection too close to the dermal layer leaves a hard lump. Release pinched tissue, aspirate, withdrawing needle slightly, then inject medication slowly. Hold a few seconds, remove needle while compressing site with a sponge. Massage is not necessary.

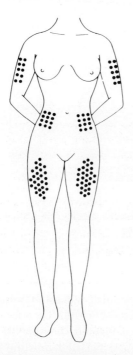

Figure B-1   Subcutaneous sites.

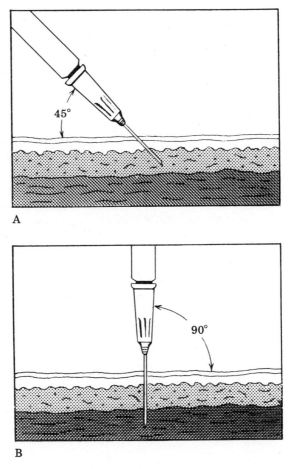

Figure B-2 (A) Angle of subcutaneous injection into a shallow fatty layer. (B) Angle of intramuscular injection.

Intramuscular Sites

Deltoid Site   The deltoid muscle is a small but actively used muscle with area limited in depth and width. Therefore, no more than 2 ml should ever be deposited. The needle should be directed slightly *upward* and inserted into the muscle no deeper than 1 inch. Stay in the center of a narrow site marked by the lower edge of the acromion process and above a line drawn around from the upper fold of the axilla. Injection should be perpendicular to the *anterior-posterior plane* of the body (Johnson and Rapton, 1965). This site can be used with great caution for infants *if* very small amounts of easily absorbable medication are ordered and *if* absolutely correct identification of site and angle of needle insertion are utilized.

Ventrogluteal Site   First described by von Hochstetter, this area has a deeply imbedded muscle attached under the iliac crest and has no large veins, arteries, or nerve tracts. It is especially useful for patients who cannot be turned, who are in pain, or who have pathology involving the back. The site is safe for children and adults (Johnson and Rapton, 1965).

Location is by three landmarks: the anterior superior iliac spine, the greater trochantor of the femur, and the top of the iliac crest, making a V shape. Insert needle in the center of the V deep enough to reach muscle tissue. Inject in a slightly *upward* direction perpendicular to the *anterior-posterior plane* of the body (Fig. B-3).

Dorsogluteal Site   The most common site for adults is the dorsogluteal area, lateral and 1 inch superior to a line drawn from the greater trochanter of the femur to the posterior spine of the iliac crest, which is located 1 inch to the right or left of the

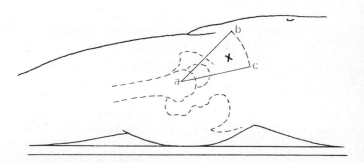

Figure B-3   Ventrogluteal site.

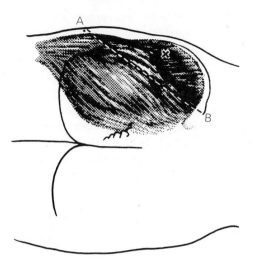

Figure B-4 Dorsogluteal site.

junction of the lumbar and sacral spine. Any injection below this line is likely to impinge upon or hit the sciatic nerve or the major gluteal arteries. Inject on a parallel course to the *anterior-posterior plane* of the body. This site is *never* used with children until active walking develops the muscle (2+ years) (Fig. B-4).

Midanterolateral Thigh Two muscles of the *quadraceps femoris* group can be used for injections for adults, children, and infants: the *vastus lateralis* and the *rectus femoris*. Since the femoral artery, vein, and sciatic nerve are grouped together, running down posterior to the femur, an injection into the anterolat-eral portion of the leg is fairly safe in any sized person (Fig. B-5).

The boundaries are the midportion of the anterolateral leg, for an adult, a hand's length above the knee and a hand's length below the greater trochanter. The needle must be directed on a front-to-back course parallel to the anterior-posterior plane of the body when using the *midrectus femoris*. The angle will change to 45° and be directed on a slightly downward course toward the knee when the alternate site of the mid or upper *vastus lateralis* is used. Volumes of medication should be kept to 2 ml or less in the muscles for adults and less than 1 ml for infants.

Technique for Intramuscular Injection   After identifying the patient by identification band and asking the patient to state name, screen and position the patient while explaining the reason for giving medication. Add the air bubble to the syringe. Locate landmarks for site, and then cleanse area with antiseptic sponge in a firm, single circular motion. Hold the syringe at midbarrel like a dart, and insert quickly with wrist movement to about one-half the needle length. A second thrust to the depth you have chosen places the tip exactly where planned. (Leave small portion of needle exposed above skin in case it breaks off.)

Aspirate and then inject all medication plus air bubble. Wait a few seconds for the medication to disperse. Place the sponge at the site, and withdraw the needle with quick reverse dart. Apply firm pressure on the site. Massaging site is not necessary and contraindicated in some cases. Reposition the patient. Remove equipment. Chart on the appropriate records. Remember to record effective action of medication in evaluation notes.

Z-Track Modification   Use a Z-track technique for any medication which could injure subcutaneous tissue. Imferon is a classic example, causing dark brown staining under the skin for up to

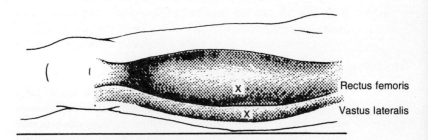

Figure B-5   Midanterolateral thigh.

6 months after an improperly administered intramuscular injection. Magnesium sulfate in fatty tissue causes a painful, inflammatory reaction. Any thick, oily medication will cause fibrosis and even some necrosis if placed in fatty tissue.

STEPS OF THE Z-TRACK METHOD

1. Draw up medication.

2. Change needle.

3. Obtain long enough needle to deposit medication in muscle. Assess depth of fatty layer.

4. Identify patient and landmarks of site. Give only in dorso-gluteal or ventrogluteal muscle (vastus lateralis for infants).

5. Pull in 0.5 ml of air before inserting needle in skin.

6. Twist or pull skin away from site.

7. Insert, aspirate, and inject slowly.

8. Wait 10 seconds.

9. Be ready immediately to slide skin surface back over site to seal off track of needle, thus preventing fluid return along track into fatty tissue after needle is withdrawn.

10. Do not massage but apply pressure to puncture site.

Adapt your technique as necessary. For example, to prepare a Z-track injection for a heavy patient when the medication is in a prepared syringe, place the needle of the prepared ampul into the lumen of the hub of a plastic syringe, slowly push the medication into the new syringe, and then add a longer needle.

Intradermal Injections

Injections into the corium of the skin are called intradermal injections. Because of fewer capillaries in the skin and because of the *wheal* raised when medication is deposited in the corium, absorption is very slow. The dorsal surface of the forearm, the lateral and posterior upper arm, and the thoracic back are used for allergens or immunizing agents.

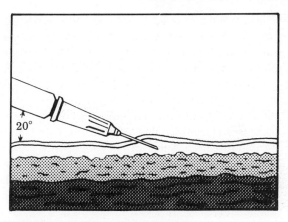

Figure B-6 Intradermal angle of injection.

Technique Using a 26-gauge, short needle, insert at a 10 to 20°
angle with hub almost touching skin. Slow injection is
important as the skin is sensitive to pressure, and pain will
usually result. Inform the patient just as you inject. Look for
the raised bump that appears to be blanched (wheal). Do not
rub area after injection. Record observations, measurement
of wheal, and patient reactions (Fig. B-6).

ADMINISTRATION OF PARENTERAL FLUIDS
Intravenous Injection

The expanding role of nurses, in many instances, includes
administration of some medications by intravenous route, as
well as drawing blood samples and starting infusions. It is
expected that a nurse will have gone through an in-service
program of supervised experience, since most basic nursing
curricula do not provide learning experiences in these skills.

Intravenous Medication

Circulation time from arm to tongue (via the superior vena
cava and heart) is approximately 16 seconds in the adult.

Thus, medications and fluids injected directly into the vein produce rapid results. The main advantage of intravenous medication is the rapid onset of effect. The main hazard is also the rapidity of effect should it be toxic to the patient.

Precautions for intravenous medications include accurate needle placement in vein prior to administration to prevent infiltration into surrounding tissue, accurate dose in a solution acceptable for intravenous use, and using a test dose first of an undiluted drug before proceeding with very slow intravenous push. (Note time limits carefully. Some drugs must be given as a bolus to be effective.) Because concentrated liquids irritate the intima of the vein, medications are best administered by "piggyback" line, which directs the medication to the main intravenous line to be mixed at the juncture with isotonic fluids. (Always check compatibility of medications and the intravenous fluids.) In this way, medications can be given via an existing line by push, or by using a set containing a controlled volume drip chamber (Soluset, Buretrol, etc.) or by mixing medication into a 100 ml intravenous bag and running the secondary tubing into the existing line (Egan, 1974).

Fluid Administration

Fluid needs of the patient are determined by the physician, but the responsibility for maintaining safe infusion belongs to the nurse. Control of the infusion rate and of the side effects of infiltration, thrombophlebitis, and infection continue to be major problems in nursing practice.

Methods to control infusion rate are listed below:

1. Position the patient so that the intravenous line is free of kinks and compression and see that the vein is not constricted.

2. Select the gauge of needle according to the fluid viscosity and size of vein. A large-bore needle or a polyethylene intracatheter should be used when blood or blood fractions are administered. The needle size should not occlude the vein or else the blood distal to the needle may form a clot.

3. Fill one-half of the drip chamber and all the tubing with fluid before attaching the needle. If air bubbles appear subsequently in the line, either separate the line from the needle and run fluid through or take an empty, sterile syringe and a 25-gauge needle and, inserting the needle (with bevel up) into the rubber connection, draw out air bubbles as they pass down the tube. Air in the tube may not injure the patient. Some suggest that small bubbles coalesce to form emboli; others do not agree.

Air embolism is rare unless the tubing enters a vein under negative pressure. A situation where this might occur is when the jugular or subclavian vein is used for a CVP line. Loose connections or unclamped stopcocks are dangerous in these situations. (Mitchell, 1975, p. 353)

The amount of air for a lethal embolus has been calculated from animal studies to be about 350 ml for a 150 lb male. The IV line contains less than 5 ml. (Mitchell, 1975, p. 353)

4. Place the intravenous solution just high enough on the pole to overcome venous (0.5–1 meter above the heart) pressure and ensure a steady rate of flow. Too much hydrostatic pressure will cause the intravenous to infiltrate because fluid will enter the vein at a pressure damaging to the vein wall (Jensen, 1960). As the intravenous is absorbed, the bottle height can be raised slightly to compensate for the difference in fluid level.

5. Every order for intravenous fluids should contain the rate of flow. For an adult, the usual rate of flow is 1000 ml/8 h (125 ml per hour). The top limit for a patient is 500 ml per hour for isotonic fluids, and 200 ml per hour for hypertonic solutions (Dudrick, 1971; Martin, 1969). If a patient has cardiovascular disease, burns, fluid and electrolyte imbalance, or is aged, "normal rates" are not valid, and fluids are titrated with patient condition and output. The toxic effects of poor rate control include:
   a. *Circulatory overload* demonstrated as symptoms of headache, tachycardia, tachypnea, venous distention, increased blood and venous pressure, and shortness of

breath, progressing to pulmonary edema and oxygen deprivation.
   b. *Drug overload* will occur when too much of a drug is administered because speed of the intravenous is not controlled. Effects will be specific to excessive levels of drug in the receptor sites.

6. Attach an infusion control pump or a controlled volume infusion set whenever an intravenous contains dangerous medication or the patient is in fragile cardiovascular balance, as well as for every infant and child (Beaumont, 1977).

7. Label the bottle with hourly levels (flow tapes) and enlist the cooperation of alert patients to notify nurse if the flow rate changes.

Methods to prevent infiltration are listed below:

1. Do not allow fluids to run too fast or too slow.

2. Instruct patient not to hang arm in a dependent position. When ambulating with intravenous pole on wheels, instruct the patient to "hold intravenous pole with IV arm," keeping arm and tubing above waist.

3. Secure needle and tubing to site using splint if necessary. Do not constrict vein with tape. Be sure to maintain joints in good alignment.

4. Observe site for early signs of infiltration:
   a. Swelling above site, coolness of tissue.
   b. Slow fluid flow despite changes in bottle height or open valve.
   c. Pain, blanching of the skin at site.
   Do not attempt to flush intravenous. Only acceptable method is to take syringe and try to aspirate blood back through needle to draw out clot.

5. Use nursing judgment if infiltration has begun. Rotate needle bevel and pull needle back several millimeters to see if good flow can be again assured. Watch intravenous carefully, or damage to tissue will result. Elevate the part and place warm

compresses on the site to speed absorption of fluid. If toxic medication has infiltrated, stop flow and obtain medical assistance and antidotes at once.

6. Change intravenous site every 48 hours when a needle is in place and every 72 hours when a cannula is used. (Godwin, 1975). Mark time on tape and Kardex.

7. Make frequent, regular inspections of intravenous flow rate and site.

Methods to prevent infections and thrombophlebitis are listed below:

1. Use strict aseptic technique when starting infusions. Prepare site with: soap and water, and then with 70% alcohol and 10% acetone solution, allowing it to dry, rub with iodine preparation, allowing it to dry, and finally wipe with 70% alcohol solution (Snider, 1974).

2. Use in-line filters especially for any solution which has added medication.

3. Apply antibacterial, antifungal ointment after venipuncture, following particular hospital procedures.

4. Apply sterile gauze square over and under needle and tape securely in place to prevent friction of needle movement and protection from external contamination.

5. Change this dressing while changing tubing set and in-line filters daily. Rotate bevel of needle each day.

6. Give most intravenous medications intermittently, diluted in isotonic fluid, and run through a piggyback line (exceptions occur, e.g., heparin).

7. Neutralize acidic intravenous solutions only on physician's orders, with 1% sodium bicarbonate solution.

8. Prevent damage to vein by avoiding traumatic puncture and infiltration. Do not allow clot formation because of poor flow. Be careful to prevent infiltration of hypertonic solution.

9. Observe for signs of thrombophlebitis:
   a. Tenderness and pain rising along line of vein.
   b. Edema and redness, increased temperature of part.
   Apply warm compress after discontinuing intravenous to encourage circulation to part.

HYPODERMOCLYSIS

Slow infusion of isotonic fluid into subcutaneous tissue is an alternate method of providing fluids to dehydrated or debilitated patients or for those whose veins are inadequate for or injured by repeated intravenous infusions. The rate of infusion is ordered by the physician and adjusted by the rate of absorption from the patient's tissues.

For adults, the needle is inserted into subcutaneous tissue at a 20 to 30° angle. The 2 to 3 inch needle is placed into the subscapular area or into the subcutaneous tissue over the mid-thigh. The needle is then attached to intravenous tubing and a solution which must be isotonic. *Hyaluronidase*, an enzyme which acts on the polysaccharide *hyaluronic acid* (intercellular cement in body tissues), may be ordered to be added to the infusion to speed spread and absorption of fluid. Hyaluronidase is available as 150 U/ml. The usual dose is 150 U added to 1000 ml of intravenous fluid. The site is observed for absorption rate, and the fluid is charged as intravenous intake on the fluid intake-output record.

Precautions Because there is occasional hypersensitivity to this agent, a test dose is usually given. If infection is present in the site, this agent may facilitate its spread.

BIBLIOGRAPHY

*Beaumont, E.: "The New IV Infusion Pumps," *Nursing* '77, **7**(7):31–35, 1977.

*Denotes particularly pertinent references

Demoruelle, J. L., W. L. Harrison and R. E. Flora: "Flow Rate and Maintenance of Output of Intravenous Fluid Administration," *American Journal of Hospital Pharmacy*, **32**:177–185, February 1975.

Dudrick, S. J.: "Rational Intravenous Therapy," *American Journal of Hospital Pharmacy*, **28**:82–91, February 1971.

Egan, A.: "Perfecting Piggyback Techniques," *Nursing '74*, January 1974, pp. 28–33.

Godwin, H. N.: "Intermittent and Direct IV Push: Rationale and Procedures," *American Journal of IV Therapy*, **2**:27–30 December-January 1975.

*Greenblatt, D.J., and J., Koch-Weser: "Intramuscular Injection of Drugs," *New England Journal of Medicine*, **295**(10):542, September 2, 1976.

Hanson, R. L.: "Heparin Lock or Keep-Open IV?" *American Journal of Nursing*, **76**(7):1102, 1976.

Hays, D.: "Do It Yourself the Z-track Way," *American Journal of Nursing*, **74**(6):1070, 1976.

Jensen, J.T.: "*Introduction to Medical Physics*," J. B. Lippincott, Philadelphia 1960, p 76.

*Johnson, E.W., and A.D. Rapton: "A Study of Intragluteal Injection," *Archives of Physical Medicine*, **46**:167, 1965.

Lang, S.A., A.M. Zawacki, and J. Johnson: "Reducing Discomfort from IM Injection," *American Journal of Nursing*, **76**(5):800, 1976.

Lewis, M.J.: "Skin Preparation Before Injection," *Nursing Times*, **75**(5):786, May 15, 1975.

*Lowenthal, W.: "Factors Affecting Drug Absorption," *American Journal of Nursing*, **73**(8):1391, 1973.

Martin, E.W.: *Techniques of Medication*, J. B. Lippincott, Philadelphia, 1969, p. 120.

Mitchell, C.: *Concepts Basic to Nursing*, McGraw-Hill, New York, 1975.

Pitel, M., "The Subcutaneous Injection," *American Journal of Nursing*, **71**(1):76, 1971.

Snider, M.A.: "Helpful Hints on IV's," *American Journal of Nursing*, **74**(11):1978, 1974.

U.S. Center for Disease Control: "Recommendations for the Insertion and Maintenance of Plastic Intravenous Catheters," The Center, Atlanta, 1972.

*Watson, J.: "Research and Literature on Children's Response to Injection," *Journal of Pediatric Nursing*, **2**(1):7, January 1975.

Index

Index

Aarane (*see* Cromolyn sodium)
Aaro on incidence of thromboembolic problems during pregnancy and recovery from birth, 134 – 135
Abortion due to maternal ingestion:
of aminopterin, 21
of chlorambucil, 21
of cyclophosphamide, 21
of ergonovine maleate, 22
of LSD, 24
of mercaptopurine, 21
of methotrexate, 21
of quinine, 20
Abramson, D.:
on effect of general anesthesia due to fetus, 212
on effect of maternal meperidine usage on neonate, 195
Abscesses, sterile, at IM sites in neonates due to semisynthetic penicillins, 284
Absorption:
in drug utilization during pregnancy, 28 – 33
of dermatomucosal medications, 32 – 33
of oral medications, 29 – 30
of parenteral medications, 30 – 32
following parenteral injections, conditions affecting, 320
of oral medication by neonate, 234 – 235
Acetaminophen (Datril, Liquiprin, Tempra, Tenlap, Tylenol):
containing ingredients not recommended during pregnancy, 58

Acetaminophen (Datril, Liquiprin, Tempra, Tenlap, Tylenol):
excretion of, in breast milk and effect of, on infant, 71
prohibition of, during pregnancy, 48
use of, in neonates and infants, 283
Acetazolamide (Diamox):
cautions against, during pregnancy, 174
contraindication for, during pregnancy, 143
excretion of, in breast milk and effect of, on infant, 73
Acetohexamide (Dymelor), dosage and comments on, 182
Acetonalid:
containing ingredients not recommended during pregnancy, 58
prohibition of, during pregnancy, 48
Acetylcysteine (Mucomyst) for meconium aspiration syndrome, 258
Acetylsalicylic acid (Aspirin):
to delay preterm labor, 221 – 222
effects of, on fetus and neonate, 17
excretion of, in breast milk and effect of, on infant, 71
interaction of: with coumarins, 139
with insulin, 178
with penicillins, 122
use of: in neonates and infants, 280, 292
during pregnancy, 58 – 59
Acid rebound due to calcium carbonate, 18, 48

Danthron (Dorbane, Dorbantyl, Doxan, Doxidan):
  excretion of, in breast milk and effect of, on infant, 75
  use of, in pregnancy, dosage and comments on, 57
Daraprim (*see* Pyrimethamine)
Darcel (*see* Potassium phenethicillin)
Darvon (*see* Propoxyphene hydrochloride)
Datril (*see* Acetaminophen)
DBI (*see* Phenformin hydrochloride)
Decadron (*see* Dexamethasone)
Declomycin (*see* Demeclocycline)
Decortin (*see* Desoxycorticosterone acetate)
Deladumone OB (*see* Testosterone enanthate with estradiol valerate)
Delivery, drugs used during, 191–231
Deltoid site for parenteral injections, 322
Demeclocycline (Declomycin), use of, during pregnancy, 129
Demerol (*see* Meperidine hydrochloride)
Dependence potential:
  of benzodiazepines, 198
  of flurazepam, 203
  of meprobamate, 199
  of oxycodone with APC, 194
  of pentazocine, 197
Depo-Provera (*see* Medroxyprogesterone acetate)
Depression:
  fetal (*see* Fetus, depression of)
  neonatal: due to maternal ingestion of barbiturates, 60, 191–192
    due to meperidine, 195
  neurologic, in neonate, due to maternal use of psychotropic drugs, 269–270
  respiratory (*see* Respiration, depression of)
Dermatomucosal medication, absorption of:
  by neonate, 235–236
  in pregnancy, 32–33
DES (*see* Diethylstilbestrol)
Desoxycorticosterone acetate (Doca, Dortate, Decortin, Percortin, Percorten), use of, in neonates and infants, 295
Dessicated animal thyroid, dosage and comments on, 184
Dexamethasone (Decadron):
  effects of, on fetus and neonate, 22
  use of, in neonates and infants, 295
Dexedrine (*see* Dextroamphetamine sulfate)
Dextroamphetamine sulfate (Dexedrine), effects of, on fetus and neonate, 24
Dextrose:
  administration of, in resuscitation of newborn, 262
  use of, during pregnancy, 54
DHT (*see* Dihydrotachsterol)

Diabetes:
  aggravation of: due to corticosteroids, 153
    due to thiazides, 169
  drugs for (*see* Antidiabetic agents)
  maternal, effects of, on newborn, 264–268
Diabinese (*see* Chlorpropamide)
Diamox (*see* Acetazolamide)
Diazepam (Valium):
  as antianxiety agent during labor and delivery, dosage and comments on, 203
  effects of, on fetus and neonate, 22
  excretion of, in breast milk and effect of, on infant, 76
  maternal ingestion of: chronic neonatal withdrawal due to, 271
    effects of, on neonate, 269–270
  for neonatal withdrawal syndromes, 275
  use of: during labor and delivery, 199–200
    in neonates and infants, 289–290
Diazoxide (Hyperstat IV) for hypertension during pregnancy, 165–166
Dicumarol (*see* Bishydroxycoumarin)
Dicyclomine hydrochloride, use of, during pregnancy, 53
Dienstrol (DV, Restrol, Synestrol) for prevention of lactation, 102
Diethyl ether, use of, during labor, and delivery, 213
Diethylstilbestrol (DES, Stilbestrol):
  for contraception, 101
  effects of, on fetus and neonate, 21
  maternal ingestion of, vaginal adenocarcinoma due to, 8
  for prevention of lactation, 104
Digitalis:
  interaction of: with amphotericin B, 111
    with thiazides, 169
  use of: in neonates and infants, 280, 292
    during pregnancy, 155–157
Digitoxin:
  interaction of phenobarbital with, 144
  use of, during pregnancy, 155–157
Digoxin (Lanoxin):
  for cardiac failure in neonates, 260
  use of: in neonates and infants, 280, 292
    during pregnancy, 155–157
Dihydrotachsterol (DHT), excretion of, in breast milk and effect of, on infant, 79
Dilantin (*see* Phenytoin)
Dilor (*see* Dyphylline)
Dimenhydrinate (Dramamine), use of, during pregnancy, 152
Dimensional analysis in dosage calculations, 307–311
Dindevan (*see* Phenindione)

Hetacillin (Versapen, Versapen-K), use of, during pregnancy, 125
Hexamethonium bromide:
effects of, on fetus and neonate, 19
excretion of, in breast milk, effect of, on infant, 73
Heymann, M. A., on indomethacin for closure of patent ductus arteriosus, 280
Hill, R. M., on relation of birth defects to anticonvulsant therapy, 140
Hormone(s):
adrenocorticotropic, use of, during pregnancy, 153—154
for contraception, 89—102
combined, 95—99
estrogens as, 89—92
medroxyprogesterone acetate as, 102
mini-pills as, 10
morning-after pills as, 100—101
progesterone and progestins as, 92—94
effects of, on fetus and neonate, 21—22
excretion of, in breast milk and effect of, on infant, 75
female, used during pregnancy, effect of, on fetus, 7
maternal use of, effects of, on neonate, 269
to prevent lactation, 103—104
use of, in neonates and infants, 294
Horsdof, A., on effect of propranolol on labor, 161
Household system of measurement, 305—306
Howel, F., on administration of intramuscular injection to infant, 250
Human chorionic gonadotropin for stimulating evaluation, 87—88
Human menopausal gonadotropins (Menotropine, Pergonal) for stimulating evaluation, 88—89
Huppert, L. C., on clomophene citrate therapy, 86, 87
Hutchinson, J. R., on glycosuria during pregnancy, 176
Hyaline membrane disease related to maternal diabetes, 265
Hyaluronidase, use of, in hypodermoclysis, 332
Hydralazine (Apresoline) for hypertensive crises during pregnancy, 164—165
Hydrochlorothiazide (Esidrix, Hydrodiuril, Oretic) for hypertension during pregnancy, 171
Hydrodiuril (see Hydrochlorothiazide)
Hydroflumethiazide (Saluron) for hypertension during pregnancy, 171
Hydrolose (see Methylcellulose)
Hydromox (see Quinethazone)

Hydroxyzine hydrochloride (Atarax, Vistaril):
as antianxiety agent during labor and delivery, dosage and comments, 203
in drug mixtures for asthmatics, 150
use of: during labor and delivery, 198
during pregnancy, 152
Hygroton (see Chlorthalidone)
Hyperbilirubinemia in neonate:
due to excessive maternal ingestion of vitamin K, 23, 296
due to maternal ingestion of novobiocin, 20
related to maternal diabetes, 267
Hypercalcemia:
due to estrogens, 90
in neonate: due to excessive maternal ingestion of vitamin D, 23
due to excretion: of dihydrotachsterol in breast milk, 79
of vitamin D in breast milk, 78
Hyperglycemia:
maternal, effects of, on neonate, 265
in neonate: due to dexamethasone, 295
due to furosemide, 294
due to glucagon overdose, 294
due to maternal ingestion of diazoxide, 166
Hyperpnea in neonate, due to withdrawal syndromes, 273
Hyperpyrexia in neonate:
due to atropine sulfate, 296
due to withdrawal syndromes, 273
Hypersensitivity states, drugs used for, during pregnancy, 147—154
Hyperstat IV (see Diazoxide)
Hypertension:
chronic, management of, during pregnancy, 160—162
due to circulatory overload, 329
drugs for (see Antihypertensives)
due to ergot alkaloids, 223
in neonate: due to desoxycorticosterone acetate, 295
due to dexamethasone, 295
due to pentazocine, 197
due to promazine, 204
Hypertonia in neonate:
due to excretion of bromides in breast milk, 77
due to ketamine hydrochloride, 217
due to maternal ingestion of bromides during pregnancy, 23
Hypertonus, uterine, due to oxytocin, 227
Hyperviscosity in neonate related to maternal diabetes, 267—268
Hypnotics, excretion of, in breast milk and effect of, on infant, 77

Pancreatin (*see* Pancreatic enzymes)

Pancrelipase (*see* Pancreatic enzymes)

Pan Heparin (*see* Heparin)

Panmycin (*see* Tetracycline)

Para-aminophenol derivatives containing ingredients not recommended during pregnancy, 48, 58

Paracervical block, use of, during labor and delivery, 209

Paraldehyde:
effects of, on fetus and neonate, 23
use of, in neonates and infants, 290

Paregoric (*see* Camphorated tincture of opium)

Parenteral alimentation total or supplementary use of, in infants, 298

Parenteral fluids, administration of, 327–332
hypodermoclysis for, 332
intravenous injection for, 327
methods for, 328–332
precautions for medication in, 327–328

Parenteral injections, administration of, 317–334
intracutaneous, 326–327
intramuscular sites for, 322–326
preparations for, 317–319
selection of site for, 319–320
subcutaneous sites for, 320–326

Parenteral medications, absorption of: by neonate, 236–237
in pregnancy, 30–32

Penicillin G (Benzathine penicillin G, crystalline), use of, in neonates and infants, 283–284

Penicillins:
excretion of, in breast milk, effect of, on infant, 74
use of: in neonates and infants, 277–278, 283–285
in pregnancy, 122–126
(*See also* Amoxicillin; Ampicillin; Benzathine penicillin G; Carbenicillin; Hetacillin; Potassium penicillin V; Potassium phenethicillin; Potassium phenoxymethyl penicillin; Sodium cloxacillin; Sodium dicloxacillin; Sodium methicillin; Sodium nafcillin; Sodium oxacillin)

Pentazocine (Talwin):
excretion of, in breast milk and effect of, on infant, 71
maternal use of, chronic, neonatal withdrawal due to, 271
use of, during labor and delivery, 197

Penthrane (*see* Methoxyflurane)

Pentothal (*see* Thiopental)

Pen-Vee (*see* Potassium penicillin V)

Pen-Vee-K (*see* Potassium phenoxymethyl penicillin)

Percodan (*see* Oxycodone with APC)

Percorten (*see* Desoxycorticosterone acetate)

Pergonal (*see* Human menopausal gonadotropins)

Pericolace (*see* Casanthranol, dioctyl sodium sulfosuccinate with)

Peridural block, use of, during labor and delivery, 210

Permitil (*see* Fluphenazine)

Pernicious anemia, masking of symptoms of, by ingestion of folic acid, 62

Pethidine (*see* Meperidine hydrochloride)

Pethoid (*see* Meperidine hydrochloride)

Petrolatum, liquid, avoidance of use during pregnancy, 57

Pettifor, J. M., on contraindications for coumarins during pregnancy, 139

Phenacetin prohibited during pregnancy, 48, 58

Phenergan (*see* Promethazine hydrochloride)

Phenformin hydrochloride (DBI), action of, 182

Phenindione (Dindevan, Hedulin), excretion of, in breast milk and effect of, on infant, 72

Phenobarbital (Luminal):
in drug mixtures for asthmatics, 150
interaction of progesterone with, 94
maternal use of, effects of, on neonate, 270
for neonatal withdrawal syndromes, 275
for preeclampsia, 159
use of: in neonates and infants, 289
in pregnancy, 143–144

Phenolphthalein (Evaculax, Ex-lax), excretion of, in breast milk and effect of, on infant, 75

Phenothiazines:
as antianxiety agent during labor and delivery, dosage and comments on, 203–204
effects of, on fetus and neonate, 23
excretion of, in breast milk and effect of, on infant, 77
maternal ingestion of, effects of, on neonate, 269–270
use of: during labor and delivery, 200–202
during pregnancy, 152

Phensuximide (Milontin), contraindication for, during pregnancy, 143

Phenylbutazone (Azolid, Butazolidin):
excretion of, in breast milk and effect of, on infant, 71
interaction of: with coumarin, 139
with insulin, 178

Viral infections in pregnancy, 107
Vistaril (*see* Hydroxyzine hydrochloride)
Vitamin(s):
   effects of, on fetus and neonate, 23
   excretion of, in breast milk and effect of,
      on infant, 78
   K (AquaMephyton, Konakion, Phy-
      tonadione): as antidote for coumarin
      overdose, 138
      use of, in neonates and infants, 296
      requirements and preparations of, for in-
         fants, 297
   use of, during pregnancy, 62, 64–65
Vivonex, contents of, 300
Volume of fluid for parenteral injections,
   318
Vorherr, H.:
   on adverse effects of maternal ingestion of
      barbiturates, 60
   on blood-milk barrier to drug transport, 38
   on dangers of antacids in pregnancy, 48

Walchtes, E., on administration of intramuscular injection to infant, 250
Wallach, E. F., on clomiphene citrate therapy, 86, 87
Warfarin sodium (Coumadin):
   effects of, on fetus and neonate, 19
   excretion of, in breast milk and effect of,
      on infant, 72
   interaction of, with chloral hydrate, 61
Water-soluble drugs, absorption of, 28–29
Waziri, M., on risks of phenytoin use during
   pregnancy, 5
Weight loss in neonate, due to excretion of
   ergot preparations in breast milk, 76
Weiss, J. B., on effect of local anesthetics on
   neonate, 208
Wentz, A. C., on progesterone for threatened
   abortion, 93
White, P., on perinatal risk in diabetic pregnancy, 176
Wilson, J. G.:
   on categories of teratogens, 9–10
   on environmental effects on fetal develop-
      ment, 6

Wilson, J. T., on inadequacy of information
   on maternal and child drug safety,
   3–4
Withdrawal from drugs in neonate, 271
Withdrawal symptoms in neonate, due to
   excretion of heroin in breast milk, 71
Woods, J. R., on adverse effects of methyldopa, 164
Wu, P. Y. K., on effect of phototherapy on absorption of drugs by neonate, 236
Wycillin (*see* Procaine penicillin G)

Xanthines:
   prohibited during pregnancy, 48, 56
   use of, during pregnancy, 174
Xylocaine (*see* Lidocaine)

Yaffee, S. J.:
   on drug distribution in newborn, 237
   on effect of elevated bilirubin levels on
      drug distribution in newborn, 239
   on effect of maturation of excretion mech-
      anisms on drug administration, 246
Yalom, I. D.:
   on behavioral defects due to female hor-
      mones, 7
   on effect of maternal ingestion of diethyl-
      stilbestrol on male offspring, 89
Yeager, A. M., on fetal alcohol syndrome,
   220

Z-track technique:
   for intramuscular injections, 325–326
   modified, for infants and young children,
      250–252
Zarotin (*see* Ethosuximide)
Zaroxolyn (*see* Methlazone)
Zawacki, A. M., on controlling infusion volume during intravenous administration of fluids, 330
Zinc and protein insulin suspensions, characteristics of, 180
Zuckerman, H., on effects of indomethacin
   on labor, 221–222